R.n

Community practice

R. Madden.

Community practice
a text for occupational therapists and others involved in community care

edited by

Eileen E. Bumphrey

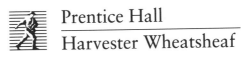

Prentice Hall
Harvester Wheatsheaf

London   New York   Toronto   Sydney
Tokyo   Singapore   Madrid   Mexico City   Munich

First published 1995 by
Prentice Hall/Harvester Wheatsheaf
Campus 400, Maylands Avenue
Hemel Hempstead
Hertfordshire, HP2 7EZ
A division of
Simon & Schuster International Group

Typeset in 10/12pt Sabon
by Create Publishing Services

Printed and bound in Great Britain by
T.J. Press Ltd, Padstow, Cornwall

Library of Congress Cataloging in Publication Data

Available from the publisher

British Library Cataloguing in Publication Data

A catalogue record for this book is available from the British
Library

ISBN 0-13-433046-3

1 2 3 4 5   99 98 97 96 95

Dedicated to –
Those we seek to serve

Contents

Preface

During the past seven years since *Occupational Therapy in the Community* was published British society has seen many fundamental changes not only in the plethora of legislation and the technological revolution, but also as a result of increased unemployment, poverty and homelessness. All have had profound effects on people's attitudes, expectations and lifestyles. Despite all 'the advances', disabled people still remain disadvantaged with many striving to become integrated citizens within our society. Whilst the Citizens' Charter, together with the Patients' Charter, empowers people to make this happen, major problems still exist for the disabled person and often require help of occupational therapists and their colleagues of other disciplines. Thus therapist and other community practitioners need to be fully conversant with all the changes, the new legislation and adapted professional philosophies. It is in response to these changes and the many requests received, that this second edition has been written so that therapists and others can be helped to practise effectively within the new scenario.

It has been necessary to virtually re-write the book and include further chapters to support the major presenting problems of today, such as 'Health promotion' and 'The head injured adult'. I am therefore grateful to the publishers for allowing us to extend the text so that these could be explored. With the new legislation has come a new language and we hope that the Glossary will help readers through the maze of 'management speak'!

The major change affecting community practice since the first edition is the whole approach and philosophy of purchasing and providing health and social care – the purchaser/provider split. More attention is now being given to patient focus care; empowerment; general management; integrated plans; flexible working; with less emphasis on professional focus; functional management; segregation; and the 'status quo'.

The impact of the NHS and Community Care Act 1990 has been profound, with the ethos of the reforms being to transfer the majority of care into the community and to encourage everyone to take greater control of their own lives.

No longer can we talk about community services being the prerogative of Social Services with 'patients' being seen in GP surgeries and hospitals and 'clients' by Social Service personnel. These terms often relate to the same person as they transfer from GP, to hospital care, to social care; therefore throughout this book both terms have been used and in some places are synonymous, and should be read as such. (Similarly, the therapist or practitioner is referred to as 'her' and the disabled person as 'him' in order to achieve flow of language.) Never before has so much emphasis been placed on health, family health services authorities and Social Services working together to provide 'seamless' care. This may seem an extravagant goal and, perhaps, a better phrase would be a 'well-seamed' service. Complementary or integrated community services are now the aim for all districts and Health Commissions and will develop through the Joint Community Care planning process.

The way in which services are now delivered has changed dramatically. For example, in many places home helps have had their roles widened to become 'home care assistants'. The growth in day care, 'hospital at home' schemes and day surgery also have major implications on the future pattern of health care in the community. In consequence there is a shift in working practices, with many health care employees now working in the community rather than the protective environment of the hospital. A subsequent decentralisation of management has resulted in isolation for many of them, often with little professional support.

In 1986 the Audit Commission in its report *Making a Reality of Community Care* (1986) stated that 'the skills of Occupational Therapists are in many ways central to the implementation of community care ... these skills should be at the forefront of an "enabling" service'. Thus, as the shift of practice takes place there is the need for more flexibility in working practices, opportunities to advance multidisciplinary teamwork and acceptance of critical evaluation. Naturally, all this has a profound effect on accepted and traditional methods of working. It is hoped that this book will enable the community practitioner to make a start to achieve these goals and stimulate them to explore further. For these reasons it is hoped that this book, while aimed primarily for the occupational therapy profession, will be of help to many other disciplines working alongside their occupational therapy colleagues.

There is also a gradual move away from the 'medical model' of care to the 'social model' which is often more realistic, relating to the real needs of the individual and transferring power from the professional to the disabled person. Within these models emphasis is being placed on 'quality care' but what is really meant by this when so much assessment and intervention is based on subjectivity. Since qualifying in their respective disciplines, care workers have striven to provide a quality service which in most cases has been very effective and efficiently delivered. But there is little doubt that accountability of these services to the general public – who indeed pay for them through their taxes – has to improve.

The NHS and Community Care Act 1990, with its internal market, has encouraged the development of the private and voluntary sectors and this has added another dimension to the delivery of service and options available for future care.

Throughout this book the emphasis has been on the therapist working *with* the disabled person, *enabling* them to achieve what *they* want to do. Occupational therapists are in a unique position of being catalysts and enablers who help disabled people to achieve their personal goals by presenting options and then facilitating the decision, so that they are able to achieve optimal interaction with the environment of their choice. This does not imply that solutions can be found to all the problems, but it forms a framework for thinking – the 'problem-solving sequence'. If disabled people are to become participating members of society, they need advice and guidance in how this might be accomplished. The family, or other carers, are often the primary support for them and it is essential that they too are fully considered.

Educational changes have also taken place within the past 7 years. All the paramedical professions have moved to degree status and National Vocational Qualifications are making inroads for the assistants. These moves are also having implications in the delivery of services with general managers looking critically towards skill mix, role blurring and multiskilling. At the same time paramedical educational philosophies have moved away from the disease–pathology–treatment model (WHO 1980) into the impairment–disability–handicap model of disablement. Shared learning, whether at pre- or postgraduate level, is increasingly being recognised as a valuable means of achieving interdisciplinary understanding and practice.

It will take time for some practices to die, old and entrenched traditions to go and different relationships to build up. For example, GPs will still consider it their responsibility to act as advocates for their patients whereas the social worker may see this as explicit within case management. The clash of values will continue, especially between free health care and means tested social care.

I would like to thank most sincerely all the contributors who have so willingly agreed to share their expertise while leading very full professional lives and struggling to implement changes at the same time. Their contributions are not intended to be comprehensive but, within the constraints imposed, have hopefully conveyed to the reader the essence of their topic taking them through the process of change. Thanks must also go to the very many readers who gave invaluable advice and criticism throughout and to all those who have supported the project in many different ways, including my own husband, whose patience and support have been immeasurable.

We all feel that we have been writing on shifting sand for, as the weeks have passed, so the philosophies have developed – and they will continue to do so. We would like to see this process slow down a little between these chapters being written and final publication date, so that the book will not again be out of date by the time you pick it up and start delving into it. As Denise Platt said when President of the Association of Directors of Social Services: 'After almost 10 years of perpetual revolution ... nothing is needed more than a period of stability so that the beneficial and far-reaching reforms currently being implemented can be thoroughly and effectively put in place'.

The changes, then, pose many questions, demand many adjustments and yet provide opportunities and challenges. This book is simply an *introduction* to community practice and hopefully it will inspire many to explore further so that those whom we seek to serve will attain their desired goals, adapt to new situations, achieve maximum independence and quality of life.

Eileen E. Bumphrey
Norwich
August 1994

Chapter 1

Introduction

DR MONNICA C. STEWART
*Formerly Principal Medical Officer (Adult Health), Basingstoke and
North Hampshire Health Authority*

The 1990 National Health Service and Community Care Act is on the statute books. Implementation structures have been ratified, guidelines gush forth in many guises. Community care, longed for by so many patients/clients, has arrived, blessed and encouraged by the Departments of Health and Social Security.

Despite it all, however, people craving support in the struggle to remain viably independent in their chosen settings, and who are not in a crisis situation, see no revitalising hurricane of change sweeping over their lives. For those in severe crisis, seemingly, a great deal of help can be mobilised from many sources, but for those gallantly trying to fend off dependency there is, puzzlingly, very little support. One wonders why this should be and reflects on what community care means and how our particular society has come to fashion this strange tapestry of services labelled health and welfare. In short, what *is* community care?

Community care can have a multitude of meanings to a myriad of people. It is an imprecise term, in some contexts being akin to a dirty word, in others indicating the best way of doing things. It would be worth considering how this polarisation may have come about and whether there is a way of eliminating some of the gloomier thoughts and highlighting the positive aspects of the subject which is now a priority on the agenda.

The 'medical model' was previously much used as the basis for all the concerned disciplines, loosely referred to as the greater medical profession, and if one considers the conventional training of doctors, especially that of the general practitioner, the lynchpin doctor of community care, then perhaps some of the strengths and weaknesses of the system become easier to understand.

One of the more cheering events of recent years in the National Health Service has been the introduction of vocational training for general practice. The necessity for doctors to spend specific periods in preparatory training, not only in general practice itself supervised by selected and experienced trainers, but also in relevant hospital specialities such as elderly care, psychiatry, obstetrics, paediatrics or accident and emergency, to name but a few, makes for a much more rounded practitioner. As these 6-month appointments are arranged by trainees rotating through different clinical specialities, it means that lateral mobility has begun to permeate the service.

The inception of the NHS in 1948 unexpectedly tipped the delicate balance of relationship between hospital consultant specialist – mainly teaching hospital based – and the family doctor who had beds at his disposal either in local voluntary hospitals or private nursing homes. He also usually had some specialist expertise himself in a chosen area of work. Pre-NHS, the teaching hospital was the centre for more esoteric consultant opinion; simpler problems were dealt with locally by fellow general practitioners who had made a particular study of their own speciality: for example, obstetrics, surgery or anaesthetics.

After 1948 there followed a very positive drive to spread excellence to every part of the country so that every health district, whether it had a medical school or not, would have the same access to expert specialist help when needed, locally available, and the patient would not need to travel to centres of learning, particularly London, where the greatest concentration of talent was found in the 12 great teaching hospitals, which are gradually being reduced in number.

Inevitably, therefore, money was channelled towards the big hospitals and, where there was none of adequate size in a health district, plans were made to build one or bring together smaller and more isolated units to make a corporate district general hospital. At the same time the various colleges of medical specialities began to require that their members achieve measurable standards of expertise by postgraduate training and examinations similar to those of the Royal Colleges of Physicians and Surgeons.

It became less easy for the family doctor to become a specialist as well as being a general practitioner, and without the relevant qualification and formal appointment and grading he would receive no extra remuneration. Gradually tension became apparent between the specialist hospital doctor with considerable sophisticated resources at his command and the non-specialist family doctor with very few resources to call upon. Some of the hospital fraternity began to view the general practitioner as one who had failed to become a specialist and for whom there was no other opening but to descend into general practice and to end his days merely treating the dross of health problems, while the more exciting, glamorous work was dealt with by the *real* doctors, the hospital-based giants. These giants were also the gatekeepers for that much-prized and valuable commodity, the hospital bed, for private nursing homes and small community-based voluntary hospitals had by and large been phased out in the name of clinical expediency and economy.

The recent regrowth of private hospitals, nursing homes and private insurance schemes, the resurrection of community hospitals and the realisation that big is neither beautiful nor very comfortable, have brought about a change of some consequence in the creative tensions in the medical hierarchy. The advent of fund-holding practices plus the Royal College of General Practitioners' firm grasp on the training of its members has not only gained greater respect for the qualifiers but the lateral mobility of trainees mentioned earlier has brought change into the walled-off hospital communities previously blissfully unaware of what was really going on in that nebulous entity, *the community*: the place where people live and cope with disability, ill health and handicap 99.5 per cent of the time, aided and abetted (or not as the case may be) by their families, friends, neighbours, primary health care teams, social services and voluntary organisations.

This being the case a future historian would be forgiven for asking why the monolithic Department of Health, with all its resources and power, had not concentrated more effort sooner into building up properly structured support services for the 99.5 per cent of the population in the place where it was most needed – that is, in their own homes; in other words, *the community*.

It would be easy to attribute any happening to only one cause, but there does appear to be a key element in the construction of this top-heavy hospital hierarchical edifice which may indeed be at least one of the root causes, if not the main one. That is the fact that all the major disciplines comprising the greater medical profession: doctors, nurses, physiotherapists, occupational therapists, radiologists, dentists and so on, receive the greater part of their clinical training in a hospital rather than in a community setting. At the most impressionable time, the imprint of the hospital hierarchy is stamped upon them and remains indelibly fixed, even if subconsciously, for life. The hospital is the apex of medical life and its workers are the cream. This impression is inevitably passed on to the media and the general public. Hence the easy capitulation to the philosophy that it is right to be born and die in hospital, rather than in one's own home; though the latter would, common sense and instinct suggest, be the best possible place for such natural and inevitable events to occur. Usually, people function best and most comfortably in the security of a known environment. Therefore, when one is in a negative state of health one needs all the reinforcement of normality and familiarity to help redress the balance. Any move into unfamiliar territory with unknown personnel to minister to one requires profound thought before such a radical upheaval is embarked upon.

A trainee in general practice presented a situation to the weekly tutorial group which still remained clear in his mind many years later. It went like this. During a Friday afternoon's surgery he was called out to deal with a home emergency. A 60-year-old woman had returned home a few days previously, having had an operation (a hysterectomy) in the local district hospital. It was clear to the doctor that she had a bowel obstruction and needed urgent readmission for further surgery of a life-saving nature. This was straightforward: a telephone call to the surgical firm at the hospital who immediately accepted her. The real problem, however, was the patient's 95-year-old mother who was almost blind and deaf, with whom the patient shared a house. Another daughter, who lived some distance away and had organised her life and family to come and look after her mother while her sister was in hospital, had gone home and could not be brought back in time for this emergency. What was the trainee GP to do? He reported to his trainer that he had had to suspend his other activities in order to deal with the crisis. The trainer wisely held his counsel but stayed available when he heard the course the trainee was proposing, which was a request to the Social Services to take over the care of the old lady. Discussions between the trainee, the duty officer and the social worker for the deaf and the social worker for the blind brought no solution as the lady was not a client known to them. No vacancy existed in the residential home and there were no emergency cover services to spare to go into the home to help. The next move was to contact the consultant in elderly care for a hospital bed to cover the crisis period. After endless telephoning to hospital departments eventually a consultant was found, who was certainly willing to help – but there was no empty bed available.

The situation seemed impossible. The time was now 5 p.m. The trainer then offered the telephone number of the organiser of the local church community help group, who willingly agreed to help by arranging a rota of members to go in and help the old lady in her own home, where she was able to remain among familiar surroundings and known hazards, able to follow her usual routine without the extra help she would have needed in a strange territory.

The best possible solution was found to enable this person to continue living as independently as possible. Someone almost blind and deaf is severely handicapped in strange surroundings and among strangers; in addition, her obvious great age would inevitably colour the attitudes of new carers and the odds are that this very vulnerable woman would have been reduced to a totally dependent (even incontinent if she could not work out the geography or special routines of the institution) 'geriatric', with all the connotations that this word has come to have. In hospital her needs would have ranked low as she had no illness; in a residential home with low staffing levels and shortage of trained personnel she would also have been at grave risk of being a name and room number and little else. It is alarming to think how close she came to losing dignity and independence.

This whole situation was viewed by the assembled tutorial group of doctors as yet another instance of the inability of the statutory authorities to cope properly with a simple crisis and how yet again voluntary services had had to bail them out. Such is the insidious nature of professional training which causes the mind to run along well-travelled grooves – in times of crisis there must be an institutional solution to the problem. Yet the ordinary human being and non-professional would see that in this case the right and optimal solution had been found. 'Surely prison is an exclamation point and every asylum is the question mark in the sentences of civilisation', as the sage S. W. Duffield commented. Such reactions are modifying but it is a woefully slow process.

This may seem a long-winded way of introducing a book on occupational therapy in the community but it is relevant, as will be seen. Occupational therapy training has been one of the sanest disciplines, keeping firmly in sight the need to treat both mind and body as a whole and ensuring that students acquire as varied a clinical experience as possible in the time available. As a result the trained therapist has had the experience of at least four quite disparate clinical settings and meeting many styles of management, both clinical and administrative; whereas some of the students of other disciplines may never have had to move away from their own health district, let alone hospital, throughout their clinical training.

The origins of occupational therapy were very much home- and community-based and the Chronically Sick and Disabled Persons Act 1970 gave the necessary impetus for therapists to move out of the hospital back to the grass roots, largely under the aegis of Social Service departments. As intensely skilled and practical professionals, the influence they have been able to exert on attitudes and thinking, both within Social Service and Environmental Health departments of local authorities, and also within primary health care teams, has been most marked, where time, opportunity and personality have been able to coincide opportunely.

None the less, from time to time institutional training may still become apparent and jar the susceptibilities of the normal independent adult, giving rise to the question: 'Is that what will happen to me if I have to seek help at some juncture of personal crisis?' These situations can arise purely from therapists working in isolation under stress and without like-minded colleagues available with whom to discuss ideas.

When circumstances become overwhelming and too much is being asked and expected of one professional and there is no time to breathe, think quietly or discuss with other disciplines, then one is forced back to known solutions and traditional ways of coping. There is no time to question whether such answers are appropriate to a specific current dilemma, and institutional answers to society's problems have been accepted by the majority of the population since Victorian times.

There are signs, however, that the climate of opinion is beginning to change. My own came in 1973 after a professional lifetime of trying to make hospital like home for elderly, disabled patients. A trip to Sweden revealed the fact that even the most sumptuous and well-designed environment could never make hospital like home for an elderly person nor indeed any age of person. Unless – and the thought is alarming – their previous environment or conditions have been so appalling that an institutional life is a welcome haven.

From 1973 onwards the inevitable route seemed to be to make the facilities and staff from the hospital available to the sick elderly person at home, in a scheme called 'Hospital at Home',[1] but when it became clear that such is the power of the institution to resist change, however logical, for me the only sensible progression seemed to be by trying to work from a base in community adult health. Consequently, for this particular health worker the last years working in the community were magical, almost like coming out of a long tunnel into the light. Suddenly to find that people, rather than patients, existed and were alive and well and functioning as members of their community, despite the fact that some were dealing with far more formidable disabilities and health problems than some of their peers languishing in nursing home beds or residential home places, was illuminating.

What makes the difference? What makes one person a resident in a young disabled unit (YDU) and another a council taxpayer living in a rented housing association's flat or owning a specially adapted property? Is it the type of disability? Is it the personality? Is it the number of family members available to help? Is it the primary health care team's input? Is it Social Services provision? Is it the part of the country in which he lives? Or is it purely the number of personnel available to help? Patently the answer lies in all these aspects, although one thing that is clear and strikes those that know, again and again, is that for every severely disabled or sick person in an institution there are many more equally so, coping somehow in their own setting in the community. The machinery to accomplish change is in place. It is being used tantalisingly and frustratingly slowly to enable anyone who wishes to be supported in their own chosen setting to be so.

It is said that many people who reside in YDUs and similar institutions have chosen to be there and would be nowhere else. This may have been so initially, when the alternative was perhaps between being a total burden on a loving relative or to live alone in unimaginable discomfort and squalor; but times have changed. Peoples' expectations of leading a full life, whatever their physical or mental disability may be, are so much higher which means that their expectations of professional advisers and helpers are also so much greater. We are being confronted daily by challenge, and all too frequently too many of us are still responding to those challenges by forcing the supplicant into straitjacket solutions of the traditional past, dredged up from training experiences. When there are too few being called upon to do too much for too many, this will be a foregone conclusion.

How do we get the equation right? So much of it currently depends on post-basic education and this book is very much part of that process. Within it, a number of exponents of the gentle art of meeting the supreme challenge of coping bare-handed with the health problems of people living in their own homes have shared their experiences with others, who may be meeting similar situations or be about to do so. This can only be good, with both sides gaining; the writer by taking stock of his practice and the underlying philosophy and rationale behind it, the reader by matching it with his own practice and experience, weighing up where to change his methods or to dispute that with which he disagrees, always bearing in mind the infinite capacity of the human mind to resist the introduction of fresh knowledge when it is already overloaded.

Meanwhile, we must press continually for medical education based soundly on the promotion and maintenance of good health in the community and for emphasis to be put on organising the necessary support in times of health crises in the individual person's own choice of setting. A similar approach should be made for support of long-term disability or illness. Finally, such situations that can be dealt with only in a special place such as a hospital or a particular type of residential home should be so arranged. If training is based on such a premise and carried out from normal bases of education, with the institutional side forming only a *small* part of a wide spectrum of clinical experience, then we will reach the time when every professional will be motivated into considering how we can support this person in his or her own home and what resources are necessary to call in to help, rather than 'How do I get this person into an institution to be looked after and his crisis coped with'.

It is not only lack of financial resources that is presently blocking this forward path – but also it centres around *attitudes*. The separation of health and Social Services into differently funded entities began the decline and subsequent reorganisations of both have done little to right the matter; even the brilliant idea of joint financing has only scratched the surface of joint co-operation and co-ordination. Funding for community care still comes from many different sources, ranging from central government to local fund-raising events. Nowhere as yet in the whole country is there a total, fully fledged structure and functioning community care service (available by telephone call for anyone who suddenly required it) to act as a model for all to see and gain faith that it can be done.

In 1985 the Prince of Wales's Advisory Group on Disability convened a working party with representatives from over 30 voluntary organisations and individuals from the statutory side. The task was to formulate guidelines for those planning services for people with severe disabilities. Interestingly, although it had been the original intention only to look at the age group 16–64 years, when *Living Options*[2] was eventually published it was clear that age was not the relevant component: disability was, and that the starting point in any consideration must be to:

1. *Recognise* that those who are affected by disability are people first and disabled second and have individual attitudes, likes, aspirations, fears and abilities.

2. *Understand* that although there may be special areas of need, people with disabilities wish to have the opportunity to live in the same way as other people.

If one takes these two statements together and applies them to all the sections of this book, be it the chapter on learning disabilities, mental health, head injuries, elderly care or children, then one can use them as a sort of litmus paper.

For an occupational therapist to function at such an individual level all the time may seem initially to be an exhausting way of working, but it is the only effective way of achieving agreed goals, and the compensations that accrue are tremendously rewarding.

Having become really person-at-home orientated and determined to help that person achieve whatever autonomy of daily living he or she is striving for we have to guard against our training once more, when the person asks for help to move outside their four walls and *do* something. The gradual move, over recent years, from a hospital patient lying passively in bed has followed a predictable path to the patient sitting in a chair beside the bed, to a table in the middle of the ward, to a day room off the ward; and from day room to out-patient department, then to day hospital, exchanging bed in ward to bed at home en route. From the day hospital the moves progress to day centre, social centre, work rooms, luncheon clubs, sheltered complexes of one type or another with centralised transport and facilities being provided for specific ages or groups of disabilities. Leisure, work, education, housing and counselling all need the same mode of application. One 15-year-old may not have the same interests as another 15-year-old, just as one 90-year-old does not necessarily have the same affinity with another nonagenarian. On the other hand, a 15-year-old and a 90-year-old, both ardent philatelists or cellists, might have a great deal in common even though one might have spina bifida and the other be an amputee.

As we move out of institutional bricks and mortar thinking, we must beware of still thinking institutionally about ways of providing activities for large numbers of people, seemingly in need of professional help. It is amazingly easy to set up, unwittingly, community institutions in order to rationalise scarce expertise or provide transport to get immobile people out of the house. In one's eagerness to provide answers it is possible to overlook all the natural everyday resources that are available to the ordinary citizen, both for education and leisure and recreation. It may take longer to set up individual programmes based on existing facilities, but in the long run a more satisfied person will be the result, who is less likely, therefore, to continually reappear on one's caseload.

We listen and read daily about the three million or more unemployed people in the land, but there are also many thousands of people (perhaps 2.5 million), who are in need of the sort of help that requires another human being, or several human beings in rotation. To solve both problems costs money; yet if there were universal conviction and faith that institutional care can and should be slimmed down, the revenue released from maintenance of buildings would more than pay for the needed human hands, thus leaving few institutional problems and much less unemployment.

Dr Geoffrey Spencer demonstrated this many years ago on Phipps Ward at the South Western Hospital: given two willing, although untrained, care attendants working in rotation, a person in a tank respirator could live alone in the community, provided that there were the needed expert back-up facilities. It is amazing how long it is taking to obtain similar freedom for less heavily dependent people such as para- or tetraplegics. The community service volunteers took up the challenge and have been able to show how efficacious the system can be. It can be done. What stops it? The answer must lie within the professional will, or lack of it, to unravel and use the plethora of new legislation and funding sources available to accomplish realistic community care.

So we are back at the beginning again – doctors' training is more reality orientated. Students are being encouraged to take their electives abroad, preferably in developing countries to see how other people cope and live, and all are being encouraged to question the relevance of some of their training. The remedial professions, too, have come out of the hospital hothouse into universities for their academic education. Occupational therapy has been in the forefront of leaving its sheltered clinical precincts to face the stress and strife of life among the Social Services, and there are now numerous experiments for incremental and collaborative training and practice.

Meanwhile, this book will help many people in various disciplines not only to understand what occupational therapists are striving for and accomplishing in the community, but also how the readers may adapt their own customs and practice towards giving much more customised help to the patient/client or person with whom they are in a professional relationship, or who may just be a neighbour or family member.

We are living in a new era and our working methods must reflect this, not only for those already mentioned but rather as a matter of enlightened self-interest. We shall all become old one day, and this is still a disadvantaged condition in our society. It would be heartening to think we might be able to retain our independence and individuality right to the end, whatever form of disability we accrue along the way.

References

1. Clarke, F. *Hospital at Home: The Alternative to General Hospital Admission*, London: Macmillan, 1984.
2. Prince of Wales Advisory Group on Disability, *Living Options, Guidelines for those planning services for people with severe physical disabilities*, 1985, Living Options Partnership, Kings Fund Centre, 126 Albert Street, London NW1 7NF.

Chapter 2

The disabled person within the family and community

JENNY CASSAM
District Manager Adult Care (Purchasing), Social Services Department, Norfolk County Council, Southern District

The term 'disabled person' is an extremely general one which is used to describe a state of not being able to function in life as well as one would wish for oneself or family or, to quote from the *International Classification of Impairments, Disabilities and Handicap*[1] by the World Health Organisation, 'a disability is a restriction or lack (resulting from an impairment) of ability to perform an activity in the manner or within the range considered normal for a human being'. There are many and varied ways to arrive at this state and indeed the end result may be very different, with functional loss varying according to the expectation and aspirations of the individual concerned.

One example of this is to be born with a disability: the baby has different parameters and goals to their development than someone born without such a handicap. Indeed, through their explorations of their abilities they can develop ways to overcome the functional loss very successfully. This was seen and well publicised in the studies carried out on children born with disabilities caused by thalidomide during the 1960s.

Other people, now described as disabled, have grown up to varying stages of their lives before suffering from an accident, injury or illness which results in the state of disability. The degree of disability may remain as at the time of their immediate recovery or they may improve their function as a result of treatment or by their own endeavours over a period of time.

Some people suffer from disease which causes functional loss, such as rheumatoid arthritis or multiple sclerosis. The nature of the disease can be sudden or cause progressive deterioration in the person's functioning and therefore in the way that they are able to adapt and cope with the resulting disability. Similarly, the disabled person who suffers from sensory impairment may do so from birth or as a result of disease or injury later in life and the sense of loss and their previous knowledge of their environment, if any, are factors in their ability to function as a result of the impairment.

Another group of people who by definition will become disabled by varying degrees and lengths of time are those who are suffering from a terminal illness. Their functional loss or disability becomes an added dimension to the situation with which the individual and their family have to cope.

Despite people having similar diagnoses and conditions they must not be regarded as 'the same as' one another. All the factors leading to their present level of functioning will have a bearing on the outcome in terms of how they cope, such as personality make up, family support and environment; nor should the effect of a disability on close relatives, friends, partners, siblings and children be ignored or underestimated. As discussed earlier, there are many ways in which the state of disability is arrived at and each one can have a different and profound effect on the other members of the close network. They may experience a deep sense of loss and bereavement as their previous expectations of life in the future are altered by the effect of the accident, injury or disease. This can take the form of grief or anger which needs to be acknowledged and worked through with them, if possible, in the same way that they would need to after an actual bereavement through death.

Parents of children born with a congenital condition or who have been recently diagnosed as having a disabling condition often experience the same kind of emotions, while siblings may feel that they are not given as much attention as the brother or sister with the disability. As an example, the mother of a 4-year-old disabled child recently arranged a week's respite care for that child as part of a care plan so that the rest of the family could go away on holiday. She asked her 6-year-old daughter if she would like to take a friend with her. The child did not answer at once, but at bedtime she politely said 'no thank you, mummy, because I hardly ever see you on my own'.

The emotions experienced by the people described above are interdependent with those emotions being experienced by the loved one who is the disabled person. This interaction can be even more pronounced when the person has a terminal illness and the inevitable result of the condition is known to them all.

Fear of the unknown often lies behind people's anxiety in the face of all disability. Human beings tend to have certain expectations of their lives, such as growing up, leaving home, becoming independent; when it becomes apparent that this natural progression through life is going to be prohibited or contracted in some way by disability, fears about the future and what is going to happen to them or their loved ones can become very real. It is through the process of understanding and exploring both the limitations and opportunities available in the care planning process that some of these emotions can be uncovered and some of the worries and fears alleviated.

Legislation

The NHS and Community Care Act 1990 is a major piece of primary legislation that has enormous implications on the way that statutory services (health, Social Services and housing) should be working with the voluntary sector in order to provide care in the community. Prior to this the Chronically Sick and Disabled Persons Act 1970 section 2 gave disabled people a statutory right to assessment for services which would provide them with access to what most people would regard as basic necessities, such as going to the lavatory and keeping themselves clean.

The Disabled Persons Act 1986 reinforced this duty on Social Services departments to decide about the needs of disabled people. It also included the need to take into account carers' ability to continue to care; and to work closely with Education departments to organise the assessment of state-mented children. A checklist of the rights and duties contained in this Act are set out in Fig. 2.1, although they have not yet all been implemented (for further information, see Appendix I).

The Children Act, which became law in 1989, builds on the need to minimise the effect of disability and give children the opportunity to live within the family and community as normally as possible (Fig. 2.2). This empowerment does, of course, need to continue as the child grows to adult-hood and their needs change and is acknowledged in *Caring for People – Community Care in the Next Decade and Beyond* (Fig. 2.3).[2]

Sir Roy Griffiths was appointed to review community care in 1987 after some criticism of policies at the time and reported the following year. There followed a great deal of professional and political debate and *Caring for People* was published in November 1990. The NHS and Community Care Act 1990 received royal assent on 29 June of that year. This was the basis for

1	A disabled person has the right to have an advocate ('authorised representative')
2	An advocate has rights to information and of access to meetings
3	A disabled person has a right to make his/her views known to the Social Services and have account taken of those views
4	Social Services has a duty to decide about the needs of disabled people for welfare services
5	Education and Social Services must work together to organise the assess-ment of 'statemented' children leaving full-time education
6	Education must keep under review the leaving date from full-time education of 'statemented' children
7	Health managers and Social Services must co-operate in organising the discharge from hospitals or long-stay patients with a mental illness or mental handicap
8	Social Services has a duty, when assessing a disabled persons' needs for services, to take into account the carer's ability to continue to care
9	Social Services has a duty to give disabled people information about relevant services

Source: *Caring for People – Community Care in the Next Decade and Beyond.*[2]

Fig. 2.1 Disabled Persons Act 1986

DEFINITION

'A Child is disabled if he is blind, deaf or dumb or suffers from mental disorder of any kind or is substantially and permanently handicapped by illness, injury or congenital deformity or such other disability as may be prescribed.'

(Children Act, Section 17(11))

PROVISION FOR DISABLED CHILDREN

'Every local authority shall provide services designed:

a   to minimise the effect on disabled children within their area of their disabilities; and
b   to give such children the opportunity to lead lives which are as normal as possible.'

(Children Act, Schedule 2, Part 1(6))

Source: *Caring for People – Community Care in the Next Decade and Beyond.*[2]

Fig. 2.2 Disabled children

Social Services departments, who were the designated lead agencies for community care and its funding under the Act, to prepare themselves for its implementation on 1 April 1993. The key objectives of the Act were the basis on which they had to make decisions on the structure, funding and staffing of their departments in order to carry out the statutory requirements on them. These key objectives are set out in Fig. 2.4, and further information is given in Appendix I.

The community care policies set out in *Caring for People* and the Act apply to services. There is much common ground between these policies and those which underlie the Children Act. Within SSDs and health authorities there will be a need to relate adult care policies to those for children. In both areas there is an objective of maintaining the individual within his or her family environment whenever possible. Assessment of individual needs followed by planned delivery of services subject to review or a complaints procedure with an independent element is common to both. This should provide the basis for a consistent approach to planning services for the two groups. There is a particular need to give attention to what happens when, at the age of 18, children's services are replaced by those designed for adults. This is particularly important for those who are disabled. The changing needs of both the young adult and his or her carer needs to be sensitively handled during this transitional stage. Separate guidance is being prepared on the Children Act which will address this interface in more detail.

Source: *Caring for People – Community Care in the Next Decade and Beyond.*[2]

Fig. 2.3 Links with the Children Act

Key objectives:

- to promote the development of domiciliary, day and respite services to enable people to live in their own homes wherever feasible and sensible;
- to ensure that service providers make practical support for carers a high priority;
- to make proper assessment of need and good care management the corner-stone of high quality care;
- to promote the development of a flourishing independent sector alongside good quality public services;
- to clarify the responsibilities of agencies and so make it easier to hold them to account for their performances;
- to secure better value for taxpayers' money by introducing a new funding structure for social care.

Source: *Caring for People – Community Care in the Next Decade and Beyond.*[2]

Fig. 2.4 National Health Service and Community Care Act 1990

One of the requirements on local authorities in the NHS and Community Care Act 1990 is that they should prepare and publish community care plans in co-operation with health and housing authorities. When preparing these the Act requires them:

> To consult with District Health Authorities, Family Health Services Authorities, Housing Authorities, Voluntary Housing Associations, voluntary organisations representing service users, voluntary organisations representing carers, bodies providing housing and community services in their area (this includes private and independent bodies) and any other the Secretary of State may direct.

Thus this provides for a local vehicle to be set up to enable individuals and organisations representing the views of disabled people to influence the planning process.

This was reinforced by another requirement of the Act, that local authorities and health authorities should produce joint agreed protocols on the discharge of patients from hospital. The Department of Health Circular HC(89)5[3] required Health Authorities to review their existing procedures to 'ensure that people do not leave hospital without adequate arrangements being made for their support in the community'. Local Authority Social Services departments were to be fully involved in the review process and received Circular LAC(89)7[4] to advise them of this. Health Authorities are responsible for the discharge of patients and guidance for the procedures and the roles of each staff group were set out in a booklet *Discharge of Patients from Hospital.*[5] Social Services departments were to be consulted about the role of their staff in the assessment and planning process, including the system for making referrals.

In the plans produced by Norfolk County Council Social Services department[6] in 1992 some of the philosophical bases for service for people with physical and sensory disabilities are as follows:

- Intervention, care and support should be determined in conjunction with the individual, his/her family and any other carers as a result of a professional assessment of their need.
- Services and resources should be both multi-agency and multidisciplinary and also be available to the client in his/her locality.
- Help should always aim to ensure that people with a disability have maximum choice of provision and retain full control over their lives. They must have a major input into the planning, development and delivery of services.

Philosophy

Occupational therapy has always been a profession which takes the broader view of a situation and, in the current political climate of emphasis on care in the community, there has never been a better opportunity for occupational therapists to use their skills to the full. The other element already mentioned briefly is the effect of the disability on any one member of a family and on the functioning of the group as a whole. This is something that the occupational therapist will need to be aware of during assessment and planning for packages of care.

The background to the philosophies which uphold the concept of the disabled person leading as full a life as possible, both within and without the family setting, go back a long time. In a previous textbook for occupational therapists, *Occupational Therapy in Rehabilitation*,[7] E. M. McDonald writes in her preface to the second edition: 'The basic philosophy and principles of the treatment remain very much the same as they have throughout history and right up to the present day. The primary needs of man are still for acceptance, recognition and security in home and job'. She continues in an almost prophetic statement: 'The challenge for the Occupational Therapist is to be observant, ingenious and up-to-date in outlook and practice; to be well informed, adaptable and versatile and to co-operate increasingly with other members of the rehabilitation teams and with government and voluntary agencies'. While written 30 years ago, this is still pertinent today and gives an early pointer to the need for multidisciplinary working as set out in the government White Paper *Caring for People*.[8]

Again in a specific reference to occupational therapy in the context of working to maximise individual potential, Louis Blom-Cooper QC offers a definition of the profession to the College of Occupational Therapists who commissioned his enquiry *Occupational Therapy and an Emerging Pro-*

fession in Health Care:[9] 'Occupational therapy is the assessment and treatment in conjunction and collaboration with other professional workers in the health and social services of people all ages with physical (and mental) health problems . . . in order to help (them) reach their maximum level of functioning and independence in all aspects of daily life'. Both the previous quotations lay foundations for the philosophy of the profession, which match so well with the latest concepts of care in the community that have emerged and become statutory over the last few years. Indeed, the aims of the NHS and Community Care Act 1990, as stated in the Introduction to *Community Care in the Next Decade and Beyond*[2] and which sets out the government's policy framework, are that 'the policy builds on the best of good practice which already exists. It aims to enable people to live an independent and dignified life at home, or elsewhere in the community for as long as they are able and wish to do so'. Therefore, the occupational therapist is a key player in the community team.

This brief resumé illustrates the professional and statutory philosophies underpinning the provision of care for the disabled person and their families in the community. In some instances it may seem to be stating the obvious; however, it is always worth comparing professional practice with the statutory parameters within which one has to work to ensure that the rights of a disabled person are recognised and valued.

One last quotation ends this section on a lighter note: 'The treatment of a patient is not completed until he is once again paying income tax'. This was the opinion of Dr Ludwig Gurman,[7] at the time Director of the spinal injuries centre at Stoke Mandeville. It offers a goal and presumes that there will be a neat end to the involvement, which is by no means always the case!

Assessment and care planning

The fact that the disabled person in the family and community setting is being considered in this chapter means that the emphasis must be on social, not medical, ways in which to help or alleviate the problems and burdens of the person and their families. In the majority of cases any medical intervention is at an end or, indeed, will be only a minor factor in the family's ability to cope with the situation, albeit emotionally charged.

One example is the case of Mrs F, an active 60-year-old very involved in local activities, who has cared for her husband, an arthritis sufferer for the last 5 years. She suffered a stroke, leaving her extremely weak on one side but retaining her power of speech. Her GP cared for her initially and decided that she did not need to go into hospital and certainly, she did not want to go. A district nurse came in for a couple of days and referred her to the local Social Services department for assessment. It was quite clear that Mrs F was going to need help with everyday social problems in order to maintain or regain her quality of life to her own satisfaction and would only need medical intervention if other medical problems occurred. The assessor to whom the referral from the district nurse was allocated was in this case an occupational therapist. The immediate considerations were to help Mrs F and her husband to keep up or return to the level of functioning that they had previously enjoyed. In other words, 'to get back to normal'; everyone will have a different definition or perception of 'normal'. The important thing for the assessor is to respect the standards and expectations of the person who is being assessed in each case and not to impose their own standards onto the situation (see Chapter 7). This, then, is the beginning of the process of collaboration with the client and family in order to devise a set of plans which from now on will be referred to as a 'care plan'. This care plan can be made up of several different elements in order to provide a solution to the problems as perceived by the disabled person in a way that they find acceptable. Some guidelines for this process are set out in the following extract from *Caring for People – Community Care in the Next Decade and Beyond*[2]. The assessment should:

- respond flexibly and sensibly to the needs of users and their carers;
- allow a range of options;
- intervene no more than is necessary to foster independence;
- prevent deterioration; and
- concentrate on those with greatest needs.

These guidelines should all be adhered to in every case and should reflect the following.

- A flexible and sensitive response to the needs of the users and their carers – this is not always as easy as it sounds as there may well be very different needs between user and carer and they will not have been openly acknowledged or discussed before this particular assessment. Everyone involved has to be made aware of the reason for the assessment and agree the desired outcome in broad terms. For example, the disabled person who wishes to remain at home rather than go into residential care, despite the fact that the situation may be breaking down and becoming extremely difficult for the carer.

- Range of options – these may be a few or many according to the client's wishes, desired outcomes, geographical circumstances or ethnic and religious considerations, but they should be identified and discussed clearly and openly.

- Intervene no more than necessary – sometimes a disabled person can feel extremely vulnerable and their experiences up to now may have left them feeling that they have very little personal control over their future. At this point the assessor needs to help them to understand that they do have choices and power over their destiny at both micro (time they want to go to bed and get up) and macro (possible return to work) levels.

- Prevent deterioration – this reflects the fact that people and situations rarely remain static and while an initial assessment deals with the immediate problems it is very important to review the situation regularly in order to identify and prevent deterioration in circumstances.

It can be extremely useful to involve someone in the assessment process who can represent the disabled person in a non-professional sense. This can be a friend or relative – not the carer – or someone from a local voluntary agency, and are known as advocates. The role of the advocate is to act as a catalyst for ideas, to ask questions which the disabled person does not think of or does not like to ask at the time, especially about financial aspects, and generally make sure that the views of the person being assessed are fully explored and taken into consideration. They can also often remember things about the conversation which are helpful afterwards and can telephone or write to ask supplementary questions or add other points, if necessary. Their knowledge of the locality might also be very useful when the time comes to discuss possible packages of care.

Having considered the wider concepts of assessment it is important to realise that within these there can be different levels of assessment. It may well be that the presenting problem and the wishes of the disabled person both have an input on the decision as to which level is appropriate. The table in Fig. 2.5 sets out six levels from simple to comprehensive assessment as defined in *Care Management and Assessment: Practitioners Guide*.[10]

For any disabled person the need for a particular level of assessment can change over time as their condition or circumstances change. It should not, therefore, be assumed that a review assessment is necessarily going to be at the same level as the original one; for example, the original assessment found a need for the provision of a toilet seat and rail. However, at the review or follow-up assessment the carer is saying they can no longer cope. This may

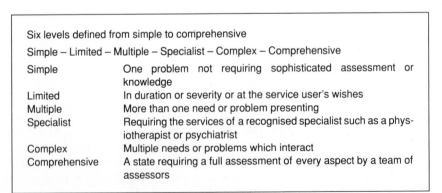

Six levels defined from simple to comprehensive	
Simple – Limited – Multiple – Specialist – Complex – Comprehensive	
Simple	One problem not requiring sophisticated assessment or knowledge
Limited	In duration or severity or at the service user's wishes
Multiple	More than one need or problem presenting
Specialist	Requiring the services of a recognised specialist such as a physiotherapist or psychiatrist
Complex	Multiple needs or problems which interact
Comprehensive	A state requiring a full assessment of every aspect by a team of assessors

Fig. 2.5 Levels of assessment

The process of assessing need is a 10 stage process

1	Deciding the scope of negotiations
2	Choosing the setting
3	Clarifying expectation
4	Prompting participation
5	Establishing trust
6	Assessing need
7	Determining eligibility
8	Setting priorities
9	Agreeing objectives
10	Recording the assessment

Source: *Care Management and Assessment: Practitioners Guide.*[10]

Fig. 2.6 The process of assessment

mean that the care plan will now need to contain home care, meals on wheels, extra equipment, respite care or any or all of the options at any one time.

Figure 2.6 gives official guidance which sets out 10 processes for assessment, beginning with the decision as to the level of the assessment and ending with the recording of the assessment. Recording the assessment is vitally important in the process. The options discussed and decisions reached should be carefully written down, preferably at the time of the assessment, and agreed and signed by all parties involved. Even where there are areas of disagreement these should be noted and the reasons clearly stated. This then becomes a record of the needs discussed and options chosen, owned and agreed by the user, carer where appropriate, and the care manager before the care plan is put into operation.

By now in any assessment process the care manager should have a very clear picture of need, what services could be provided to meet that need, and how they can be arranged in order to obtain maximum benefit and satisfaction to the disabled person and their family. This may well involve different agencies in multi-agency or multidisciplinary provision of care or services, such as the primary health care team, housing authorities, Social Services, voluntary sector agencies and specialist health services, in a fairly comprehensive care plan. It will, however, remain the responsibility of the care manager, or key worker as they are sometimes known, to co-ordinate the arrangements and ensure that they all work in a complementary way to produce the agreed outcome for the disabled person. Care plans and their possible outcomes are described in Fig. 2.7.

It will be obvious from the potential complexity of such care plans that good local multi-agency and multidisciplinary relationships are essential in order to maintain the required level of co-operation needed. These can be fostered and enhanced by the encouragement of local multi-agency training

Once needs have been assessed, the services to be provided or arranged and the objectives of any intervention should be agreed in the form of a care plan. The objective of ensuring that service provision should, as far as possible, preserve or restore normal living implies the following order of preference in constructing care packages which may include health provision, both primary and specialist, housing provision and social services provision:

- support for the user in his or her own home including day and domiciliary care, respite care, the provision of disability equipment and adaptations to accommodation as necessary;
- a more to more suitable accommodation, which might be sheltered or very sheltered housing, together with the provision of Social Services support;
- a move to another private household, i.e. to live with relatives or friends or as a part of an adult fostering scheme;
- residential care;
- nursing home care;
- long-stay care in hospital.

Source: *Caring for People – Community Care in the Next Decade or Beyond*,[2] paragraph 3.24.

Fig. 2.7 Agreeing a care plan

and staff development sessions which, wherever possible, should include local GPs who are an essential factor in care in the community.

The role of the GP in assessment and planning of care in the community is an important and unique one. The practice will have an almost universal coverage of the local population and in many cases their surgeries are a focal point in the local community. They are usually held high in public esteem and there is little or no stigma attached to going to see them. They also have an important role to play in hospital discharge planning, when further medication or treatment is necessary.

There is, however, an element of tension between their role as advocate and long-term 'provider' for their patient and some of the harder decisions which inevitably have to be made when allocating finite resources to packages of care. This needs to be acknowledged from the outset of any discussion.

It is also important to remember the fluidity and possible speed of change in any situation. It is therefore essential that good lines of communication between agencies are kept open so that potential problems can be identified quickly and acted upon to prevent the situation breaking down.

It cannot be emphasised enough that assessment must be *needs-led*. However, there will be occasions when the disabled person's preferred outcome cannot be wholly met. This could be a resource issue or a lack of availability of the type of provision they require. Clearly, the skill of the assessor in negotiating an acceptable outcome or enabling the disabled person to attain their preferred option in a different way is extremely important.

As the first year of the new legislation has progressed these skills have been developing constantly in professional assessors and some very flexible and imaginative, and not always wildly expensive, packages of care have evolved.

Enabling

The effect of having to be cared for by someone else because of a disability can be very debilitating in itself. There is a loss of personal dignity and sometimes of feelings of self-worth. There can be small but subtle ways in which the carer makes decisions for the cared-for without realising what they are doing or the effect that it can have on the disabled person; even a small thing such as putting them in slippers rather than shoes because it is easier can have a demoralising effect.

Most readers will be familiar with the phrase 'Does he take sugar?' which epitomises some of society's attitude to disability. It is therefore extremely important when assessing need and drawing up care plans to make certain that the individual and their family have access to enough information to enable them to discuss the options available and make informed choices. Whether the discussion is centred around large choices such as whether the cost of an adaptation to property is affordable or can be eligible for a grant, or smaller but equally important issues such as what time the individual prefers to get up in the morning or go to bed at night, the right to contribute to the discussions should be implicit.

Enabling and empowering people to make their own choices gives them some control over their life and a feeling that their ideas and opinions are valid and matter in the discussion which does, after all, concern them a great deal. It is possible in some circumstances that to enable the disabled person and their carer to contribute fully, some of the discussions need to take place apart from one another and this is perfectly acceptable practice, as long as everyone involved knows that the aim of the exercise is to agree a care plan which is achievable and works for all concerned.

Similarly, when discussing the most appropriate provision of service it is important that the disabled person is given enough information on which to base their judgement and equally important to make sure that the care plan is flexible enough to be changed if it does not work. The disabled person and their carers must know from the outset that changes can be made without prejudicing their right to continued help.

Sadly, the feeling of powerlessness sometimes prevents people from indicating that they are not satisfied because they fear reprisals. Instead of stating their real feelings, they then agree to things that they may not really want at all. Guidelines on complaints procedures and inspection units being set up by local authorities under the NHS and Community Care Act 1990 are designed to combat this, but it is also important for everyone working towards helping someone to live as full a life as possible in the community to make sure that their personal choices and opinions are always considered and valued first rather than last on the list.

Networks

The importance of an assessment of need reflecting the needs of the carer as well as the disabled person has already been highlighted. However, it must be re-emphasised that their needs can be substantially different from those of the disabled person being assessed. They are likely to know the disabled person a good deal better than the assessor and be able to point out areas of potential conflict of interest. Official guidelines on working with and involving carers are shown in Fig. 2.8.

For any disabled person living alone in the community or with their family there is likely to be a much wider network of people who can contribute to an overall pattern of care or better quality of life. They may include neighbours, friends, relatives not living in the same house, local organisations, churches, clubs, disability groups, the local pub, shop or school.

In order to gain the best possible outcome for the disabled person and their carer in terms of quality of life, it is important to discuss any of these wider networks as potentially being able to be included in the care plan. Sometimes where a disability pressure group exists, their support can be enlisted in order to obtain a particular service or piece of equipment which is otherwise unobtainable through statutory means. Other relatives, friends and neighbours can often help by giving the carers a break and time to themselves, either by taking the disabled person out for a while, by coming to sit with them while the carer goes out or contributing to respite care arrangements.

12	Relatives and other carers often know a great deal about the patient's earlier life, previous interests, abilities and contacts and may have personal experience of the course of his/her illness spanning many years. Wherever consistent with the patient's wishes, professional staff should seek to involve them in the planning and subsequent oversight of community care and treatment.
13	Carers often make a major and valued contribution to the support received by many people with a mental illness being treated in the community. Where a care programme depends on such a contribution, it should be agreed in advance with the carer who should be properly advised both about such aspects of the patient's condition as is necessary for the support to be given, and how to secure professional advice and support, both in emergencies and on a day to day basis. In addition, professional staff may be able to offer the carer help in coming to terms with his/her role *vis-à-vis* the patient.

Source: *Caring for People – Community Care in the Next Decade and Beyond*,[2] paragraphs 12 and 13.

Fig 2.8 Involving carers

All these things help to make the situation less fraught for carer and disabled person alike and therefore less likely to break down.

Information

With this wealth of legislation and structures to enable proper assessment for services, consultation and joint care plans, what happens when someone suddenly needs to know what is available to help them? Information is power and if the disabled person and their carers do not have information about what is available, they can feel powerless. It is therefore very important that they are given as much information as possible in an accessible form, including braille, cassette, ethnic language and signing, so that they can make informed choices.

At the time of the visit to their home for an assessment the disabled person and their family may not be able to assimilate all the information. Just as it is difficult for anyone to assimilate all the information available at the travel agent's when choosing a holiday, so it is much more helpful if that information is left with them in order that they can take it in at their own time and convenience and then decide what might be of most benefit to them. Local disability groups often produce a great deal of useful local and national material and most libraries hold the addresses of clubs and user groups who meet regularly. While the professional assessor does not need to have all this information to hand, it is very useful to be able to direct people to the place where they can obtain the information.

Another vital area for disabled people and their families to know about is their eligibility for benefits. Many benefit agencies have mechanisms for providing this service and often local Citizens' Advice Bureaux can be invaluable in helping individuals with this and other related subjects. *The Disability Rights Handbook*[11] which is published annually provides instant access to information on rights and benefits. As loss of income or the inability to obtain open employment mean the disabled person and their families may have financial worries, as well as other problems concerned with illness and disability, it can be of enormous help to them to be informed of where to go for help in order to maximise their income.

A small personal collection of miscellaneous leaflets or addresses on such things as travel, holidays and accessible entertainments can also be a useful tool for the professional as they may provide the answer to a particular expressed need as long as out-of-date leaflets are regularly thrown away!

The recent legislation and high profile of care in the community have highlighted the plight of the disabled person and their family and with it brought the hope of more choice, with budgets being devolved downwards and the ability to manage them more flexibly at local level becoming a reality. The emphasis now should be on influencing the attitudes of society. Access does not only have to be for the disabled. An accessible environment benefits everyone and prejudices none.

References

1. World Health Organisation, *International Classification of Impairment, Disabilities and Handicap*, Geneva: World Health Organisation, 1980.
2. *Caring for People – Community Care in the Next Decade and Beyond – Policy Guidance*, London: HMSO, 1990.
3. Department of Health Circular HC(89)5.
4. Department of Health Circular HC(89)7.
5. Department of Health, *Discharge of Patients from Hospital*, 1989.
6. *Norfolk County Council Social Services Community Care Plan*, 1992.
7. MacDonald, E. M. (ed.) *Occupational Therapy in Rehabilitation, 2nd edn*, London: Bailliere, Tindall and Cox, 1964.
8. White Paper, *Caring for People*, London: HMSO, 1990.
9. Blom-Cooper, L. *Occupational Therapy an Emerging Profession in Health Care – Report of a Commission of Enquiry*, London: College of Occupational Therapists, 1989.
10. *Care Management and Assessment: Practitioners Guide*, London: HMSO, 1991.
11. Disability Alliance Educational and Research Association, *Disability Rights Handbook*, London (annual publication).

Further reading/Resources

The Carer's Guide, Basingstoke: Macmillan Magazines, 1994.
Griffiths, R. *Community Care: Agenda for Action*, Report to Secretary of State for Social Services, 1988.
Wagner, G. *Report of the Independent Review of Residential Care A Positive Choice*, London: National Institute for Social Work, HMSO, 1988.

Chapter 3

Understanding ethnic groups

SHEILA EDEN

Head Paediatric Occupational Therapist, City and East London Family and Community Health Services, NHS Trust

In a relatively short period of time Britain has changed from a predominantly white homogeneous society into one that is multiracial, multicultural and multilingual. Britain now has a variety of cultures so diverse that to try to discuss them in only a few pages would do none justice. It is therefore not the intention within this chapter to look at different cultures in any great depth, but to identify commonalities of working with people from a wide range of backgrounds.

We all aspire to be part of a cultural group and to have an identity. Cultural values develop over a period of time and key people, particularly our parents and peers, play a significant role in influencing it by the messages they communicate and, more importantly, through their own behaviour. No one is neutral and none has a monopoly on wisdom, nor fully understands the subtleties that exist in cultures other than our own.

'Black and ethnic minority' is the current term used in official documentation to describe a group of individuals who consider themselves, and are seen by the community at large, as being distinct because of one or more differences, such as racial origin, skin colour, language, religious beliefs and practices or dietary customs. Unfortunately, like all labels, its frequency of use produces abuse, and to many the term implies that the user is referring only to this country's black and Asian population. This should not be the case, as any reference to a minority group includes all cultures that are different from the indigenous population.

Patterns of migration

Having some knowledge of the reasons behind immigration to Britain can assist therapists in raising awareness and give an understanding of the specific issues relating to ethnicity, and its associated health and social behaviour patterns.

This country has a long history of accepting, with varying degrees of tolerance, peaceful migration from different parts of Europe. Jewish, Italian, Greek and Cypriot communities have all become well established and can be found in many parts of Britain. Prior to the beginning of the Second World War this immigration was small and predominantly white. Immigration on a large scale began after the war as a result of the expansion of western European economies and poor economic prospects in large parts of the Commonwealth. Legislation has now virtually stopped new immigrants, and people entering the country today are usually from areas of conflict, such as Somalia and former Yugoslavia.

During the 1950s Britain was desperately short of unskilled labour for its economic revival and so actively recruited overseas workers. Many prisoners of war also chose to remain in Britain, bringing their families here to live. The influx of Poles, Hungarians, Ukranians, Italians, Czechs and Slovaks brought changes and new traditions to the British way of life. Much of the culture from these groups has now become integrated into British life.

By 1952 the United States closed its doors to people from the Caribbean Islands wishing to work in America. They consequently looked to Britain for employment and joined large employers, such as London Transport, who had opened recruitment offices in the Caribbean. During the following 10 years immigration from these islands was at its peak.

During the 1960s Asian immigration took place, particularly following the war between India and Pakistan, and the eventual partition of Kashmir, the Punjab and later Bangladesh. The loss of farms and poor prospects of jobs in their own countries encouraged Asians to look to Britain. At about the same time, the African nationalist movement caused severe economic and political pressures on the large Asian community in East Africa, particularly in Uganda. Families were forced to leave as refugees, abandoning properties and businesses, and looked to Britain and India for safety.

Initially the majority of new immigrants were young men, unskilled and often illiterate in English. Like Britons abroad, they often grouped themselves together in small communities for support. During this time Britain experienced good employment prospects and new immigrants had little difficulty in finding work, although this was mostly in the low-paid sector of large industrial cities. Once settled, they found homes and sent for their dependants. This chain of migration brought many difficulties for immigrants, including the often hostile and arrogant attitudes of some white Britons.

Contrary to some people's beliefs, black and Asian people are not a homogeneous group but represent wide cultural, religious and linguistic diversity. More recent arrivals to Britain are very different in language, dress, diet and religion; consequently, people are becoming more aware of value systems which may be different from one's own, thus creating the potential for racism. A prerequisite for counter-balancing racism is a greater understanding of one's own attitudes and of the various ethnic groups that make up our society.

Problems of adaptation

Today, it is estimated that three million people living in England and Wales are from ethnic minority groups. This constitutes 6 per cent of the total population (OPCS 1991 census).[1] The arrival of immigrants into a community brings with it inevitable stresses during the initial period of adjustment. For therapists working with them it is important to remember that families will experience culture shock. The level and severity of such shock is related to the amount of change experienced, influenced by unsympathetic officials and exacerbated by homelessness and unemployment. Adult members of a family can develop various changes in attitude and behaviour which may cause family tensions with children and other family members, the resulting anxiety and insecurity manifesting themselves in physical and/or mental illness. Fortunately, many groups have set up their own systems for supporting new arrivals, particularly where statutory services are ignoring these needs (see Photo. 3.1).

One of the fundamental problems for all ethnic groups is the ability to understand and communicate with the various statutory authorities.[2-4] Even for those born in Britain, these services can appear confusing, as confirmed by the amount of unclaimed benefits each year. Small problems can easily become major anxieties for those unfamiliar with the complexities of the

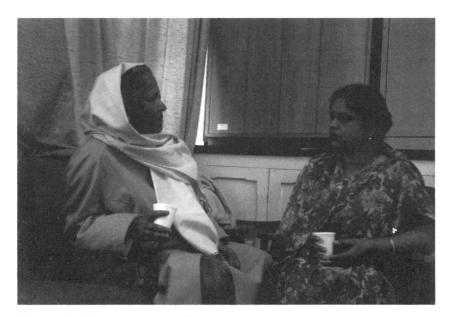

Photo. 3.1 Advocacy and counselling service

British Health, Social Security and Local Authority systems. Knowledge of statutory services is gained by contact with the various agencies and therapists should *never* use length of residency as an indicator of a person's level of understanding but be ready to give advice which is always clear, concise and accurate.

Cultural differences

Social customs and modes of behaviour need to be respected. Some religions, for example the Islamic faith, lay down a detailed code of conduct which becomes an integral part of a Muslim's social, political and cultural life. Many religions also attach great importance to personal cleanliness and methods of cooking and eating.

For many children, particularly newer immigrants, preschool years are spent immersed within their own community and culture. On reaching school age some children still have a poor command of English, which puts them at an instant disadvantage. This difficulty can vary widely among people of the same ethnic group and usually depends on the parents' educational background and their access to English. Activities may be alien for some ethnic groups and children can appear awkward in their use; for example, using a knife and fork by children from Chinese, Asian and Middle Eastern communities may not be taught at home. Therapists should be aware that an inability to produce this skill at school may be due to inexperience rather than a lack of skill. They should also learn to question whether the teaching of a skill is actually relevant to that person. Any information given, whether verbal or written, must be presented in a form that can be easily understood, is translatable and contains no ambiguities (see Photo. 3.2).

As children mature, the prominent problem is often the conflict of values that can occur between home and the community, especially school. In many ethnic communities there is a distinct cultural difference between the expected roles of men and women. Older children, particularly teenagers, often feel caught between their own culture and that of their adopted country, thus creating conflicts and difficulties in reconciling the two patterns of behaviour. For example, girls may be expected to stay at home in the evenings and not join their peers in mixed social gatherings. Therapists therefore need to use great sensitivity when integrating young disabled people into social activities.

The statutory authorities

The National Health Service was created to provide a high standard of health care to people from a fairly homogeneous culture and background. The patterns of service and staff training are still largely based on the needs of this population and often fail to take into account the multicultural nature of Britain today. This failure can affect the quality of care ethnic minority

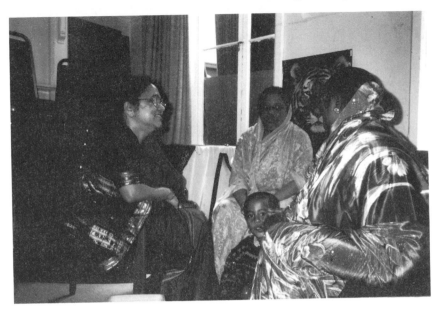

Photo. 3.2 Self-help community drop-in service

people receive, making it less accessible, equitable or appropriate to their needs.[2,3,5]

The ultimate objective in health and social care is that all minority groups are integrated into, and make use of, the existing structures of the Health and Local Authority services. However, because of the broad and complex needs of these groups there is an increasing recognition that it is impossible to supply 'the same service for all'. Several factors determine the need to change this approach relating mainly to communication, culture and religion.[2,4,6] Other factors include issues around racial prejudice and discrimination, disease variation patterns and specific conditions prevalent to different groups, such as sickle cell disease and thalassaemia. It is now recognised that services must adapt and take account of these differences so that care can be delivered in a more flexible, sensitive and culturally acceptable manner.

Recent government legislation, such as The Children Act 1989 and National Health Service and Community Care Act 1990 has put race, culture, religion and language on the agenda for the first time (see Appendix I). The challenge ahead is to ensure that all agencies and staff provide and deliver services with equity and sensitivity despite limited resources.

A challenge for therapists

Cultural and religious issues are extremely important to many people from an ethnic minority background. All vary considerably in their beliefs and lifestyles and it is important to remember that the extent to which individuals observe their religion and culture can differ greatly. Individual needs will depend on the immigrant; for example, first generation immigrants, not having adapted to a western lifestyle, often have different needs when compared with subsequent generations.[7] In addition many established ethnic groups have modified their attitudes to diet, religious observances and dress since coming to this country, the extent of which varies between generations and gender. Therapists should never assume from a person's name, appearance or religion what their needs are but always ask, using information about different cultures purely as a guide.

The broad aim of occupational therapy is to meet the needs of an individual within their own culture. Therapists have an important role in ensuring that all groups have access to good standards of health and social care. Most British-trained therapists, however, have little exposure to other cultures in any formal training situation and thus have little idea of how different cultures really perceive health and sickness. Gaining an understanding of different cultures is essential for appreciating clients' views, values and interpersonal interactions. It can also assist in understanding how lifestyles can be influenced by other cultural standards and why therapy does not always work. Obtaining training is vitally important; it helps the therapists to understand themselves and in broadening an awareness and appreciation of just how diverse communities are. It also helps to examine personal attitudes; to break down preconceived ideas about race and the fixed images so frequently attached to people in a very stereotypical and misleading manner. Training should encompass cultural beliefs, values and customs; how these shape a person's behaviour; how ethnic minority groups are disadvantaged by poor social–economic situations, social and work conditions and how these factors affect their health. Appropriate services can only be provided once therapists are fully trained and informed about the nature of the community in which they work and are able to empathise fully with their clients.

Specific issues

Probably the areas that produce the most anxiety among therapists are how to address people correctly, using interpreters and visits to homes. It is for this reason that these areas have been selected for specific comment.

Names and records

Each culture has its own naming system. For many the formal title used, for instance Mr S. Cirpan, is similar to the British system thus presenting no problem when recording a person's last name. However, others are very different which can cause serious and even dangerous confusion. For example, in some systems the first name is religious and not a personal one. In another the last name is a title which indicates religion and/or gender, and not a family surname, resulting in each family member having a different name. Yet other systems, when written, place the family name first while some have regional differences which denote caste or subcaste.

It is therefore easy to muddle records and cause offence or embarrassment by using names incorrectly. One very common error is to ask a person for their Christian name; this is meaningless to a Muslim and thus 'first name' should be used. Further complications are now arising as families adapt their traditional system to the British style, which can lead to further confusion for the therapist. They are therefore advised to ask families for assistance and to enter a clear explanation in any records. Good practice is always to check that the initial information is correct at the first meeting. Find out:

1. the client's full name;
2. the correct way to address them;
3. the person's first name rather than Christian name;
4. whether the last name is a shared family surname – if not, create a method to help identify this on the record;
5. any 'nickname' used – particularly with children, as these are often used by families in preference to the child's registered name; and
6. the correct pronunciation of the name in brackets if it is pronounced very differently.

Communication

Effective communication is essential and evidence from nursing research, such as that undertaken on pain[8] and patient recovery,[9] proves that by giving people information this has a positive affect on recovery and wellbeing. Occupational therapists may increasingly require the support of interpreters in their assessment and intervention with clients; particularly as there is now a sizeable ageing population among ethnic groups. An interpreter will not only assist those who do not speak English, but those whose command of English is affected by illness or stress. Recent surveys in Leicester and Bradford[10] support the need for multilingual literature or interpreters to enable minority groups to gain access to services (Photo. 3.3).

Where there is a language barrier the therapist is faced with three options:

1. using a professional interpreter;
2. using a friend or relative to interpret; and
3. communicating without an interpreter.

Using professional interpreters. Ideally both therapist and client should have access to an interpreter whenever necessary to facilitate com-

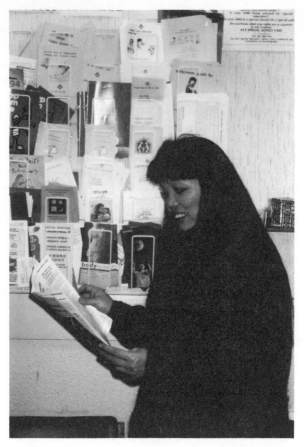

Photo. 3.3 Providing information in a format usable by all local community groups

munication. Access to such services is now recognised as a person's right and purchasing authorities are expected to pay attention to this when commissioning Health and Social Services.[11] If interpreter time is not available for every client consultation, then the therapist should plan longer sessions at key points of time – for example, when preparing for hospital discharge; at the first community visit; or when reporting back results. To interpret for someone else is a skill that should not be underestimated. To give clients good care and support the interpreter should be:

1.   trained and experienced;
2.   fluent in English and the client's mother tongue and dialect;
3.   able to understand the terminology to be used, e.g. medical terminology; and
4.   someone both therapist and client can trust.

In most cases it is neither sufficient, nor possible, for an interpreter to simply translate words. Interpreters act as advocates to clients, helping to redress the imbalance of knowledge and power that exists between a professional and client.[4,5,6] The interpreter is there to ensure that genuine two-way communication takes place and the client's comments are taken seriously by the visiting professional. This task can be extremely difficult and the interpreter plays an essential role in ensuring that the client understands what is happening; asks all the necessary questions; and has the relevant information to make informed decisions.

The therapist will need to check that the interpreter is the right one for the situation; that they speak the same language and dialect; whether gender would be an issue for both client and interpreter; that the client is comfortable about using the interpreter before starting; and confidentiality is guaranteed. In addition there are several points to consider during the interview.

1.   Allow adequate time – at least twice as much time as usual. If the situation is complicated a great deal of explaining may be necessary; thus, investing time at this stage can reduce misunderstanding and problems later.
2.   Prepare for the interview in advance. Outline the situation to the interpreter and explain the aims and any possible complications.
3.   Allow time for the interpreter and client to get to know each other. Many people find it discourteous to talk about personal issues straight away.
4.   Ask the interpreter for assistance with how to address the client and make clear that their advocacy role is understood and welcomed.
5.   Keep the language simple and free from jargon.
6.   Conduct the interview in English if the client understands English and ask the interpreter to listen for any misunderstandings.
7.   Beware of over-burdening the interpreter and never leave them alone to give clinical advice. Remember, therapists are responsible for client care.

Using a client's friend or relative. There will be occasions when a professional interpreter is unavailable and a friend or relative is used. This can be difficult for everyone but there are a few ways to minimise problems and distress.

1.   Listen to the interpreter's command of English and decide on how much can be expected from them. There may be situations where only the bare essentials are discussed or communication may be better without an interpreter at all.
2.   Find out the interpreter's relationship with the client, as this may affect what they can be asked to translate.
3.   It is unethical to use children to interpret except in simple day to day conversations or extreme emergencies.

4.   Be aware that the client may not want the interpreter to know everything. Remember, it is almost impossible to respect a person's confidentiality in this situation and some things may best be left until a professional interpreter is available.

5.   Give the interpreter the confidence to do a good job. Find out if there are concerns about how to translate any information.

6.   Make it clear that their assistance is valued and recognise that the situation is not ideal.

7.   Get a professional interpreter to check what has been said wherever possible, particularly if in doubt about the interpreter's ability and reliability. Incorrect translations can have serious consequences and cause distress to clients and families.

Communicating without an interpreter. In too many situations staff still have to communicate across a language barrier without an interpreter. Although this is unsatisfactory, there are ways in which a therapist can improve communication.

1.   Plan ahead and take one topic at a time.

2.   Speak in plain English, avoiding long words and colloquial language.

3.   Speak slowly and listen for the words the client uses; try to include these.

4.   Consider ways to assist communication when the client has difficulty in expressing themselves owing to emotional or physical stress.

5.   Avoid questions that can be answered with a simple 'yes'. This is the first word most people learn and it does not necessarily mean that they understand the question!

6.   Give any instructions in the order they are to be used.

7.   Become sensitive to non-verbal signs, e.g. body language, tone of voice.

8.   Use demonstrations where possible to illustrate points.

9.   Remember, coping with a language barrier can dramatically affect the way people behave.

10.   Leave clear notes of explanation for the client or family to read later, as listening to a foreign language is tiring and can affect a person's memory.

Visiting the home

A successful visit can always be achieved if it is well planned and the therapist empathises with the client. Meeting people from a different background to one's own can produce feelings of inadequacy and awkwardness and therefore it is important to remember that people are people irrespective of their ethnicity. It is not the differences that prevent therapists assisting clients, but *attitudes* towards these differences. If the visiting therapist is able to show respect for others, then an open approach is possible. Problems can be more easily identified once trust and understanding is established.

The initial visit is important in reaching the right relationship with the client and their family. Correct introductions must be made, with a full explanation given about the reason for the visit and who has asked for it to take place. By completing these formal introductions any confusion can be minimised. This will also assist in relieving anxieties that may be present, particularly for people inexperienced in using the statutory organisations. A right approach initially will produce positive attitudes towards receiving future care.

Assessment

Like any occupational therapy assessment, the therapist should initially assist with whatever the client and family consider to be the main area of difficulty, leaving other problems to later. However, in some situations a client may be unable to explain the true nature of the problem. Activities of a more intimate nature, such as managing the toilet without assistance, may not be readily admitted in front of others. A client may only offer the information they think the therapist wants to hear, rather than indicate their true feelings. If in doubt rephrase the question or make a note to check again at a subsequent visit.

Before offering advice or equipment therapists need to be aware that some solutions, though sensible within one's own culture, may not be acceptable in another. It is not uncommon to find clients failing to respond to previous advice. If this does occur endeavours need to be made to discover the reason behind such apparent lack of co-operation, for it may be that the client's initial response was not accurately understood. For example, a report *Asian and Disabled*, jointly published by the Asian Disability Advisory Project team, Spastics' Society and Barnardos[10] found that difficulties in providing Bradford's Asian communities with the appropriate services were related more to gender than to a person's religious belief.

When selecting equipment it is important to consider cultural factors. Occupational therapists rightly place importance on usefulness or function but acceptance within a community may well be more important to the client. Cultural affects must be considered before trying to convince a person to accept equipment that may make their disability more noticeable.

Developing or maintaining a person's independence is an important thera-peutic function. The way skills develop can be influenced by cultures. If a person's disability prevents the use of their traditional skills the obvious solution is not always the right answer. Feeding is a good example of this, as simply using the left hand may not be an acceptable solution to many people of the Muslim faith. In some situations cultural values may therefore take precedence over independence.

Rehabilitation

Attitudes towards an individual family member's disability or illness can vary among all sectors of society. Beliefs and customs sometimes cause people to be undervalued. Fear of what is strange, different or simply not understood can explain many people's negative feelings. Many ethnic groups have very strong family ties, with each member having a particular role. When a disability is introduced, whether through birth, injury or acquired, these traditions can affect a person's independence and role within the family unit. In some situations status within the family unit can change. For example, a mother with poor mobility within the home could expect other female family members to take over her duties.

For many people the sharing of feelings within a group situation can be extremely difficult. Within some minority groups this public sharing of feelings is alien and becomes even more difficult if mixed gender is involved. Physical contact, particularly in role-play situations, may also be unacceptable. Some ethnic minority groups use techniques such as meditation or relaxation to quite advanced levels and in some situations these skills can be utilised for the benefit of all.

There are no short cuts or easy answers when attempting to break down the barriers that exist between therapists and clients from minority groups. Barriers will only be broken by careful thought, planning, empathy and training. Therapists should research and evaluate their own effectiveness in providing accessible and acceptable local services. Current changes in legislation regarding minority ethnic communities is a beginning in building the necessary bridges towards integrated services that are antidiscriminatory and antiracist. Community care poses a whole number of issues for service providers and occupational therapists will be at the forefront in ensuring that sensitive and equitable services are available to everyone, irrespective of their religious, cultural or linguistic backgrounds.

References

1. Office of Population Censuses and Surveys, *1991 Census: Outline Statistics for England and Wales derived from the County Monitors*, National Monitor CEN91 CM58, London: HMSO, 1992.
2. National Association of Health Authorities, *Action Not Words: a strategy to improve health services for black and minority ethnic groups*, London: NAHA, 1988.
3. Shah, R. *The Silent Minority – Children with Disabilities in Asian Families*, London: National Children's Bureau, 1992.
4. NHS Publication, *Caring for Everyone – Ensuring Standards of Care for Black and Ethnic Minority Patients*, Cambridge: National Extension College, Cambridge, 1991.

5. Wyke, S. and Hewison, J. (eds) *Child Health Matters*, Buckingham: Open University Press, 1991.
6. Henley, A. *Asian Patients in Hospital and at Home*, London: Kings Fund, 1979.
7. Hopkins, A. and Bahl, V. *Access to Health Care for People from Black and ethnic Minorities*, London: Royal College of Physicians, 1993.
8. Hayward, J. *Information – Prescription against Pain*, London: Royal College of Nursing, 1975.
9. Boore, J. *Prescription for Recovery*, London: Royal College of Nursing, 1978.
10. Asian Disability Advisory Project Team, the Spastics' Society and Barnardo's, *Asian and Disabled: a study into the needs of Asian People with disabilities in the Bradford area*, Barnardo's Keithley Project, 1993.
11. National Health Service Management Executive, *Social Voices – the views of local people in the purchasing for health*, London: NHME, 1992–4.

Further reading

Barker, J. *Black and Asian Old People in Britain*, London: Age Concern Race Research Unit, 1984.

Barnes, C. *Disabled People in Britain. A Case for Anti-Discrimination Legislation*, Hurst and Co, 1991.

Black, J. *The New Paediatrics – child health in ethnic minorities*, British Medical Journal, 1985.

Cruikshank, J.K. and Beevers, D. G. *Ethnic factors in Health and Disease*, Wright, 198².

D'Ardenne, P. and Mahtani, A. *Transcultural Counselling in Action*, London: Sage Publications, 1989.

Fernando, S. *Mental Health, Race and Culture*, Basingstoke: Macmillan, 1991.

Henley, H. *Asians in Britain: Caring for Hindus and Their Families*, Cambridge: National Extension College, 1981.

Henley, H. *Asians in Britain: Caring for Muslims and Their Families*, Cambridge: National Extension College, 1982.

Henley, H. *Asians in Britain: Caring for Sikhs and Their Families. Religious Aspects of Care*, Cambridge: National Extension College, 1983.

Hopkins, A., Kavanagh, K. and Kennedy, P.H. *Promoting Cultural Diversity – Strategies For Health Care Professions*, London: Sage Publications, 1992.

Karseras, P. and Hopkin, E. *British Asians: Health in the Community*, Chichester: Wiley Publications, 1987.

Littlewood, R. and Lipsedge, M. *Aliens and Alienists: Ethnic Minorities and Psychiatry*, London: Unwin Hyman, 1989.

Mares, P. *The Vietnamese in Britain: A Handbook for Health Workers*, Cambridge: National Extension College, 1982.

Norman, A. *Triple Jeopardy: Growing Old in a Second Homeland*, Centre for Policy Ageing, 1985.

Pearson, M. *Black and Ethnic Elders in Britain*, University of Keele, 1988.

White, D. and Woollet, A. *Families – A Context for Development*, London: Falmer Press, 1992.

Wilson, A. *Finding a Voice – Asian Women in Britain*, London: Virago Press, 1988.

Further resources

Kings Fund Centre, 126 Albert Street, London NW1. Tel. 267 6111.
Joint Council for the Welfare of Immigrants, 115 Old Street, London EC1. Tel. 251 8706.
Commission for Racial Equality, Elliott House, Allington Street, London SW1. Tel. 828 7022.
Community Health Foundation, 188 Old Street, London EC1. Tel. 251 4076.

In addition, most communities have their own national and local organisations who are always willing to assist with information and informal lectures.

Chapter 4

The contribution of occupational therapy in the community

IRENE ILOTT
Principal Lecturer, School of Health and Community Studies, University of Derby

Occupational therapy, as the discipline concerned with empowering and enabling occupational competence,[1,2] has made an important contribution to health and social care in community settings for many years.[3–5] This was more recently highlighted in the Social Services Inspectorate report on local authority occupational therapy services[6] which contained an example in which 28 per cent of all referrals to one Social Services department were routed to the occupational therapy staff, who comprised only 1 per cent of the total workforce.

This chapter provides a general introduction to the obvious, invisible and related contributions which underpin this statistic. It also aims to set the scene for other chapters which illustrate the diversity of practice within community settings. The obvious contributions of occupational therapy span a range of interventions including treatment, habilitation, rehabilitation, prevention and health promotion. The variation emanates from a 'common core philosophy ... which gives an inner purpose to the diversity'.[7] This chapter will outline four elements of the common core: occupation, values and beliefs, the intervention cycle and clinical reasoning, all of which become explicit in the roles undertaken by occupational therapists. The range of roles includes acting as an advocate, assessor, counsellor, therapist, educator, researcher, consultant and manager. These roles, practice principles and conceptual processes are summarised within this chapter for they are critical to occupational therapy's vision of promoting 'social justice by enabling people to participate as valued members of society despite diverse or limited occupational potential'.[7]

Invisible contribution

Occupation

Occupational therapy is derived from the recognition of the 'centrality of occupation in the lives of people'.[8] 'Occupation' is a generic term encompassing the goal-directed use of time, energy, interest and attention. It is the active, or 'doing', process of people engaged in purposeful, gratifying and culturally appropriate occupations.[9]

In 1993 Wilcock[10] presented a powerful argument for considering 'occupation' as a basic human need which is essential for both survival and health. The purposeful use of time provides people with the mechanism to exercise and develop innate capacities of a biological, social and cultural nature, to adapt to environmental changes and to flourish as individuals.

'Occupation' is therefore an intrinsic part of the pattern of human life and is usually categorised as self-care, productivity and leisure. This traditional taxonomy is associated with one of the beliefs of occupational therapy: that a balance of well-chosen occupations is essential for health.[11] However, research has highlighted the limitations of these global, static categories which omit both the cultural and personal meaning of engagement in occupations and the social context, with the possibility of performing several roles or tasks simultaneously.[12–14]

The complexity of 'occupation' is the focus of study for occupational scientists and occupational therapists, both of whom aim to understand and then apply this knowledge to enhance occupational competence. The essential elements of each are contained in Yerxa's definitions:[15]

> Occupational science is the study of the human as an occupational being including the need for and capacity to engage in and orchestrate daily occupations in the environment over the life span.

> Occupational therapy is therapeutic intervention that promotes health by enhancing the individual's skills, competencies and satisfaction in daily occupations. In order to accomplish this, it applies the principles of occupational science to enable people with chronic disease or disability to act on the environment and successfully adapt to its challenges.

While both disciplines share an interest in occupation, professional practice is also guided by values and beliefs.

Values and beliefs

The values and beliefs which underpin occupational therapy have their roots in the evolving history of the profession. They are also central to one of the basic tenets of *Caring for People – Community Care in the Next Decade and Beyond*,[16] i.e. helping people to lead, as far as possible, full and independent lives.

Fundamental assumptions exert invisible influences on client-centred care and service planning. Benefits are likely to accrue from making these assumptions, and perceptions of desirable behaviour, explicit. Farnworth[17] summarises three theoretical premises which underlie practice. These are as follows.

1.   Humans are active, moving and stimulus seeking beings who act on, interact with, and seek to alter their surroundings.
2.   Through interaction with the environment, humans grow and develop skills and abilities which enable them to be competent members of a society, and to gain a sense of self and social worth.
3.   Activities used to acquire skills can be used therapeutically to restore, regain and renew skills.

These beliefs reflect the audacious values proposed by Yerxa, who reinforced the complementarity between professional and societal values.

> What occupational therapy values is what society has been seeking increasingly: a grasp of the whole picture, person and environment; encouraging persons to take responsibility for their own bodies and destinies; and recognizing the potential, dignity and autonomy of each individual.[18]

While there will be variation to respect cultural differences relating to health beliefs and lifestyle, realistic optimism about an individual's resilience and their capacity to change and adapt is a constant value (see Chapter 3).

Obvious contribution

The intervention cycle

The intervention cycle is a generic term incorporating the problem solving, treatment planning or occupational therapy processes. Pelland describes the treatment planning process as the 'core of occupational therapy practice'.[19] The cycle comprises the dynamically interdependent elements of assessment, intervention and evaluation.[20,21] It reflects a cognitive, creative and collaborative process of problem identification and solving.

A sifting process often begins the intervention cycle when referrals are prioritised on the basis of a risk and needs analysis to determine further action. This decision-making phase is subject to many influences, including local management arrangements and contracts, clinical and social policies, resource constraints and professional expertise. The outcome may be allocation to a key worker from the community team; onward referral to a more appropriate facility; or placement on a waiting list according to agreed eligibility and priority criteria (see Chapter 5).

Assessment

Assessment involves the collection, analysis and interpretation of relevant, reliable and valid information about an individual's ability to perform occupational roles, tasks and activities. It requires judgement to sift objective and subjective data gathered in different contexts (hospital, day care and home) about intrinsic motivation and stresses upon both client and carers. A comprehensive client-centred assessment will identify both deficits in, and enablers of occupational competence related to:

- occupational performance in the areas of self-care, productivity and leisure;
- mental, physical, sociocultural and spiritual components of performance; and
- cultural, physical and social aspects of the environment.[22]

Client-centred practice is an intrinsically needs-led approach, for it focuses on problems identified and prioritised by the client. It is a partnership with the therapist acting as an accurate assessor who outlines all the available options, provides necessary information and then accepts the client's decision.[23] This approach complements the Disabled Persons (Services, Consultation and Representation) Act 1986 and other recent legislation.

Assessment, whether using standardised or informal measures, involves skills, knowledge and judgement to integrate up to date clinical knowledge. This is necessary if relationships between the course and prognosis of an impairment, with societal attitudes, are to be understood; in particular how unfair discrimination can exacerbate disability.

Initial and ongoing assessments may contain a redefinition of problems related to presenting and underlying needs, wants and wishes. All assessments (and outcomes) are influenced by external factors which may create a mismatch between the rhetoric and reality of community care with the constraints and management of finite resources. Unfortunately, these can often result in long waiting lists and excessive waiting times.[6] Another is the continuous restructuring of services which limit the remit of a practitioner to purchaser or provider responsibilities. However, a welcome feature of recent community care initiatives has been increased accountability to consumers. This can be achieved by monitoring the relationship between assessment, goal setting and outcome. This process is likely to reflect quality standards and provide individual indicators of health gain.

Intervention strategies

A range of interventions may be utilised to enable clients to gain or regain their optimum level of occupational competence. This diversity in response to the 'gift' of community care is clear, whether in Lock's description of developments in a specific locality[24] or within the United Kingdom, for the rest of this text contains examples of treatment (Chapter 17), rehabilitation (Chapter 14), habilitation (Chapter 16), preventative (Chapter 11) and health promotion (Chapter 6) intervention strategies.

This stage begins with planning based upon a needs and risk assessment and includes identification of immediate goals and long-term aims. The process of negotiating and agreeing a care plan with the client and carer demands the conscious use of self to establish a therapeutic alliance. Planning, followed by implementation of an acceptable, appropriate intervention are influenced by both theoretical and practical factors, such as professional ideologies, access to resources, facilities and expertise. The occupational therapy knowledge base contributes two distinctive theoretical factors to all stages of the intervention cycle. These are:

1.   occupational analysis and synthesis; and
2.   generic and/or occupational therapy specific frames of reference.

Occupational analysis and synthesis. Nelson[25] has provided a framework for describing the complex, dynamic, individual nature of occupation within environmental contexts which incorporates both meaning and change over time. Occupational analysis may therefore be considered as a more sophisticated, client-centred form of activity analysis which is a core component of professional practice.[26,27]

Occupational analysis involves understanding the relationship between occupational form (the pre-existing structure which elicits, guides or structures) and the subsequent occupational performance, this latter being influenced by the meaning and purpose of the occupational form for each person. Occupational synthesis (i.e. modifications to the occupational form to enable satisfactory and satisfying performance), together with task analysis, forms the basis for all interventions.

Frames of reference. There is much debate about definitions; the application and value of theories; frames of reference; paradigms; approaches and models of practice. In this context a single term is used to describe a cluster of compatible theories which may guide intervention by providing a tool for thinking, prediction, action and evaluation.[28,29] Some are generic, shared with other members of the interdisciplinary team which aid teamwork and consistency. These include psychodynamic, behavioural, developmental, humanistic, biomechanical and neurodevelopmental frames of reference. The exclusive or eclectic use of these theoretical frameworks pervade the interventions described in the following chapters.

The rehabilitative frame of reference is commonly used in community settings. It 'focuses on the use of a person's remaining abilities to achieve the highest level of independence possible'[30] through the use of compensatory techniques, assistive equipment, environmental adaptations, ergonomic principles and by formal or informal carers. Visibility, cost and consumer satisfaction are high when interventions enable self-care occupations to be performed with dignity and safety.[6]

Many current occupational therapy frames of reference originate in America with its very different cultural, sociopolitical and health care context. Examples of these are Role Acquisition,[31] Sensory Integration,[32] Cognition and Activity[33] and the Model of Human Occupation.[34] While much from these frames of reference is applicable some are emerging from the United Kingdom, including a client-centred model for community practice.[35] Although these require further development, they demonstrate a dynamic pluralism and commitment to research as the basis of practice.

Evaluation

An appraisal of the effectiveness of the intervention cycle is essential and encompasses an ongoing, as well as a terminal, evaluation of both the process and outcome from the perspective of all participants. While the purchaser may concentrate upon quantitative measures of cost effectiveness and efficiency, the clients' perceptions of change and benefits, together with those of carers, are most important (see Chapter 20).

The ending of the therapeutic alliance with the closure of relationships is an important aspect of this stage. It is usually formalised in documentation to the referrers. These discharge reports should also provide a valuable source of data for researchers.

The intervention cycle, with its elements of assessment, intervention and evaluation, provides a systematic approach to problem setting and solving. However, a net linear description masks the unpredictable, uncertain reality of practice and clinical reasoning.

Clinical reasoning

Clinical reasoning, or reflection-in-action, underlies the intervention cycle and is another 'hidden' contribution of occupational therapists. It is a complex, conceptual process which underpins proficiency, particularly when working at the indeterminate zones of practice. In 1987 Schon[36] described the artistry of practitioners as they make 'new sense of uncertain, unique or conflicted situations' for which there is neither a right answer nor existing professional knowledge. The ability to reflect 'in' and 'on action' is needed to build a bank of experience from comparable situations so that original, acceptable interventions may be made to each client's situation. The interdependence of the three dimensions of clinical reasoning, i.e. scientific, ethical and artistic, are highlighted in Roger's[37] statement:

> without science, clinical inquiry is not systematic; without ethics, it is not responsible; without art, it is not convincing.

Recent research has confirmed both the complexity and multidimensionality of clinical reasoning. Fleming[38] portrays a therapist with a three-track mind who uses different forms of reasoning to solve problems, design and conduct therapy. These are:

1.   procedural reasoning which guides the therapist's thinking about physical performance problems and incorporates an understanding of the client's impairment with treatment selection;

2.   interactive reasoning, reflecting a desire to understand the client as an individual, their experience of and feelings about, disability; and

3.   conditional reasoning, an imaginative and integrative form used to construct the future, taking into consideration the constraints imposed by the impairment within the client's personal and social context.

Fleming[38] suggests experienced therapists demonstrate the ability to shift from one mode of reasoning to another in order to analyse, interpret and resolve various types of problems.

These subtle reflective skills may be enhanced through professional supervision and strategic management and both are required to optimise the contribution of occupational therapy to service planning and provision. Clinical reasoning and the intervention cycle reflect a sensitive, yet systematic approach towards community or individual care plans.

Other contributions

Occupational therapists fulfil a variety of roles in health and social care including advocate, assessor, counsellor, therapist, educator, researcher, consultant and manager.[20,39] These are the visible expressions of professional values and clinical reasoning and embody the purpose of empowering and enabling occupational competence among clients and their carers. However, roles are susceptible to external factors which influence the present and potential contribution of occupational therapy to community care. These factors provide the context for a review of roles.

Occupational therapists have a tradition of crossing the boundary of health and social care to achieve the aim of resettlement. This is facilitated by a broad curriculum demanding an integrated competency across occupational science, occupational therapy, management and research within the biological, behavioural and clinical sciences.[40]

Legislation provides a remit for occupational therapy and includes the Chronically Sick and Disabled Persons Act 1970, Disabled Persons (Services, Consultation and Representation) Act 1986, Children Act 1989, Local Government and Housing Act 1989 and the National Health Service and Community Care Act 1990. The implementation of legislation requires interdisciplinary and inter-agency co-operation to create innovative care packages that enable people to live safe and satisfying lives within their community (see Chapter 2).

Occupational therapy may contribute in a variety of ways to the commissioning or provision of services, the extent and emphasis of roles being determined by personal and organisational factors including the expertise, interests, experience and qualifications of the therapist. Although job descriptions and resource constraints provide parameters for practice, these are subject to the subtle influences of expectations, opportunities and role protection resulting in potential limitations of service. This was highlighted by clients in the recent Social Services Inspectorate report where high satisfaction levels with outcomes were reported, but more help with managing wider aspects of disability was required, and not simply an equipment and adaptation service.[6]

This, and other research relating to clients' perspectives, confirm restrictions upon their life experiences and choices when intervention is limited to performance components of self-care.[41,42] However, this can be compounded by cultural factors as disabled persons tend to be set apart, treated differently and devalued by other members of the society.[43] Attitudinal, organisational, financial and architectural barriers perpetuate this stigma and segregation. In their roles of advocate, assessor, counsellor, therapist, educator, researcher, consultant or manager, occupational therapists have a responsibility to promote equality and social justice. The following definitions encapsulate each role:

Advocate   This comprises being an ally with, and advocate for, clients in the planning and delivery of culturally sensitive, ethical and appropriate services. The role of patient advocate is controversial and may not be advisable when acting as a therapist (Chapter 2).

Assessor   A comprehensive, initial and ongoing needs-led assessment of occupational competency provides the baseline for intervention and performance indicators. It complements one of the objectives of the National Health Service and Community Care Act 1990 which aims to make the proper assessment of need and good case management the cornerstones of high quality care. Assessment may extend into needs analysis with strategic planning for community care plans.

Counsellor This role incorporates acting as a facilitator for change; assisting adaptation to the loss of something treasured or taken for granted; encouraging problem solving; sharing knowledge to enable informed choices and supporting intrinsic striving for mastery and control (see Chapter 9).

Therapist   Each practitioner has a duty to maintain and develop their clinical competence which means improving and updating their knowledge and skills. Intervention strategies, whether treatment, habilitation, rehabilitation and health promotion, need to be derived from research rather than 'custom and practice'.

Educator   This role spans participating in the initial and continuing education of colleagues; encouraging adherence to optimise the benefits from an intervention programme; and promoting occupational therapy to ensure the most effective and efficient use of scarce resources.

Researcher Evaluation is inherent in the intervention cycle and clinical reasoning. Individual or collaborative research is essential for ascertaining the effectiveness and cost effectiveness of interventions.

Consultant A number of factors have increased the opportunities for consultancy. These include the internal market with a mixed economy of care and encouragement of voluntary, private and statutory providers; an emphasis upon health promotion and disease prevention; a mixed profile of skilled staff who require support, supervision and training; and recognition of consumer rights with complaints procedures which may culminate in the occupational therapist acting as an expert witness in medico-legal cases.[44]

Manager Planning, prioritising, setting and auditing quality standards, with time and task management are essential skills of each practitioner. Clear strategic and managerial leadership, supported by documented policies underpin business plans and assist the management of change. This role demands communication, negotiating and decision-making abilities, particularly in the context of care management.

This summary of roles represents the visible and valuable contribution of occupational therapy. The following chapters provide examples of promoting occupational competency with different client groups in, and as part of, a changing society.

The contribution of occupational therapists, as members of interdisciplinary teams with clients and their carers at the core, crosses the boundaries of health and social care in community settings. The Audit Commission acknowledged their skills as being 'in many ways central to the implementation of community care'[5] and would seem to be particularly fitted for the roles of assessor and care manager. These skills are based upon a shared philosophy, values and conceptual processes which are then expressed in multiple roles and intervention strategies intended to promote occupational competency and social justice.

References

1. Stewart, A. Empowerment and enablement: Occupational Therapy 2001, *British Journal of Occupational Therapy*, Vol. 57(7), pp. 248–54, 1994.
2. Polatajko, H.J. Naming and framing occupational therapy: a lecture dedicated to the life of Nancy B, Murial Driver Lecture, *Canadian Journal of Occupational Therapy*, Vol. 59(4), pp. 189–99, 1992.
3. Bumphrey, E.E. (ed.) *Occupational Therapy in the Community*, Hemel Hempstead: Woodhead-Faulkner, 1987.

4. Richards, S.E. Community occupational therapy: past dreams and new visions, *British Journal of Occupational Therapy*, Vol. 55(7), pp. 257–9, 1992.
5. Audit Commission, *Making a Reality of Community Care – A Report*, London: HMSO, 1986.
6. Department of Health, *Occupational Therapy The Community Contribution – Report on Local Authority Occupational Therapy Services*, London: Social Services Inspectorate, Department of Health, HMSO, 1993.
7. Townsend, E. Occupational therapy's social vision, Murial Driver Lecture, *Canadian Journal of Occupational Therapy*, Vol. 60(4), pp. 174–82, 1993.
8. Clark, F. Occupation embedded in a real life: interweaving occupational science and occupational therapy, Eleanor Clarke Slagle Lecture, *American Journal of Occupational Therapy*, Vol. 47(12), pp. 1067–78, 1993.
9. Evans, K.A. Definition of occupation as the core concept of occupational therapy, *American Journal of Occupational Therapy*, Vol. 41(10), pp. 627–8, 1987.
10. Wilcock, A. A theory of human need for occupation, *Journal of Occupational Science: Australia*, Vol. 1(1), pp. 17–24, 1993.
11. Mayers, C.A. A philosophy unique to occupational therapy, *British Journal of Occupational Therapy*, Vol. 53(9), pp. 379–80, 1990.
12. Zuzanek, J. and Mannell, R. Gender variation in the weekly rhythms of daily behaviour and experiences, *Journal of Occupational Science: Australia*, Vol. 1(1), pp. 25–37, 1993.
13. Christiansen, C. Classification and study in occupation: a review and discussion of taxonomies, *Journal of Occupational Science: Australia*, Vol. 1(3), pp. 3–21, 1994.
14. Mounter, C. and Ilott, I. Occupation: the relationship between health and lifestyle, *Paper presented at the College of Occupational Therapists Conference, Health Promotion: An Investment for the Future, London*, 12 May 1993.
15. Yerxa, E.J., Clark, F., Frank, G. An introduction to occupational science: a foundation for occupational therapy in the 21st century, *Occupational Therapy in Health Care*, Vol. 6(4), pp. 1–17, 1989.
16. White Paper, *Caring for People – Community Care in the Next Decade and Beyond*, London: HMSO, 1989.
17. Farnworth, L. Understanding work, self care and leisure in human occupation, *Paper presented at the 10th International Congress of the World Federation of Occupational Therapists, Melbourne*, 2–6 April 1990.
18. Yerxa, E. Audacious values: the energy source of occupational therapy, in *Health Through Occupation: Theory and Practice in Occupational Therapy* (ed. Kielhofner, G.), Philadelphia: F.A. Davis, 1983.
19. Pelland, M.J. A conceptual model for the instruction and supervision of treatment planning, *American Journal of Occupational Therapy*, Vol. 41(6), pp. 351–9, 1987.
20. Turner, A., Foster, M. and Johnson S.E. (eds) *Occupational Therapy and Physical Dysfunction: Principles, Skills and Practice*, Edinburgh: Churchill Livingstone, 1992.
21. Creek, J. (ed.) *Occupational Therapy and Mental Health: Principles, Skills and Practice*, Edinburgh: Churchill Livingstone, 1990.
22. *Guidelines for the Client–Centred Practice of Occupational Therapy*, Report of a

Task Force convened by the Canadian Association of Occupational Therapists and the Health Services Directorate, Health Services and Promotion Branch, Ottawa, 1983.

23. Sumsion, T. Reflections on ... client–centred practice: the true impact, *Canadian Journal of Occupational Therapy*, Vol. 60(1), pp. 6–8, 1993.

24. Lock, C. Fighting for our professional lives, *British Journal of Occupational Therapy*, Vol. 57(4), pp. 131–2, 1994.

25. Nelson, D.L. Occupation: form and performance, *American Journal of Occupational Therapy*, Vol. 42(10), pp. 633–41, 1988.

26. Young, M.E. and Quinn, E. *Theories and Principles of Occupational Therapy*, Edinburgh: Churchill Livingstone, 1992.

27. Willson, M. *Occupational Therapy in Short-Term Psychiatry*, Edinburgh: Churchill Livingstone, 1984.

28. Creek, J. and Feaver, S. Models for practice in occupational therapy: Part 1 defining terms, *British Journal of Occupational Therapy*, Vol. 56(1), pp. 4–6, 1993.

29. Christiansen, C. and Baum, C. *Occupational Therapy: Overcoming Human Performance Deficits*, Thorofare, NJ: Slack, 1991.

30. Trombly, C.A. (ed.) *Occupational Therapy for Physical Dysfunction*, Baltimore: Williams & Wilkins, 1983.

31. Mosey, A.C. *Psychosocial Components of Occupational Therapy*, New York: Raven Press, 1986.

32. Ayres, J.L. *Sensory Integration and the Child*, Los Angeles: Western Psychological Service, 1979.

33. Allen, C. Activity: occupational therapy's treatment method, *American Journal of Occupational Therapy*, Vol. 41, pp. 563–75, 1987.

34. Kielhofner, G. and Burke, J. A model of human occupation: framework and content, *American Journal of Occupational Therapy*, Vol. 34, pp. 572–81, 1980.

35. Mayers, C.A. A model for community occupational therapy practice, Stage 1, *British Journal of Occupational Therapy*, Vol. 56, pp. 169–72, 1993.

36. Schon, D. *Educating the Reflective Practitioner: How Professionals Think in Action*, New York: Basic Books, 1987.

37. Rogers, J.C. Eleanor Clarke Slagle Lectureship – Clinical reasoning: the ethics, science and art, *American Journal of Occupational Therapy*, Vol. 37(9), pp. 601–16, 1983.

38. Fleming, M.H. The therapist with the three-track mind, *American Journal of Occupational Therapy*, Vol. 45(11), pp. 1007–14, 1991.

39. Craik, C. What could occupational therapists not achieve? *British Journal of Occupational Therapy*, Vol. 57(6), pp. 217–18, 1994.

40. Curriculum Framework for Occupational Therapy, *Standards, Policies and Proceedings*, London: College of Occupational Therapists, 1993.

41. Greveson, G. and James, O. Improving the long-term outcomes after stroke – the views of patients and their carers, *Health Trends*, Vol. 23(4), pp. 161–2, 1991.

42. Sutherland, A. and Chesson, R. The needs of physically disabled people aged 16–65 years and service users in Grampian, *British Journal of Occupational Therapy*, Vol. 57(5), pp. 171–6, 1994.

43. Gething, L. Generality vs. specificity of attitudes towards people with disabilities, *British Journal of Medical Psychology*, Vol. 64, pp. 55–64, 1991.

44. Harris, I. Occupational therapy in personal injury litigation, *Paper presented at the 10th International Congress of the World Federation of Occupational Therapists, Melbourne*, 2–6 April 1990.

Chapter 5

The practitioner in the community

EILEEN E. BUMPHREY
Consultant/Adviser in Occupational Therapy and Rehabilitation

Occupational therapists have been working in a variety of community settings for many years. Traditionally this has mainly been within Local Authority Social Service departments following the introduction of the Chronically Sick and Disabled Act 1970, but with the advent of the NHS and Community Care Act 1990 further opportunities are being given to Health Service Trusts to respond to the thrust of Care in the Community. In consequence they, together with general practitioners (GPs), are initiating a variety of services with some employing occupational therapists to work within health centres and GP practices and alongside their Social Service colleagues. There are now legislative reasons for purchasers of health and social services to work more closely together in order to achieve a 'seamless' service for those patients transferring from hospital to community care, and especially for those with permanent or progressive conditions requiring long-term care.

Hospital discharge policies are an essential part of achieving a 'seamless', or rather 'well-seamed' service; however, hospital-based therapists are often encouraged to discharge patients home as early as possible, sometimes before they feel it is right, and perhaps before all the necessary support systems are in place. Community colleagues then have to respond quickly to these discharges and often need to continue rehabilitation programmes at home. However, hospital discharges form only a minority of those requiring assistance to make life manageable within the community and their home. Consequently general practitioner fund holders (GPFH) are taking opportunities for purchasing services to meet the clinical needs of their patients, including alternative therapies. Unfortunately, many are unaware of the variety of skills that are available to them, although opportunities do now exist for occupational therapists to inform them of their skills[1] and the contribution they can make to health and social care.

The past few years have also seen the decentralisation of services as general management together with the development of primary care teams, have taken the place of many district-organised services. The majority of clinical disciplines now find themselves working in the community either on a contractual basis from NHS Trusts or directly employed and, as few professional networks continue to exist, they are often left feeling isolated and vulnerable without professional support.

While the health service reforms and the Community Care Act give opportunities for initiatives, individuality and NHS Trust and GP autonomy, many constraints still exist but the *focus of Community Care* remains the same – that is, to provide the right intervention for the disabled person, whether it be assessment, advice, treatment or retraining; in the right place, be it institution, home, work, school, health centre or community centre; and whenever possible at the right time.

Primary care teams

The new GP contract (1990), together with the health service reforms, have had a tremendous impact on the way in which people work in the primary care setting. Never before has there been such an opportunity for all disciplines to work together to develop a wide range of services within the community. Most teams are based within health centres or GP practices and they develop their own methods of multidisciplinary practice and liaison. To participate effectively, all team members need to:

- be clear about the team's purpose; its vision for the future, and the need for working towards the same goals;
- have a clear understanding of their own role and responsibilities;
- understand the roles and responsibilities of other members in order to integrate their own effectively and to agree acceptable working patterns;
- try to understand the internal dynamics between members of the team which affect the whole's performance;
- encourage multidisciplinary and whole team learning and continuing education activities.

Core skills

At one time only senior grade occupational therapists were employed within the community setting; however, with increasing demands and diversity of interventions, lower grades and support staff are now employed, each contributing in differing ways. While all need core skills, senior staff have the responsibility of providing support, specialist skills and supervision. Some functions require postqualifying experience while in other situations the therapist will act as a co-therapist alongside other professional colleagues. As community occupational therapists acquire different competences, these need to be shared with others, and a network of expertise established which may well include colleagues within specialised hospital settings.

There may also be overlapping skills between professions (or role blurring) which give rise to confusion among colleagues, managers and the practitioners themselves. It is essential, then, that within the multidisciplinary team individual professional skills and roles are identified.

The ever-increasing awareness of economic restraints and the need to provide 'value for money' make it increasingly imperative that managers and those negotiating contracts have a firm understanding of what to expect from each level of practitioner, especially as occupational therapy, like most other community services, is expensive with the majority of treatments being individually tailored interventions.

Ellis[2] believes that there is no generally accepted definition of 'competence' related to skills, however, the practitioner of whatever discipline needs to state what their perceived competences are and how these can contribute towards health and social care. For the majority of those working in the community, these contributions will include:

- reducing dependency on others;
- reducing discomfort and distress and thus the call on medical help;
- protecting and supporting carers;
- preventing secondary pathology and promoting health;
- acting as a catalyst for the client;
- addressing issues that are the key concern for the client and their carer;
- facilitating discharge from hospital;
- preventing readmission to hospital.

Many of these, and others, are elaborated within the following chapters.

Role expectations from the uninitiated non-occupational therapy manager, medical practitioner or colleague will vary according to their knowledge and experience. Variations may also occur according to the perceptions of colleagues, supervisors and those self-imposed. In consequence these expectations need to be realistic, agreed and attainable.

Communications. The task of all community workers is to restore the client's autonomy and to encourage good citizenship, individuality and self-esteem. The essential element in achieving this is clear communication with the patient, their family and carer. It is not only fundamental in establishing a good rapport, but an essential part of the therapeutic process. The practitioner must choose her words carefully to ensure that no misunderstanding occurs when discussing the patient's condition, the proposed treatment regime and the choices for them to make. Jargon must be avoided and particular care taken when giving technical instructions.

To be effective the practitioner needs to exercise good interpersonal skills which include:[3]

Empathy: showing empathetic understanding and allowing themselves to merge with the experience of the client and be able to communicate this understanding to them.

Respect: positive regard for the client's worth and his/her rights as an individual.

Genuineness: showing genuine concern for the client's needs.

Time needs to be given within the intervention process for adequate communication, especially to those who are slow or have difficulty in comprehension. It is also needed for gaining the person's confidence, developing rapport and the involvement of the family and other carers.

Liaison with others. Interpersonal skills are also essential for establishing co-operative effective working relationships with colleagues. All community workers need to work together, discuss their individual contributions and plan integrated treatment regimes together. Although getting to know colleagues, strengths and weaknesses, skills and working practices can be time-consuming, it is worthwhile, and indeed essential, if integrated practice is to be achieved together with happy working relationships.

Senior staff, with experience and development of personal interests, all develop further skills which may not be directly attributed to one's own profession. However, it must be remembered that the occupational therapist's contract of employment will be for an 'occupational therapist' and therefore it is these skills that the manager will expect to receive. Effective communication and liaison can obviate any problems that may arise from these situations.

Specific role of the occupational therapist in the community

The role of the occupational therapist is extensive, as is described in Chapter 4, but the primary one remains the same – that is, to develop the optimum level of function and independence of the person in the physical, psychological and social aspects of life considering their age, handicap and environment.[4] The optimum level of functioning can be achieved by therapeutic programmes designed to:

> promote and maintain health;
> optimise functional abilities;
> diminish or correct pathology; and
> facilitate the learning of new skills.[5]

The occupational therapist working in the community now needs high technical skills as well as problem-solving ones owing to the multiplicity of arenas in which they may find themselves, and the diversity of clinical situations with which they need to be familiar. While precise competences are often difficult to specify, purchasers will wish to know what skills will be provided for their 'customers' in order for them to make informed judgements about whether or not to purchase.

Community occupational therapists will also portray a variety of roles if the needs of the disabled person living at home are to be met and, in many cases, this will only be determined once all the services involved with the case agree with the individual concerned, the goals to be achieved and subsequent programme. In consequence the community occupational therapist will more often than not assume a generic role, for they may well be required to continue therapeutic programmes commenced in hospital; undertake treatment programmes at home to achieve maximum independence and prevent further disability or dependence; teach coping skills; train carers in the safe ways of managing disability; intervene to prevent admission to hospital; evaluate the need for adaptations to the environment; and offer advice on employment, leisure and social activities.

Other contributions occupational therapists can make are as follows.

1.   Schools: e.g. therapeutic programmes for individual children whether they be in special or mainstream schools, and advising teachers and others on specific problems, equipment and architectural needs.
2.   Residential homes for elderly and handicapped people: by advising staff on specific and purposeful activities.
3.   Day centres: providing advice for individual problems and group activities.
4.   Self-help groups: promoting these and offering advice.
5.   Housing projects: giving appropriate advice on those specifically designed to meet the needs of handicapped people.
6.   Group homes and hostels for mentally ill people and those with learning disabilities: advising on the planning and management of these and assisting with individual clients.
7.   Health promotion programmes.

The generic community occupational therapist needs to have a fund of knowledge if she is to meet all the demands referred to her. This can be overwhelming and encourage the notion of being 'Jack of all trades and master of none'. However, this must not be the case. There are very special skills needed by community occupational therapists which embrace shrewdness in identifying the person's *real* problem as early as possible and discerning whether help is needed and in what form.

Case loads

Coping with a large number of referrals is all too common and apart from identifying priority groups, different ways of meeting the demands need to be explored. Examples of this might be the establishment of clinics in various locations for the assessment of such tasks as bathing needs, hoists or wheelchairs; and direct access centres where disabled people can call for assessment, advice and to obtain special equipment. Home visits can always be arranged following these appointments if indicated.

Referrals

Local Authorities are required to publish their criteria for client eligibility for assessment and service provision. Referrals are made to the service and where appropriate, allocated to the occupational therapist for attention. Within the health service it is different, with referrals often being made directly to occupational therapy. While these can be initiated by medical practitioners, key worker, care manager, colleague, or in some cases the patient himself, they should be viewed as a referral to the employing authority or NHS Trust. Private practitioners will have their own criteria. At all times the referral must be supported by the name of the GP, consultant or care manager being the ones who are ultimately responsible for the care of that person.

Prioritising referrals is acknowledged to be a difficult process, as often the reason given on the referral form may not in fact be the real problem for the patient. The actual problem may be very sensitive and therefore will only emerge after confidence in their therapist is gained. However, prioritising is essential and the agreed format made known to clients/patients, colleagues and referring agencies.

The priority agenda should be simple, but not simplistic, concentrating on urgent needs, recognising that these may only be perceived, and those where intervention may provide positive results, even if this be acceptance of the status quo. An example of such an agenda is as follows.[6]

1.   Acute conditions requiring intervention to prevent hospitalisation.
2.   Those who are perceived to be at risk, for whatever reason.
3.   Those whose discharge from hospital is imminent and dependent on intervention from community workers.
4.   Those who are unable to reach their maximum potential without intervention.
5.   Those requiring early intervention and review for a condition that is changing such as motor neurone disease, rheumatoid arthritis or psychological states.
6.   Those requiring educative and prophylactic programmes to prevent ill health.

A simpler three-point system may be one way of achieving this.[7]

Priority 1.   Immediate action required: e.g. those whose health could be seriously impaired for whatever reason without immediate action.
Priority 2.   Urgent: e.g. those who are unable to sustain their level of independence without intervention, such as the sudden deterioration of their condition or the breakdown of essential equipment.

Priority 3.   Non-urgent. (In these instances it is important that an agreed waiting time is made known to all concerned.)

Some areas are using client assessment forms to assist them in prioritising referrals.[8] This often helps the client and their carers to see their own difficulties in a different way and may highlight other problems that they may have thought a nuisance, but not important. Assistance may need to be given to those unable to complete such a form, for whatever reason. Such a system has the advantage of assisting in the initial assessment especially if the client is hesitant to identify their problems; however, they should *only* be used as a guide and not as a definitive document.

Records

There are many ways of keeping records. Some areas are moving towards joint disciplinary records, or client-held/parent-held records. These systems enhance multidisciplinary practice and communication; reduce confusion to the patient and their carers about differing approaches to treatment techniques; and enable all involved with the client to be aware of instructions given by other professionals.

Individual patient records must be kept for all patients referred to the practitioner and be accessible to both managers and patients. The location of these may present problems to the community worker, especially when covering a large rural area, or involving multidisciplinary care plans. Client-held records solve many of these problems and few seem to be lost. The purpose of any documentation is to:

- provide a systematic progressive record of the patient's condition; relevant family/carer factors influencing the long-term care of the patient; and the intervention applied;
- ensure legal requirements are met;
- provide a means of communication between all disciplines involved with the patient's care;
- provide line managers with relevant information and data especially as they apply to quality assurance requirements.

The basic information required for all patients or clients should include:

> full personal details of the person referred;
> details of the carer if appropriate;
> name, address and telephone number of therapist responsible; and
> details of colleagues involved.

Records should only contain information regarded necessary for specific purposes with no subjective opinions and should never be used without appropriate authorisation. Where confidential matters need to be recorded separate personal notes can be kept, although these must be placed in a secure location. The practitioner should also make sure that legal requirements are met by ensuring the following.

1.   Records are written as soon after the event as possible and dated. It is imperative that the practitioner does not leave the recording of events to their memory.
2.   Reports made by helpers, care assistants, students and others are countersigned by their supervisor.
3.   Entries made by non-case holders are dated and signed (initials can be confusing).
4.   Errors are corrected and countersigned with the signature and date of the person altering them. They should not be obliterated by liquid paper or some other means.
5.   They are factual and do not contain any subjective opinions unless these are substantiated.
6.   The terminology used is understandable by all and common abbreviations only are used.

Reports need to be brief and succinct so that others will not only read them, but are able to act on their colleague's behalf should sickness or other untoward occurrence warrant it. It is important that all practitioners are familiar with the Data Protection Act and the local arrangements by which clients and their carers can access their records.

Resources

Resources available to the community practitioner can be numerous but the key ones are as follows.

1.   *Personnel*: including colleagues within the community team from all agencies, and others such as volunteers.
2.   *Technology*: this is an expanding area that can be exploited. Hand-held computers and light pens using bar codes can assist in the immediate recording of events. Computer networks assist in communicating with others.
3.   *Facilities*: such as
        (a) hospital departments which are available to community staff for treatment programmes, or as a managerial base. Many of these are now available 'out of hours' so that late afternoon or evening sessions can be held which are more conducive to clients;
        (b) health centres for individual consultation or group work;
        (c) local authority residential homes for specific activities; and
        (d) church/village halls which may be suitable for community-based activities.
4.   *Budgets*: for equipment, materials, travel; hire of rooms, training, books and other needs. Community care is an expensive service,

therefore before specific developments can take place purchasers will not only wish to know the benefits expected of such proposals but how much it will cost and the proposed number of patients to be seen – or 'cost per case'. These charges will need to include the above items, as well as staff salaries and any overheads. Determining the cost is difficult given the enormous variations of need between each client and the various methods of calculation used. It is important, though, that the practitioner is aware of just how much the service costs so that they can act responsibly.

There are other hidden financial implications which need to be considered, such as *time costs*. These include such factors as:

- using a room for only part of the time it has been hired;
- non-attendance for treatment; and
- careful planning of routes for home visits so as to keep mileage to a minimum.

Good time management is an essential quality for the community practitioner in keeping these costs to a minimum.

There is also a price to the patient. Some may need to take time off work in order to see the occupational therapist which could well result in loss of earnings. Minimising the *time costs* for these people is not only courteous but essential in obtaining their full co-operation. Satellite clinics, where these are feasible, are a useful means of bringing the service nearer to them, thus helping to reduce their hidden costs and encouraging full co-operation. More importantly fatigue from long journeys, which might well negate treatment, can be kept to the minimum. Such a clinic will also enable the therapist to see more patients within the vicinity, thereby making use of their time more effective. Weekend visits may also be attractive to the patient's family if the therapist needs to discuss the management of the disabled person with the family when they are not so tired after a day's work. Flexible working times for domiciliary visits are therefore important.

Home visits

These need to be well planned. Patients may be apprehensive about the first meeting, and therefore by making and keeping an appointment; taking all the known patient information, and showing an identity card (ID) on arrival, some apprehensions may be dissipated. The therapist, however, needs to be prepared for the unexpected as awkward situations will arise and they will need to know how to deal with them. Learning to talk one's way out of such situations and taking advantage of any training opportunities will help prepare for such occurrences. However, when one is very apprehensive being accompanied by a colleague will often defuse the situation and give the community worker confidence and access. Sadly, violence is a very real occupational hazard for community workers and therefore all precautions need to be taken and well rehearsed.

Good interpersonal skills, as outlined earlier, and sensitivity regarding the client's lifestyle are requirements for successful interventions which start with the recognition that the therapist is a guest in the client's home. The ability to relate effectively, particularly in the initial interview, is also a skill to be acquired, for without this it is unlikely that the client will relate their real concerns.

It is important to go well equipped with all that one anticipates may be needed, such as a basic set of tools, assessment equipment, first aid kit and, perhaps, a high-pitch device to deter dogs!

Ethics

> As we get to know more about the complexity of the human mind, so we try to make our shades of responsibility finer and more complex, and so I think we get into deeper and deeper muddles
> Baroness Wootton of Abinger, House of Lords, July 1962.

Ethics is a very complex subject and much has been written about it. The debates surrounding perceptions, philosophies and ideals will never be completed. Much is based in tradition with social anthropology identifying a bewildering variety of customs and behaviour patterns which are often completely contradictory in different places, such as the place of women and girls within differing cultures. In spite of this, every community has their own accepted minimum code of behaviour which is usually embodied in the common law of that community. Individuals may also hold personal convictions which may differ from the majority view but, overall, the community does expect, and in fact often demands that all should conform. This is particularly pertinent to the community practitioner who sees clients from differing backgrounds, cultures and traditions.

Ethics relate to morals – those matters that are morally correct and honourable. The layman thinks of it as a set of principles relating to behaviour, or rules of conduct, i.e. what is socially acceptable, and as such ethics governs the relationship between two people, creating and maintaining a mutual trust between them and setting the boundaries for their relationship.

Ethics also refers to identifiable statements about norms and values that guide professional practice. Codes of practice and standards in professional practice are examples of this and practitioners are expected, both by colleagues and society, to adhere to these.[9,10] Indeed the possession of corporate ethics, or the codes/standards of practice, is an essential mark of that profession and professionalism.

Codes of practice are statements of principles. They are not rules which are applicable in all instances, but embody the standards by which each practitioner should behave and apply her skills. They also influence her capacity for moral reasoning and so govern practice. Some principles are given legal embodiment in the form of statute law while others are embodied in rules of etiquette. Most, however, are carried in the practitioner's own professional consciousness and become 'natural' to them.

Ethics and the law are not synonymous. While much of what is ethically acceptable behaviour is embodied in society's law, much is not and therefore the practitioner should not presume that what is legal is ethically correct or what is ethically the norm is legal. Case law sometimes sets the ethical scene, but the implications are usually extremely narrow relating to one specific case or incident. Nevertheless, it does influence ethical thinking and action.

Moral reasoning

While ethics relates to the structure or system of standards of practice, morals relate to individual beliefs and actions with regard to what is right and wrong.

Moral reasoning refers to a more philosophical inquiry about norms and values and about how therapists make moral decisions in their professional work. Many issues have to be resolved through reflective thinking and problem solving, as guidelines to ethics cannot relate to specific instances. Here dilemmas may occur as practitioners become concerned about the consequences of any recommendations they make or actions taken and seek guidance for.

Conflicts will occur on occasions between one's duty as a therapist on one hand and respecting the wishes and rights of the client on the other, as is illustrated in Fig. 5.1.[11]

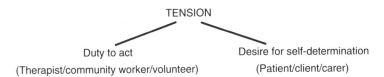

TENSION

Duty to act — Desire for self-determination
(Therapist/community worker/volunteer) — (Patient/client/carer)

Fig. 5.1

Some dilemmas

Conflicts of claims. Conflicts between practitioners, clients, management and society may arise from time to time, such as when a patient disagrees with the recommendations offered by the therapist and challenges moral rules; for example, agreeing what is acceptable social behaviour by the psychopathic patient. These conflicts can be summarised as those between:

- client's wishes and self-determination and the practitioner's judgement;
- the duty to the client and duty to society;
- what the client requests and the practitioner's conscience which may forbid her to provide it.

In these conflicts the practitioner has to make up her mind and act as she thinks right, taking into account any relevant law and general guidance from professional codes of practice and advice from colleagues and line managers. However while they cannot impose their recommendations, this may well lead to cognitive dissonance.

Conscience. This is a difficult concept, especially when the practitioner's and patient's consciences differ. Nevertheless, by discussing the problem and accepting the existence of differing values, both will be able to understand each other's difficulties.

Varying opinions between team members can also occur and this is where the case conference is a very useful milieu in which opinions can be debated and conclusions made. Ultimately in such conflicts, the final decision lies with the case manager or doctor.

Risk taking. Occupational therapy and rehabilitation is about helping people to cope within their own environment with all it hazards and problems, and therefore risk taking is an essential element of leading to independence; but what about accountability for 'risk taking'? For example, who will take responsibility for the patient discharging himself from hospital against all advice? Although the medical practitioner has the overall responsibility for medical care they will often accept and act on the therapist's opinion, who in consequence may well feel totally responsible for any resultant action. However, ultimately the responsibility must rest with the patient himself or his advocate and as such the practitioner, while feeling duty-bound to protect the patient from impending danger, has a duty to respect their wishes. Making them aware of all the risks and recording these may obviate this dilemma, and where the patient does not fully understand the implications others, including the family, must be informed of the seriousness of the situation.

Doctors, practitioners and clients all have differing views regarding taking risks because of their varying perceptions and the implications of what may be involved. In resolving such difficult dilemmas the equation of *risk versus benefits* can be applied with the client participating fully in the decision making. Where there is the likelihood of others being in danger as well as the client, then this must be considered within that equation.

All risk situations should be referred along the line management route in case of future complications, especially if there is the potential for legal action.

Veracity. Practitioners sometimes find themselves in a dilemma when faced with a difficult situation involving veracity – is it kinder to tell the client and their loved ones the full facts; to act as a 'gatekeeper' of the facts gradually relating them at appropriate times; or to withhold them altogether?

For example, how much should a father be told about his daughter's feelings when she is no longer able to look after him knowing full well that he would be devastated about this decision, especially as to him she appears perfectly fit and able? By finding another reason for resettling him into a residential home which satisfies all concerned, the relationship between father and daughter can be maintained despite his initial anger about the change.

It is essential that the truth is told at all times even if some of the facts are withheld at the time. In this way the consequences of any actions and comments made can be justified. Patients and carers, also, must be encouraged to be truthful concerning the problems under discussion so that the therapist has the full picture and can give realistic advice.

Such decisions around veracity should not be taken alone but after full discussion with the person in charge of the case, one's supervisor and colleagues, bearing in mind who has the ultimate responsibility for the patient. This is a complex debate between all health and social care professionals, and often carers, with no easy answers.

Resources. Sometimes the practitioner's role of contributing to the patient's good health and welfare is hindered by insufficient time and the lack of resources. Varying opinions within the care management team about what is best for the client and what is possible within the resources available may arise and compromises have to be made. The practitioner will need to be clear about her boundaries so that unrealistic promises are not made to patients or carers.

Confidentiality. This is complex as the failure to report information could be actionable in law. Confidentiality embraces the idea of trust between two people and the majority of clients expect and indeed believe that what is told 'in confidence' means exactly that and will not be repeated or recorded.

Confidentiality, though, can be a major problem for all practitioners of whatever discipline – from home carers to care managers. Some believe that it does not equate to secrecy, while dictionary definitions do. If the former principle is accepted, sharing confidential information with one's superior or the person in charge of the case makes the practitioner feel comfortable. However, if the latter is accepted – then what? Different disciplines within health and social services apply different principles which confuse the issues even further. Professional codes of practice often state that the practitioner should safeguard confidential information about the client. What does this actually mean when the sharing of information is essential for integrated treatment programmes? It is important then that the community team reaches agreement on the practice of confidentiality that will safeguard the client and practitioner and yet not violate professional codes of practice. Gaining permission from the client or their advocate can always be requested which will ease this path, although if it is refused, further complications can arise.

There are exceptions to the above guidelines, as follows.

1.   Statutory requirements such as seen in child abuse.
2.   Orders of court.
3.   Disclosure in the public interest.[12]

In these situations the legal instructions will need to be followed.

A fully reasoned approach to these dilemmas and others is essential if actions are not to be questioned. Opinions are too pragmatic and subjective and consequently unacceptable. It is therefore essential that patients, if they are to gain autonomy, are made to feel they are respected; given all the facts; encouraged to participate in the treatment regime and make their own decisions, as well as understanding their responsibilities. They should be helped towards their own realistic goals, which could include refusal to co-operate or, indeed, the right to end their own life. Practitioners will have particular problems when the latter decisions are taken and the client cannot benefit from their intervention because of their organic or psychosocial disability. This is where advocacy is helpful (see Chapter 2).

Ethics is complex – there are no easy answers, but by discussing issues among colleagues, agreeing and deciding on principles and practice, the occupational therapist will be given the framework within which to practice.

Professional negligence and litigation

With an increasing number of cases being resolved within the legal system, practitioners need to be aware of what this may involve. On the other hand, the fear of litigation should not in any way influence professional activities and create defensive practices. Gaining expert advice from professional organisations and through line managers will help to keep things in perspective.

There is an important link between ethical decisions and litigation, for if the practitioner is ever challenged about their actions there is the expectation that they will have carried out an acceptable professional procedure, followed their professional code of practice and is able to justify the action taken as seen in the eyes of professional colleagues, the client and others involved in the case.

Supervision and support

Working in isolation and without direct supervision is not helpful to anyone and should be avoided wherever possible; however, if the practitioner does find herself in such a situation, steps need to be taken to find one's own peer, mentor and supervisor. Supervision serves two functions.

1.   It ensures accountability by monitoring and evaluating the work undertaken and communicating important administrative decisions from senior managers.
2.   It provides for professional development by understanding of the

clinical and social problems in hand and by encouraging further training.

Practitioners need to look to their supervisors for support, advice and personal professional growth. They should therefore expect from their manager:

- accessibility on a regular basis in person and at other times by telephone;
- informal feedback on performance with a formal performance review at least annually;
- well-defined guidelines and job description which include such guidance as expected case load, and priority of referrals;
- clarification of the occupational therapist's responsibilities, including those related to working with other agencies;
- formal induction at the commencement of a new job;
- regular formal supervision.

Caring for oneself

In the community the experience of isolation and loneliness by virtue of the nature of the work is real. The practitioner sees herself continually as a 'giver' with little reward and support not readily at hand. Consequently there is a real danger of emotional exhaustion which is not always realised by the person concerned. The therapist often has a strong conviction that 'I can cope', 'I can take care of myself'. This self-perception of competence and control leads to self-imposed constraints which in turn not only lead to professional limitations but encourage further loneliness, failure and lowered self-esteem – or sheer arrogance! No one can endlessly give to others without finding ways of replenishing the emotional resources used. Sometimes this results in excess stress.

Stress. Feeling stressed at times is normal and does not indicate weakness. However, not practising self-care constitutes self-neglect. 'Coping' is used widely in this context but is an ill-defined construct. It is frequently used to explain individual differences to stressful situations or to covering it up rather than its acknowledgement. Everyone has a different level of functioning and the shrewd manager will be aware of this rather than expecting everyone to function at the same level according to experience.

Stress occurs when the demands made on the individual exceed their resources, be these personal abilities, such as time management, or practical ones such as insufficient equipment to issue to clients. Positive work features reduce stress whereas negative ones exacerbate it. These latter ones include role ambiguity; large case loads; insufficient resources; and lack of support and supervision. Continued stress can lead to poor performance, complaints and eventual ill health and therefore action needs to be taken to rectify the causes through discussion and revised priorities and practices.

The practitioner needs to apply the same principles for stress management as that given to their patients and evaluate regularly their own personal stress level, accepting limitations and emotions. It is also important to get to know what factors cause stress to colleagues, understand these and consider ways of helping each other.

Social and professional support from one's peers can mitigate the effects of stress through catharsis, practical advice and support at times of conflict. Regular support meetings and supervision encourage the ventilation of feelings, sharing of problems and constructive plans to resolve them and these need to be built into one's programme.

Every therapist needs to know themselves, their high and low points and set their own parameters for self-survival. For those employed full time it is important that some personal space is built into each day's programme with 'time out' from the working environment and from direct client contact. A 'cut-off' point at the end of the day is also important to enable the emotional change from the work role to the social and domestic role to take place. In this way the practitioner will find their work within the community not only manageable, but worthwhile and hugely satisfying.

References

1. Greenhill, E.D. Are occupational therapists marketing their services effectively to the fundholding general practitioners? *British Journal of Occupational Therapists*, Vol. 57(4), 1994.
2. Ellis, R. (ed.) *Professional competence and Quality Assurance in the Caring Professions*, London: Croom Helm, 1988.
3. Lloyd, C. and Maas, F. Interpersonal skills and occupational therapy, *British Journal of Occupational Therapists*, Vol. 55(10), 1992.
4. College of Occupational Therapists, London.
5. Bumphrey, E.E. *Occupational Therapy in the Community*, Hemel Hempstead: Woodhead-Faulker, 1987.
6. *Occupational Therapy Specifications*, Norwich Health Authority, 1990.
7. Leonard, C. An evaluation of the prioritisation of referrals by Leeds Social Services senior occupational therapists, *British Journal of Occupational Therapists*, Vol. 56(12), 1993.
8. Mayers, C.A. A model for Community Occupational Therapy Practice, Stage I, *British Journal of Occupational Therapist*, Vol. 56(5), 1993.
9. *Standards, Policies and Proceedings*, London: College of Occupational Therapists.
10. *Code of Professional Conduct*, London: British Association of Occupational Therapists.
11. Barnitt, R. *Yes Please, I'll have the treatment: Informed consent in Therapy*, London: World Federation of Occupational Therapists Congress, 1994.
12. Anderson-Ford, D. *Legal and Safe Seminar*, London: College of Occupational Therapists, 1994.

Further reading

Bumphrey, E.E. *Occupational Therapy and Primary Care: Connections*, London: Royal College of General Practitioners, 1991.

Charlesworth, E. and Nathan, R. *Stress Management*, London: Souvenir Press, 1993.

Cox, C. Practical aspects of stress management, *British Journal of Occupational Therapists*, Vol. 51(2), 1988.

DHSS Advisory Committee, *Violence to staff*, London: HMSO, 1988.

Handbook of Medical Ethics, London: British Medical Association, 1981 (currently being revised).

Finch, J.D. *Aspects of Law Affecting the Paramedical Professions*, London: Faber and Faber, 1984.

Hollis, V. Core Skills and Competences Parts 1–4, *British Journal of Occupational Therapists*, Vol. 56(2, 3, 4, 5), 1993.

Occupational Therapy, The Community Contribution Report on Local Authority Occupational Therapy Services, London: Social Services Inspectorate, Department of Health, 1993.

Rees, D.W. and Smith, S.D. Work stress in occupational therapists assessed by the Occupational Stress Indicator, *British Journal of Occupational Therapists*, Vol. 54(8), 1991.

Ward, C.D., Crates, P. and Skeates, S. Development of a disability team in general practice, *Clinical Rehabilitation*, Vol. 7, pp. 157–62, 1993.

Wright, R.A. *The Practice of Ethics: human values in health care*, New York: McGraw-Hill, 1987.

Chapter 6

The role of occupational therapy in health promotion

EILEEN E. BUMPHREY
Consultant/Adviser in Occupational Therapy and Rehabilitation

Health promotion is not a new idea, as every generation seeks to rediscover the benefits of preventing disease and handicap. However, it is only recently that occupational therapists have been encouraged to become actively involved with these specific programmes and to make a valuable contribution.

Over the last century significant improvements in health within western countries have taken place, much of this being due to environmental and public health measures rather than to advances in medicine, despite how significant these have been. During the 1800s Medical Officers of Health were required by statute to provide an annual report on the state of the health of the population for which they were responsible. These reports were to serve as a 'Community Diagnosis' upon which appropriate public health action – 'the Community Treatment' – would be based. Sadly, in time, these became rather tedious listings of services provided and events that happened during that year. With the abolition of Medical Officers of Health in 1974, annual reporting ceased and in consequence the real needs of the local populace failed to be identified. Localised annual reports were reinstated in 1988 'as an epidemiological assessment which will serve, within limits of available resources, to inform strategic plans and short term programmes'.[1]

What is health?

In 1946 the World Health Organisation (WHO) defined health as 'A state of complete physical, mental and social well-being and not merely the absence of disease or infirmity'. It has also been defined as 'the ability of the individual to function in a manner acceptable to him/herself and to the group of which he or she is a part'.[2] The *Concise Oxford Dictionary*, however, defines it as 'soundness of body or mind'.

Health embraces physical and mental well-being and a recognition that alongside these there is something about human nature which calls out for spiritual fulfilment. Being tripartite beings all these aspects need to be satisfied to provide health. It is also related to an overall balance between work/occupation, play, rest and self-care.

Health also embraces 'quality of life', which is often used in a glib way as there is no precise definition for it and everyone has their own interpretation of what it actually means. However, one thing is certain: it has little to do with the person's own handicap or disability as these carry significant subjective elements. It could, however be defined in terms of a combination of some objective measures such as pain, disability and functional mobility.

Health therefore is about feeling good, a perceived quality of life embraced by an acceptable environment. This can be illustrated thus (Fig. 6.1).

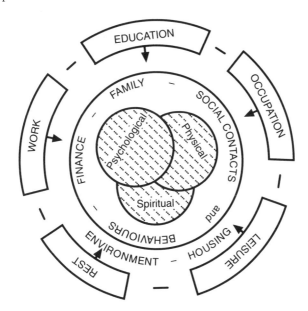

Fig. 6.1 Influences on health

Health, however, can be affected by many factors apart from environment, disease, accident and self-induced afflictions. Marc Lalonde, the Minister for National Health and Welfare for Canada, introduced the concept of 'health fields' which affect and determine the individual's health.[3] These are:

1.   Human biology
2.   The environment
3.   Behaviour/lifestyles
4.   Health care facilities

Human biology includes all those aspects of health, both physical and mental, which are determined as the basic biology of the individual, i.e.

genetic inheritance, maturation, ageing. The health implications of human biology are numerous and wide ranging, from minor nuisances to chronic disease and disorders. Many health problems originate from a disturbance to human biology.

Environment includes all those factors without the human body. Many of these factors the individual can control; however, much cannot, such as air pollution, safe food production and sewage disposal.

Behaviour and lifestyles within the health field concept consist of the decisions individuals make which affect their health. Personal decisions and habits that are bad from a health point of view create self-imposed risks, such as smoking, whereas positive decisions can enhance health, as is seen with regular exercise and a good diet.

Health care facilities relate to national and local provision for health services and resources. Screening for disease, immunisation, medical and paramedical facilities, together with locally based health care systems including health promotion programmes, form part of these resources.

Health has also been seen as a multidimensional concept with the following components:[2]

- the absence of chronic disease;
- freedom from illness (illness being the subjective state and not necessarily medically defined);
- behaviour in relation to activities and relationships;
- fitness as expressed in terms of physical well-being; and
- psychosocial well-being, i.e. happiness.

As can be seen, health is achievable through the partnership of the individual with those who are responsible for the environment and medical personnel. In essence, it is a collective responsibility involving everyone. Examples of this were seen with the introduction of the Clean Air Act and the legislation on sewage treatment, both of which had an enormous impact in improving health. Clean water has even a greater impact than all that medicine can achieve, as has been seen in some developing countries. Together with the improvement of the environment much is now done to improve the nation's health through medicine, especially with the many advances in medical technology, drugs and genetic research. Human biology is improving overall as is evident by the dramatic decrease of infant mortality and the increasing elderly population. The combining of biological and socio-cultural needs help to improve health, and here the therapist can influence this for those whose disability make it more difficult to achieve.

It is in the areas of behaviour and lifestyles where much of the success of health lies, as it is the individual who must take on much of the responsibility for their own health. However, without being made aware of potential ill influences, the individual is unable to make informed judgements. Health promotion programmes aim to help people in this.

Health promotion and preventative medicine

Health promotion: the Ottawa Charter[3] defined health promotion as 'the process of enabling people to increase control over, and to improve, their health. To reach a state of complete physical, mental and social well being, an individual or group must be able to identify and to realise aspirations, to satisfy needs and to change or cope with the environment'. It also states that 'changing patterns of life, work, and leisure have a significant impact on health'.

Preventive medicine applies western medical and social science and knowledge to preventing disease, promoting health by intercepting disease processes such as immunisations and prolonging life to all races.[4] Research has found high levels of sickness among ethnic minority groups with high prevalence of common symptoms of ill health and a higher proportion of long-standing conditions, such as asthma and diabetes.[5]

Health promotion and prevention of disease are consequently affected by many influences such as the following.

1.   Preventing disease through changes of lifestyle, manipulating the environment and altering human biology where possible. The scope for such interventions is wide and will involve many agencies such as environmental health, housing departments, health and safety executives.
2.   Reducing disability/handicap through the restoration or compensation of loss of function by intervention of health and Social Services, housing and other agencies.
3.   Improvement in quality of life by a mixture of intervention, relating particularly to the relief of distress and reduction of disability.

Health for All

In 1977 WHO launched the *Health for All* movement. The aim of this was to enable all citizens of the world to reach a level of health which would allow them to lead a socially and economically productive life by the year 2000. It is based on six major themes – equity; health promotion and disease prevention; community participation; multisectoral co-operation; and international co-operation. From this initiative emerged the European strategy, which has set itself 38 targets and the *Health of the Nation* White Paper for England.[6]

Following this came the *Healthy Cities* project[7] which offers a vision of pulling together much of what was already happening within cities to improve the health of their citizens. Through this initiative many cities around the world have formulated their own 'community diagnosis', identified their needs and begun to bring together all the agencies concerned with health.

Social problems such as violent crime, poor housing and unemployment are seen as the greatest threat to health within the inner cities. Racism has also been identified as having a bad effect on health. This project is an attempt to encourage the different agencies within a city to work together in tackling these issues in the same way the Victorians did a hundred years ago, using civic pride as a motivator. Local health would then undoubtedly improve.

Health of the Nation

In June 1991 the government issued its White Paper *The Health of the Nation: A Consultative Document for Health in England*[6] as part of its health service reforms. The major theme of this consultative document is the prevention of ill health and the promotion of good health. Within it there is considerable emphasis on empowering people to take charge of their health; giving them the knowledge of what this means, and encouraging them to change their behaviour where appropriate.

The report lists its main objectives as:

- to identify the main health problems;
- to focus on promotion of health and prevention of disease; and
- to recognise that health is determined by a number of different influences.

Wishing to be proactive, it has set five key target areas for action which are as follows.

1.	Causes of substantial morbidity:	coronary disease strokes cancers accidents
2.	Causes of substantial ill health:	mental health diabetes asthma
3.	Causes that contribute to both morbidity and mortality and to healthy living:	smoking diet and alcohol physical exercise
4.	Areas where there is scope for improvement:	pregnant women children rehabilitation services for people with physical diseases environment
5.	Areas where there is a great potential for harm:	HIV/AIDS communicable diseases food safety

These targets do not fall within the responsibility of any single agency but as the *Health of the Nation* White Paper stresses, there is the need for healthy alliances between each of the following:

health services	voluntary sector
social services	industry; commerce; trade unions
education	local government
environmental health	leisure centres
housing	the media

Co-operation between all these is essential if success and changes are to materialise. In practice, however, working together is not easy with each having their own management structure; demographic areas; differing goals, ideals, and priorities; and financial constraints. The Department of Health encourages some essential components such as a shared vision, a common agenda, agreed priorities, openness about self-interests, mutual respect and trust, the ability to learn from others and accepting cultural sensitivities.[8] Consequently, many and varied local initiatives are being carried out of which the community practitioner should be a part. Health authorities and general practitioners now have specific responsibilities for the overall health of their population and in meeting targets outlined by the government for health gain and, as GP contracts now include many health promoting activities, several programmes are being based within their practices or health centres.

Health for All 2000

In 1978 the United Kingdom, alongside many other countries, became a signatory to the Declaration of Alma Ata which stated that to improve public health, it was necessary to reorientate medical care in order to achieve much more public participation in health. It challenged these countries to attain health for all by the year 2000.

The *Health for All* project and philosophy is much broader than the *Health of the Nation* document as it relates to local views about their own needs, rather than the more medically orientated latter document. *Health for All* follows the lead of the WHO and sets out ambitious programmes for shifting the focus of health care from sickness to health.

While *Health of the Nation* with its clear targets for health gain has become government policy, *Health for All* has not. It is seen as an application of management by objectives to health care and aims to provide health care rather than a health service that responds to ill health, providing treatment and care services. It has, however, been the stimulus for local joint working between many agencies and formal alliances have arisen from community care planning. In consequence, some exciting community developments are taking place such as staff being appointed specifically to implement local *Health for All* initiatives; the demolition of unsuitable tower blocks within some inner cities so as to improve housing; and the Age Well programme which is designed to empower older people to look after themselves as well as encouraging them to continue to make a contribution to society. The Health

Education Authority (HEA), a special authority within the NHS, provides information and advice to the public, as well as assisting organisations and professionals in designing their programmes. They too have initiated some interesting national projects, such as 'No smoking' days and 'Look after your heart' projects.

Attitudes

People vary in their response to health and illness. Some tolerate ill health with dangerously stoical indifference or arrogant non-acceptance, while others show concern over the most trivial symptom – from the martyr to the hypochondriac. Good health is not seen as a high priority among many people as they tend to take it for granted and only think about their health when illness comes. For example, young people are far more concerned about enjoying themselves and responding to peer group pressures, even if this does mean taking drugs, and achieving their ambitions. Professional groups are more concerned about reaching their personal goals, clambering for acknowledgement and winning contracts over a glass of beer. Their own well-being comes a poor second. On the other hand, older people tend to give more importance to health and are more conscious about their weight, diet, physical and mental fitness.

Those who live full lives tend not to think too much about their health – which in fact is a healthy attitude to have, as boredom and inactivity affect both physical and mental well-being. However, over-occupied lives lead to tensions, stress, depression and physical problems as balanced diets, relaxation and rest are ignored.

Health has also been directly related to wealth. Low levels of family income not only affect what families are able to purchase, but the resulting problems can swamp their thoughts to such an extent that actions necessary for preserving the health of the family are overlooked. Alternatively, too much wealth can lead to over-indulgence!

Many people have a low level of awareness of what GPs and paramedical staff, including health promotion staff, can offer them. This is in part due to lack of information which all can understand. By improving knowledge, health providers can help to change attitudes and expectations; however, the cardinal focus must be to do things 'with' people and not 'to' them.

Various projects have been undertaken to try to identify attitudes among various groups of people regarding their health.[9] In South Derbyshire a survey found that there was an absence of local knowledge about the prevalence of mental health problems and that there was a distinct relationship between mental health and social deprivation. Stress and lack of money proved to be barriers to improving a healthy lifestyle. The authorities in Sheffield also found that those areas that suffered the greatest deprivation had the poorest life expectancy. Another survey carried out in Leicester among

Asians found that 97 per cent preferred not to use English but their own language, and as many as 18 per cent required an interpreter. In consequence health promotion literature and other information needed to be in their own language.

It is therefore important that social issues are dealt with alongside medical ones in order to achieve improved health.

The occupational therapist's contribution

Occupational therapists take a holistic approach in the total functioning of the individual within society and as such are well placed to be fully involved in this field. Their role includes a number of health-promoting activities although traditionally they have tended to concentrate on prevention of disease. In fact, some argue that the whole ethos of occupational therapy is to promote well-being and thus health, although concentration has been given to those already known to be needing medical care. Opportunities now exist for their skills to be applied to many other areas related to primary care (preventing problems from happening) and secondary care (preventing a problem from becoming worse) as well as tertiary (continuing) care.

Occupational therapists can contribute to both the *Health of the Nation* and *Health for All 2000* programmes in many ways, although their involvement will vary considerably and be dependent on locally designed initiatives. Briefly they include the following.

Coronary heart disease	• programmes designed to prevent further episodes of illness, and promote rehabilitation to enable the patient to live a more balanced life by adapting their lifestyle and physical fitness
Strokes	• therapeutic programmes to enable patients to relearn everyday activities including perceptual and cognitive problems
	• adaptation of the environment
Mental health	• providing wide-ranging programmes to help those who are the 'worried well' as well as for those with chronic psychoses. Individual programmes and group work to improve self-esteem, confidence, social and work skills
Accidents	• assessing the person's performance of certain activities and general working practices
	• advice given on safe practices within the home or working environment
	• preventing accidents to carers such as teaching lifting and handling techniques
HIV/AIDS	• providing special equipment that may be

	required to enhance the quality of life, and support to the sufferer and their family
Cancers	• providing equipment to make life more tolerable
	• counselling and support to both patient and their carers
Diet/alcoholism	• resolving any problem relating to food preparation
	• providing a balanced diet and budgeting
Asthma	• helping with adapting the environment
	• advice on work and leisure activities
Smoking	• anxiety and stress management programmes to ease the need for smoking
Physical exercise	• provision of specialised equipment to enable a wide variety of activities to be attainable
Health of pregnant women and children	• a special contribution can be made for the disabled woman and mother
Rehabilitation services for people with a physical disability	• help with all life skills to enhance the health of these people
Environmental quality	• advice in those aspects relating to housing and access to public buildings and transport
Communicable diseases	• advice on sexual behaviour
Food safety	• general advice for those activities relating to shopping, food preparation, cooking and serving

As will be seen, the occupational therapist needs to work closely with colleagues of other disciplines for, in many instances, a multidisciplinary approach is important if the same goals are to be achieved. For example, when considering food safety where diets are important, the dietician will need to be involved.

There are many other areas in which the therapist can contribute towards promoting well-being. These include the following.

The elderly. Assisting GPs with their screening programmes and responding to identified problems; assessment for functional and cognitive ability; encouraging mental well-being and continued independence.

Rheumatoid arthritis. Joint protection programmes which are vital in all stages of the disease.

Operative conditions. Preoperative assessments for conditions such as hip replacements, help to alleviate anxiety as well as maintain maximum functional ability and reduce pain, while awaiting surgery.

Admissions to hospital. Teaching patients the management of self-care and activities of daily living at an early stage of disease can, at times, preclude the need for admission to hospital. Early referral to the therapist is essential in these instances.

Work-related incidences. Advising employers in helping those employees who have encountered problems in some way and thus help to reduce the number who need to take time off work because of work-related illnesses such as back pain, musculoskeletal disorders and stress. The cost to society is estimated as over one billion pounds, but the cost to the individual and their family is often inestimable.

The use of *occupation*, in whatever guise, is a major part of the occupational therapist's contribution to health. 'Occupation', in this context, is a fundamental part of human survival for it influences a person's well-being, health and personal growth – be it the child at school, or the retired engine driver fully engrossed in his hobby. It gives purpose to life, encourages movement and thereby agility, gives motivation and alleviates boredom. A healthy mind is an occupied mind. Occupation therefore is one of the means by which everyone is able to realise their potential; cope with their environment; and live as healthy a life as is possible. Thus the occupational therapist is able to use all forms of occupation as therapeutic measures to promote health and satisfying lifestyles.

References

1. Health Circular HC88 (64) London: Department of Health, 1964.
2. *On the State of its Health, Volume 1*, Norwich Health Authority, 1988.
3. *A new perspective on the Health of Canadians*, The Canadian Government, 1976.
4. Wilcock, A.A. Health promotion and rehabilitation work, *Journal of Prevention, Assessment and Rehabilitation*, Vol. 2(3), pp. 15–20, 1992.
5. Bristol and District Health Authority.
6. *The Health of the Nation: A Consultative Document for Health in England*, London: HMSO, 1991.
7. *Healthy Cities, Concepts and Visions*, University of Liverpool: Department of Community Health, 1988.
8. *Working Together for Better Health*, London: HMSO, 1993.
9. Roberts, H. and Dengler, R. *Trent Health Lifestyle Survey: Interim report to Trent Regional Health Authority*, University of Nottingham: Department of Public Health Medicine and Epidemiology, 1991/2.

Further reading

Baxter, M. *Health and Lifestyles*, London: Tavistock Routledge, 1990.

Rothman, J. and Levine, R. (eds) *Prevention Practice – Strategies for Physical Therapy and Occupational Therapy*, USA: WB Saunders, 1992.

Smith, A. and Jacobson, B. (eds) *The Nation's Health, A Strategy for the 1990s*, London: King's Fund, 1988.

Chapter 7

Achieving independence

JEAN J. MACLEAN
Lecturer, Department of Occupational Therapy, Queen Margaret College, Edinburgh

Many professionals working in community and other settings would define attainment of a person's independence as a major aim of their involvement with them, if not the main one. Indeed, many definitions of occupational therapy, in particular, those of the World Federation and the British Association of Occupational Therapists identify the attainment of independence as a key component of them. The Blom-Cooper Report[1] also reinforces this aim, stating that occupational therapy intervention helps people to 'reach their maximum level of functioning and independence'.

The notion of promoting independence is not unique to occupational therapy and it is one of the major aims identified in the National Health Service and Community Care Act 1990. The handbook, *Care Management and Assessment: Practitioner's Guide*,[2] which offers guidance on the operationalisation of the Act, suggests that 'the fundamental aim of community care is to promote independence of individuals so that they are able to live as normal lives as possible'. It must, however, be remembered that the concept of independence is not easily definable and that there are many individual interpretations of it. In reality very few people are entirely independent of all others; most have some degree of reliance on tools and equipment and interdependence on others in order to complete satisfactorily the widely differing array of tasks and activities in daily life. Nor is the degree to which people are dependent on others constant, for there are times during their lives when all members of society are more or less reliant on others for some level of support.

People who suffer from illness or handicap may find themselves in a situation where they have to be proportionately more reliant on assistance in enabling them to achieve their desired level of independence. This reliance is often viewed in a negative light rather than as a point on a normal independence–dependence spectrum. People with special needs are often encouraged in the direction of achieving independence in a somewhat hierarchical manner, starting with personal activities of daily living, the attainment which to many may not be particularly fulfilling and working up to independence in social and cultural aspects of life which, in many instances, represent the most fulfilling elements of it.

A number of authors[3-5] suggest that professionals have for too long assumed that they know what the needs of their clients actually are and that they in turn have tended to be passive recipients of the treatment and services offered to them. Many occupational therapists would argue that they work from a client-centred base, taking their opinions into account, but the fact that such criticisms are made means that careful analysis should be considered of what occupational therapists and others exactly mean by 'client-centred practice'.

It is true that many occupational therapists initially focus on aspects of activities of daily living with which clients have problems and assume their wish to be independent in all aspects of these. For many people, this may well be so but, as Campbell[5] warns, care must be taken not to disempower people by professional help. She states that 'for many disabled people the effort of achieving such physical independence traps them in a lifestyle of unceasing hard work'. This idea is supported by French[6] who goes so far as to ask what is so important about being independent; she further suggests that striving for physical independence in terms of every day skills when, for that person, there are better things to do, may seriously reduce their independence by restricting the person's freedom of thought and action.

Oliver[7] and Zola[3] also suggest that there is a need to scrutinise long-held beliefs and assumptions about desire for independence, and that community services are often dealt with in such a way that they can actually reinforce dependency. Zola[3] argues that there must be an expansion of the 'notion of independence from physical achievements to sociopsychologic decision-making'. These thoughts are echoed by Campbell[5] who advocates the use of the expression self-determination, rather than the term independent living.

Such a move involves a change in the notion of control, the locus of which has, in the past, largely tended to rest with professionals but which more equitably should belong with each individual. The focus of achieving independence should therefore relate to those areas identified by the individual as important to them. This view is supported by the National Health Service and Community Care Act 1990 which advocates the use of needs-led assessment and service provision. Even within this framework there is still a danger that concepts of independence and need may be viewed too narrowly.

Law,[8] Oliver,[9] Dunn,[10] Sumsion[11] and others suggest that for therapists and other professionals to meet the needs expressed by clients they must be willing and able to consider a wider view of disability and illness in society. Oliver[9] proposes that professionals must view problems from more sociological, political and anthropological perspectives, thus diverting the focus of attention from a reductionist view of disability, concentrating solely on the individual, to a wider environmental and contextual view.

Within that type of framework the expectation of what can be achieved should be much higher. Mayers[12] argues, however, that even when clients are given the freedom to identify areas of need they still tend to focus narrowly on aspects of activities of daily living. This means that people with special needs will probably be required to reconsider their expectations of themselves as well as those of a range of professionals and they may have to learn, in some instances, and after time to take control over their own lives rather than having other people acting as decision makers on their behalf. Oliver again argues that there is a real need for further development towards social change which enables people with disabilities more opportunities for autonomy and decision making.

However, this process will not occur overnight. If clients are given 'permission' to have the main say in what areas and by what means they wish to achieve independence then gradual changes can be made on an individual, local, national and international level. Therapists and others will also need to see the consumers of their services as the experts on what they want from it. This is not a new concept; indeed, almost two decades ago, McKnight[13] suggested that 'modern heretics' were those professionals advocating consumer control and direction while at the same time demystifying their own role.

Few professionals would deny the attractiveness of these arguments. However, Corbett[14] warns that there is a significant theory/practice divide between what is desirable and what is available and/or practical. For example, problems may exist when dealing with those clients who have significant difficulties in personal decision making, motivation and self-confidence and those who have clinical features which affect their ability to view themselves in a realistic manner. This may include clients who are anxious or depressed and those who suffer from delusions or hallucinations. Placing requirements on them to identify their own needs may well be counter-productive and destructive. It is important to consider all interventions in both a positive and realistic light and in relation to each individual client and his presenting problem.

The foregoing arguments are relevant to a client-centred, holistic approach which arguably has always been a key feature of occupational therapy intervention. It is important for all community workers to continue to adopt and develop such approaches in all their dealings with clients.

Assessment

Having established that need should, where possible, be identified by individuals, the next stage is to consider the process of assessing that need.

Most intervention begins with a referral to a service or professional and there is a subsequent assessment of the client and his circumstances. Occupational therapists use a vast array of assessment tools including standardised and non-standardised assessments focusing on a very wide range of functions, skills, abilities, competencies and attributes. Indeed, there are assessment tools available to collect data on virtually all aspects of human life and performance, in fact it is one of the core skills of the occupational therapist.[15]

The main purpose of assessment is to form a baseline for future intervention. It is important that the process is viewed as a means to an end and not, as can sometimes appear, as an end in itself. The assessment process requires skill in collecting, collating and interpreting information. Since this information will shape the future input for any client, every effort must be made to ensure that it is as accurate as possible. Occupational therapists and others must be able to utilise a range of interpersonal skills effectively in order to reduce anxiety in clients which could, in turn, lead to poor performance. The significance of verbal, non-verbal physical and emotional responses must also be viewed as an integral part of the assessment process.

The first stage of this process is to establish whether or not the referral is an appropriate one. This can be achieved by gathering initial information which will also help to determine the level of assessment required and its urgency. The use of a standardised form, rather like an expanded referral form, is recommended for use in obtaining this information and it is important that this stage of intervention is carried out thoroughly in order to minimise delays in ensuing assessment and service provision. Occupational therapists in the community will be involved with people at the levels of assessment as outlined in the *Care Management and Assessment: Practitioner's Guide*[2] – see Chapter 2.

As noted previously, one of the main features of current practice in community care is that assessment should focus on identification of need. Some clients may, however, require help in defining their personal needs because there is a danger that they could do this by relating them to what services they believe to be available. This could lead to problems since one of the key findings of the Social Services Inspectorate report: *Occupational Therapy the Community Contribution*[16] was that users' and carers' knowledge about what services are available is very restricted. If people only define need in relation to those services for which they believe they are eligible and this knowledge is limited, then a vicious circle could be established. Need should be defined in relation to what people aspire to achieve rather than what they believe to be possible in terms of service provision.

The other major problem in assessment is that for it to be entirely comprehensive, clients would have to be exposed to a range of tests and assessments covering all aspects of their lives and functioning. This would, however, be entirely impractical, potentially intrusive and more time consuming than is reasonable as well as generate more information and data than could be used realistically. It is, therefore, necessary to adopt a flexible and realistic approach when assessing need keeping at the centre of the process the aspirations of the client.

Areas for assessment

Although the potential range of areas for assessment is very extensive there are several major elements which are most likely to be dealt with by occupational therapists and others working with people in the community.

The World Health Organisation[17] recommends a range of domains for assessment of elderly people, these are as follows.

1. Activities of daily living: including mobility and physical and instrumental activities of daily living.
2. Mental health functioning: considering cognitive factors and psychiatric symptoms.
3. Psychosocial functioning: including emotional wellbeing in the individual's social and cultural context.
4. Physical health functioning: covering self-perceived health status, physical symptoms and diagnoses, levels of activity and incapacity.
5. Social resources: relating to accessibility to and availability of family, friends and significant others in normal and in changing circumstances.
6. Economic resources: particularly focusing on income relative to external norms.
7. Environmental resources: assessing in particular appropriate, adequate and affordable housing and access to transport, shopping and public service. (Adapted by permission from '*Health of the Elderly*', report of a WHO expert committee.)

The Royal College of Physicians and the British Geriatric Society[18] have agreed the adoption of these areas when assessing the elderly in hospital. With some additions and modifications they could be equally suitable for others with special needs and fit a community context. To make a more comprehensive list which could be more widely applicable a number of other sections could be included such as:

A   Education and training: considering the individual's potential and aspirations as well as availability of suitable courses and locations.
B   Work: taking account of skills, preferences and availability.
C   Leisure: dealing with how clients wish to use their time and those activities or pursuits in which they want to participate.
D   Quality of life: focusing on life satisfaction overall.
E   Carers and family needs: which could in many instances lead to viewing carers as service users in their own rights (see Chapter 2).

The assessment process

One of the purposes of assessment is to obtain information about the client and his/her lifestyle as well as identifying problem areas which can be tackled in care management. A number of issues in assessment should be borne in mind when carrying out the process.

Interviews. Assessment is essentially an information collection process, which can be carried out in several ways. The most common initial step is the interview which is usually carried out at the time of the first contact with the client. Interviews may be formal or informal and follow a semi-structured or structured format. In the context of community care the use of a semi-structured format with a mixture of open and closed questions allows for the collection of a range of information and at the same time permits exploration of clients' needs and aspirations. Interviews should be a two-way process with opportunities for the therapist and the client to both give and obtain information. The skill of the therapist at this stage is crucial in putting the client at ease and in the establishment of an effective communication network/rapport.

Information gathering. Information can also be obtained by carrying out one or several assessment procedures. Denton[19] questions whether or not it matters if assessments are standardised and suggests that it both does and does not. She outlines the advantages of standardised assessment as minimising error in results as well as gaining some assurance that the results do indeed reflect the client's performance rather than have bias related to test development, administration, scoring or interpretation. This is supported by Foster[20] who defines the two major advantages of standardisation as being that it 'provides a valid and reliable standard or "norm" against which to measure individual performance' and that 'it sets out the content of the test and explains how it is to be carried out to achieve maximum validity and reliability'.

Both Denton[19] and Eakin[21,22] support the notion of using standardised assessments and argue that through their use occupational therapists and others can have greater confidence in assessing clients accurately and providing data for quality assurance purposes.

In relation to activities of daily living assessments, Eakin also points out that standardisation does not mean that all occupational therapists should use the same scale, but that they utilise assessment instruments which have been evaluated for reliability and validity. This approach could be adopted in all aspects of practice.

Non-standardised tests are widely used and many have been developed to meet a local need. However, their use and the interpretation of the findings should be approached with a considerable degree of caution because of the potential problems associated with bias in evolution and execution of the test and evaluation of the results.

Information can also be collected from a range of non-client sources including existing case files, other professionals or agencies and when appropriate from relatives or carers. Sharing information with others involved in case management ensures that there is little repetition of work already carried out and that everyone concerned is informed about what is happening and what future plans are. Information should also relate to wider issues concerning the client, such as available services; community policies and resources; education and leisure facilities; local housing policies and so on. The nature of this type of information will depend very much on the individual client.

Skill required in assessment. Many skills are required in effective assessment including those of effective interpersonal, listening, analytical and evaluative skills. However, the skill which pervades all aspects of assessment is that of observation. Therapists must be alert at all times to cues and clues which can be observed as well as those responses which can be heard or measured. Observation used in conjunction with other information and clinical reasoning can help to complete a picture of the client and his circumstances. They may reinforce other information or raise suspicions about the accuracy of it. For instance, a client may state that he can cope independently in a large supermarket but on observation, difficulties in reaching and lifting items are identified.

Approaches to assessment: self-rating/report scales. If an entirely client-centred approach is considered to be desirable the logical method of assessment would be to use self-report or rating scales. Garbutt[23] suggests that the potential benefits of such self-assessments are that they are client-led and involve their active participation, at a pace which suits them. Other possible advantages are that there is time for reflection and potential to improve the quality of services offered. On the other hand, Edwards,[24] on reviewing a range of activities of daily living, self-rating scales and literature, suggests that caution is necessary when using these because there is a tendency to overrate their abilities, especially among the elderly and those with cognitive deficits. There are also those who would be excluded from independent completion of a self-rating format such as those who are very young, demented, blind or illiterate. Those with limited skills in the language of the form would also have difficulties in interpreting and completing it without help.

Self-report and rating scales may well be helpful as part of an assessment process and when the results are used in collaboration between the client and the therapist they can form a very useful basis for additional assessment and intervention.

Collaborative/client-centred assessment. Much assessment involves the client and the therapist working collaboratively towards identification of problem areas and the establishment of intervention goals. Different assessments involve varying degrees of therapist direction. By their very nature, standardised assessments tend to have higher levels of therapist direction and therefore they should only be used as part of a total assessment package, thus encouraging procedures with higher levels of client control.

In recent years a number of authors[10,25-27] have suggested that many assessments are fine as far as they go, but that in many instances their focus is often too narrow, relating to limited aspects of function and failing on occasion to take account of both the context in which the activity is carried out and the psychological and emotional components of it.

Trombley[25] suggests that occupational therapists have all too often adopted a bottom-up approach concentrating on aspects of function which are thought to be prerequisites to successful overall functioning. She advocates a top-down approach, starting with consideration of role competency and meaningfulness, thus meaning that roles most pertinent to the individual are the major focus of the assessment and subsequent interventions. It is suggested that by adopting such an approach the initial assessment provides a complete framework upon which to build case management. This is entirely in line with the recommendations of the National Health Service and Community Care Act 1990.

Dunn[10] and Pollock *et al.*[28] also support this notion of broadening the concept of assessment to include environment and social role expectations. Dunn proposes the use of a contextual approach where the environment in which a task is to be performed is scrutinised in order to consider factors within it which might enable an individual to perform a desired task.

The Canadian Occupational Performance Measure 1990, which is based on the Model of Occupational Performance,[29] is a format for assessment, designed to assess clients' perceptions of their occupational performance. It considers three major areas, i.e. self-care, productivity and leisure, each being examined for performance ability, satisfaction and level of importance to the individual. This method is very useful in identifying problem areas, assisting in goal setting and measuring change in performance over time. Although the actual measure may not be universally applicable, this type of approach goes a long way to considering the client in context and highlighting what he can do, needs to do and wishes to do, as well as the relative importance of each task for the individual.

Function in context should be addressed and also, within a holistic approach, psychosocial factors which may affect function must be accounted for.[27]

If the current research on assessment is linked with that on independence, several suggestions emerge.

1.   Assessment should start with the individual being assessed.
2.   It is not sufficient for the assessment to focus entirely on individual function, as it must take account of the context in which the person lives as well as psychological and social circumstances which influence that individual.
3.   Assessment should be made of wider social and political issues which influence how people are either enabled to achieve or prevented from achieving personal goals.

Goal setting and intervention planning

This process will in most instances be carried out by the therapist in collaboration with the clients and where appropriate their family or carer, along with any other relevant professionals. Although it may be desirable for people to set their own goals it is likely that many people will in fact require help with this process. The therapist can, however, act as a facilitator rather than a leader in helping the client to understand the nature of the presenting problems. It is important to examine the main locus of the problem, which may be with the individual, in the immediate environment, support network or lie within a wider environment or social structure. Awareness of this allows for realistic goal setting. The goals to be achieved should then be identified and prioritised in order of importance to the client.

After this stage options available need to be identified, solutions considered and their feasibility explored. It is likely that, in seeking means of achieving identified goals, both the client and the therapist will be frustrated by factors outside their control (see Chapter 5). All possible options will need to be discussed fully and careful analysis made of the implications and consequences of each. In this way the client can make an informed decision about the preferred solution.

Solutions should focus on the locus of the existing problem. If this lies with the individual, personal limitations may be overcome by changing a method of achieving a task, learning to use a piece of equipment safely, or agreeing that someone else can assist in or be responsible for accomplishing it. A rehabilitation programme may be established focusing on specific treatment areas, this being of particular significance when clients are discharged quickly from hospital. In this situation the ideal would be for a programme to commence in hospital and be continued in the community. If the locus of the problem lies in the immediate environment, solutions may involve property adaptations or the opportunity to move house. If the problem lies within the client's support network it may be that alternative arrangements will resolve the problem. It could also be that the solutions lie with assisting carers in their role and may involve training them in safe use of equipment; counselling them with regard to coping with their new role or arranging for additional support. If, on the other hand, the problem is located in the wider environment or structure of society resolutions may be much more difficult to find. It is important that such problems are not regarded as lacking solutions. Those involved with clients in the community should encourage them to voice their difficulties and bring them to the attention of those responsible for policy making, with a view to instigating change.

Once the agreed interventions have been implemented time should be allowed for clients and, where appropriate, carers to adapt to them and then the situation should be reassessed, when comparisons can be made between goal setting and attainment. It may be that if initial solutions are unsatisfactory a change will have to be made to the programme.

In helping clients to identify need, assess priorities and set and attain goals therapists must be flexible and imaginative in their approach and at all times remember that each client is an individual with his or her own personal goals, the attainment of which the therapist has the skill and expertise to assist him to achieve.

References

1. Blom-Cooper, L. *Occupational Therapy: an emerging profession in health care*, London: Duckworth, 1990.
2. Department of Health, Social Services Inspectorate, Scottish Office, Social Work Services Group, *Care Management and Assessment: Practitioners Guide*, London: HMSO, 1991.
3. Zola, I. Social and cultural disincentives to independent living, *Archives of Physical Medicine and Rehabilitation*, Vol. 63, 1982.
4. Swain, J., Finkelstein, V. and French S. *Disabling Barriers: Enabling Environments*, London: Sage Publications in association with the Open University, 1993.
5. Campbell, J. Equipped for independence or self determination, *British Journal of Occupational Therapy*, Vol. 53(3), pp. 89–90, 1994.
6. French, S. What's so great about independence? *New Beacon* (Royal National Institute for the Blind), Vol. 74(886), pp. 153–6, 1991.
7. Oliver, M. Disability and dependency, in *Disabling Barriers: Enabling Environments* (eds Swain, J. *et al.*), Sage Publications, 1993.
8. Law, M. The environment: a focus for occupational therapy, *Canadian Journal of Occupational Therapy*, Vol. 58(4), pp. 171–9, 1991.
9. Oliver, M. *The Politics of Disablement*, London: MacMillan Press, 1990.
10. Dunn, W. Measurement of function: actions for the future, *American Journal of Occupational Therapy*, Vol. 47(4), pp. 356–9, 1993.
11. Sumsion, T. Reflections on . . . client-centred practice: the true impact, *Canadian Journal of Occupational Therapy*, Vol. 60(1), pp. 6–8, 1993.
12. Mayers, C. A model for community occupational therapy practice Stage 1, *British Journal of Occupational Therapy*, Vol. 56(5), pp. 169–72, 1993.
13. Knight, J. Professionalized service and disabling help, in *Disabling Professions* (eds Illich, I. *et al.*), Marion Boyars Publishers, 1977.
14. Corbett, J. The quality of life in the independence curriculum, *Disability, Handicap and Society*, Vol. 4(2), pp. 145–63, 1989.

15. Hagedorn, R. *Occupational Therapy: Foundations for Practice, Models, Frames of Reference and Core Skills*, Edinburgh: Churchill Livingstone, 1992.
16. Social Services Inspectorate, *Occupational Therapy the Community Contribution*, London: HMSO, 1993.
17. World Health Organisation, *Health of the Elderly*, Technical Report Series No. 779, pp. 34–5, Geneva: WHO, 1989.
18. Royal College of Physicians and the British Geriatrics Society, *Standardised Assessment Scales for Elderly People (a report of joint workshops)*, London: Royal College of Physicians and the British Geriatrics Society, 1992.
19. Denton, P.L. *Psychiatric Occupational Therapy: a workbook of practical skills*, Boston, Massachusetts: Little Brown Co, 1987.
20. Foster, M. Assessment, *Occupational Therapy and Physical Dysfunction* (eds Turner, A. *et al.*), Edinburgh: Churchill Livingstone, 1992, pp. 179–203.
21. Eakin, P. Assessments of Activities of Daily Living: a critical review, *British Journal of Occupational Therapy*, Vol. 52(1), pp. 11–15, 1989.
22. Eakin, P. Problems with Assessments of Activities of Daily Living, *British Journal of Occupational Therapists*, Vol. 52(2), pp. 50–4, 1989.
23. Garbutt, J. An introduction to self assessment, *British Journal of Occupational Therapists*, Vol. 52(2), pp. 47–9, 1989.
24. Edwards, M.M. The reliability and validity of self-report Activities of Daily Living Scales, *Canadian Journal of Occupational Therapists*, Vol. 57(5), pp. 273–8, 1990.
25. Trombley, C. Anticipating the future: assessment of occupational function, *American Journal of Occupational Therapy*, Vol. 47(3), pp. 253–7, 1993.
26. Pollock, N. Client-centred assessment, *American Journal of Occupational Therapy*, Vol. 47(4), pp. 298–301, 1993.
27. Bonder, B.R. Issues in assessment of psychological components of function, *American Journal of Occupational Therapy*, Vol. 43(3), pp. 211–16, 1993.
28. Pollock, N. Baptiste, S. and Law, M. Occupational performance measures: review based on the guidelines for the client-centred practice of occupational therapy, *Canadian Journal of Occupational Therapy*, Vol. 57(2), pp. 77–81, 1990.
29. Law, M. *et al. Canadian Occupational Performance Measure*, Toronto: Canadian Association of Occupational Therapy Publications ACR, 1992.

Examples of standardised assessment tests

The Barthel ADL Index
The Bay Area Functional Performance Evaluation
Canadian Occupational Performance Measure
Chessington Occupational Therapy Neurological Assessment Battery
The Craig Handicap Assessment and Reporting Technique (CHART)
The Functional Independence Measure

The Morningside Rehabilitation Status Scale
Reintegration to Normal Living Index
The Rivermead Perceptual Assessment Battery
The Role Activity Performance Scale
Satisfaction with Performance Scaled Questionaire
The Short Form 36 (SF-36)
Guttmann Scale
Quality of Wellbeing Scale
Nottingham Health Profile

Chapter 8

Maintaining dignity

GILLIAN ASPINALL
*Head Occupational Therapist, Elderly Directorate, Norfolk Mental Health Care
NHS Trust*

Living in the community means more than being able to care for one's personal needs independently or having a care programme to attend to them. Individuals have additional facets to their lives which will be different for each person. The meanings and values attached to these activities make up a person's 'reason for living' and as such professionals must not overlook the importance of understanding these meanings and their impact on the client and their family.

It is interesting to reflect on the meaning of the phrase 'maintaining dignity'. What is dignity? What does loss of it represent to an individual? Dignity encompasses notions of an individual's uniqueness and a sense of worth and identity as a person. The antithesis of this might be dehumanisation or a loss of personality. Hilgard and Atkinson[1] define personality in terms of an individual's unique adjustment to their environment.

> We stress particularly those personal traits that affect the individual's personal adjustment, in his maintenance of self-respect. Any description of the individual personality must take into account appearance, abilities, motives, emotional reactivity and the residues from experiences that have shaped the person as we find him ... it refers to the individual and the unique organisation of traits that characterise him and his activities.

If a person's sense of worth or selfness, their dignity, is linked to their interaction with the environment, then professionals who help to create or modify this environment must accept some responsibility for helping to maintain dignity. Placing a commode in the corner of someone's living room may be a necessary change to the environment, but what affect does that have on that person's sense of dignity?

A fundamental concept is that of civil liberty and the rights of an individual to be treated with respect – in other words, to maintain his or her own dignity. Those who have their liberties reduced or removed are invariably in vulnerable situations. Due to illness, frailty or disorientation they are dependent to a degree on others to have their wishes, views and rights fully satisfied. All too often they have to trust in goodwill and the advocacy of their carers. If a person has their rights taken away from them, even unintentionally, the result is abuse. Vulnerable adults do not have the long established and detailed legislation that children have to protect their rights. There are no detailed investigative procedures to ensure that abuse can be identified and dealt with. In law, adults are considered independent and therefore able to protect their own rights; thus, being cared for in some way may rob a person of this ability. Most carers and professionals have the wellbeing of the client at heart and it might be disturbing to consider that their best intentions may lead to infringement of rights, loss of dignity or even abuse. It is therefore important to reflect regularly on areas of practice in order to learn to promote dignity.

Decision making and consent

It is a basic common law principle that a person's body is inviolate and that any intentional touching of it without consent is a trespass. Thus any medical procedure involving touch performed without consent is, in legal terms, a tort or civil wrong. This rule has been modified by what is termed the 'doctrine of necessity'. Necessity provides a justification for intervention, such as emergency treatment, for which consent cannot be obtained.

Professionals and carers should be clear that they need to obtain consent from a client for any intervention, however straightforward it might seem to the person undertaking it. Many procedures become second nature to a carer and the sense of intimacy or the invasion of privacy may be dulled by repetition. Carers should be sensitive to the wishes of the client, particularly taking account of what the procedure means to that particular client. It may take time to establish this, but it is vital if the client is to be treated with respect.

Giving consent to treatment means that the person should be fully and properly informed about the suggested procedure, its risks and the consequences of refusing it. For consent to be valid it is important to establish that the client understands in broad terms what is involved. Again, this may take time. It is not acceptable to assume that consent is given if a person does not object to his treatment – opportunity must be given for the person to object. The caring relationship places the client in a most unequal position where the professional holds the power. While many clients feel grateful to their carer or practitioner and feel unable to question a procedure, others feel that to question it will jeopardise his or her future treatment. Too often medical language simply does not allow the space for the client to participate in the decision-making process.

An important issue is the question of how to proceed if a person is incapable of giving consent to treatment. A legal incapacity arises whenever the law provides that a person is incapable of taking a particular decision or engaging in a particular transaction. Under law the general approach has been that it is presumed that the person is capable unless proved otherwise, and capacity is judged in relation to the particular decision to be made at that particular time. Incapacity to make a decision may be due to a variety of causes. People under 18 years of age, for example, are considered incapable of voting. However, certain illnesses or disabilities may give rise to an incapacity to make certain decisions. Some mental health problems or learning difficulties may, at some time during their course, involve this. This is obviously not to suggest that everyone with a mental health problem or indeed everyone with Alzheimer's disease is incapable of making their own decisions. The Mental Health Act 1983 is extremely specific in its scope for using its powers to give compulsory treatment or detention.

The policy of community care has resulted in more people with a mental health problem or a learning disability being cared for in the community rather than an institution. The benefits of living as normal a life as possible are recognised as being preferable to the restrictions of an institution. Life in the community does, however, render people with these difficulties more vulnerable and possible targets for abuse or exploitation. In responding to this there is a very real danger that such people have their dignity stripped away through over-protection by their carers. What must be considered is that the risk of institutionalisation may be much greater than the risk of occasionally being open to making an unwise decision. Living in the community means being free to experience normal risks. Part of ensuring dignity is to allow some risk in order for the person to learn and maintain independence. Dignity encompasses making mistakes and sometimes getting things wrong, rather than being shielded from these experiences in the name of the person's best interests.

For those people unable to make an informed decision, the 'doctrine of necessity' may be used to determine what treatment may be administered without the person's consent. This is not always helpful as some procedures are desirable, rather than necessary. An alternative principle in law is that of best interests – that is, treatment may be given if it can be demonstrated that the procedure is in the client's best interests. The concept of what is or is not in someone's best interests is open to many interpretations. This is never straightforward, as a case in 1990 demonstrated where, as there was no legal precedent, the House of Lords was asked to decide whether or not a woman with a learning disability should be sterilised. Was it, for example, in the woman's best interests, or society's, that she be sterilised? In other words how should a person's best interests be assessed?

Traditionally it has been medical staff who have decided what is in a person's best interests. Increasingly, however, family members or carers are becoming involved in this decision making. To ensure good practice a client should have an advocate appointed to look after their best interests. This is important, as family members may have an agenda which is different or opposed to the client's. Although not yet implemented in some areas of practice, this was recommended by the Disabled Persons (Services, Consultation and Representation) Act 1986 and by the NHS and Community Care Act 1990.

Advocacy

Advocates may assist professionals in the important job of determining what is in the client's best interests but may also suggest what the client might have wanted had they been able to speak for themselves. This is particularly valid in the case of a person who has previously had capacity and may have expressed opinions on the subject, or left evidence of what his wishes might be. In such a case it might be preferable to adopt the 'principle of substituted judgement', by which decisions are decided in the way the person would have acted, taking full account of any idiosyncratic views they may have held. For example, in order to achieve an individual's definition of a dignified death some people are drawing up 'Living Wills'. While not yet a legal document in England, these set down the person's wishes beforehand regarding their treatment in the event of a serious illness. In order to address this important area of civil rights Age Concern has drawn up a 'Charter of Rights to Community Care for Older People'[2] which contains the following statement of purpose:

> Each older person has the right to a life which maintains personal independence, safeguards privacy, offers genuine and informed choices, provides opportunities to enjoy and contribute to society as fully as possible and meets his/her social, cultural and individual needs. If such an independent life involves a degree of risk which the older person accepts, the authority will respect such a wish and endeavour to support the individual wherever possible.

While concentrating on the rights of elderly people this work does illustrate the importance of non-statutory agencies and pressure groups in maintaining the dignity of vulnerable people. Personal dignity cannot be separated from the position of disabled people in our culture. The empowerment of disabled people, their initiation of and participation in policy making are vital steps towards their dignity in society. Current legislation in Britain still does not tackle the discrimination which occurs from the barriers encountered by disabled people in many areas of life, including employment and access to public buildings. How dignified can it be for a person in a wheelchair to be refused access to a theatre or night club, or be informed that they are a fire hazard?

Further to the importance of personal right and representation, some practical aspects of dignity follow.

Communication

The ability and opportunity to convey one's feelings or intentions and to have these understood in return can be seen to be a fundamental need for the individual. A breakdown in effective communication is frustrating, distressing and leads to a loss of dignity. The tendency of people to communicate with the carer of a disabled person rather than the person directly is well illustrated by the 'Does he take sugar?' situation. Some conditions lead to speech difficulties and expert assessment by a speech and language therapist is vital in order that the client and their family receive the advice and treatment needed to promote effective communication. Not listening to an individual or ignoring their attempts to communicate can be damaging and abusive. Carers and professionals must be aware that their style of communication has an impact on dignity. For example, the simple act of repeatedly finishing another person's sentence can be destructive.

The caring relationship can be intense and the demands unremitting. Carers often need someone with whom they can share concerns, and sadly, if this is not available, verbal or emotional abuse of the disabled person or the carer may be the result. Carers' groups and counselling services are much needed to prevent this type of abuse, which largely goes undetected.

Pain management

Although the sense of pain serves the important function of signalling danger, prolonged pain can be physically and emotionally draining. Maslow's[3] hierarchy of needs suggests that protection from pain is a basic human need. At the base of his pyramid are physiological needs, such as hunger and thirst. Once these have been satisfied the individual is able to turn their attention to safety needs. Among these is the need to be free from fear and pain and to be out of danger. Human rights may feel much less important to an individual who is in severe pain.

Pain is a variable phenomenon and is felt in very individual ways. The distress it causes may often be due to the sense of being out of control that ensues. To counter this some methods of pain management aim to give the sufferer a greater sense of control over their body, therefore reducing the pain. Teaching techniques of relaxation have been effective in reducing pain, for example in childbirth and back pain. Giving information and explanations about the causes of pain also reduces the feelings of lack of control. Education, therefore, may be helpful in reducing pain associated with some conditions such as arthritis.

Research has demonstrated that the brain itself produces substances known as endorphins that reduce or eliminate pain by affecting the body's pain receptors and inhibiting pain signals from the spinal cord to the brain. Physical exertion or stress can activate this process, leading to the body's own mechanism to work against pain. A runner, for example, will not feel pain until after the race is over. Some forms of pain management aim to harness this natural process.

In Britain the hospice movement has contributed to a greater body of expertise in the management of pain, especially that associated with terminal illnesses. Expert help from an oncologist or anaesthetist will be able to determine the most effective means of controlling pain with the participation of the client and carers. Macmillan nurses have a vital role in the community to ensure that terminally ill clients are able to remain pain-free and in their own homes for as long as possible, as well as providing support and counselling for the whole family.

Pain clinics are multidisciplinary centres where comprehensive assessment of pain can be undertaken and a management programme initiated.

Incontinence

The lack of dignity caused by incontinence is distressing and embarrassing. It can lead to social isolation, as its effects are social as well as physical. A number of medical conditions can lead to incontinence in people of all ages; it is a symptom which is often curable and usually amenable to improvement through correct management.

Assessment and diagnosis of the medical problem should be carried out by the client's GP or, if necessary, by admission to hospital. Correct treatment of the underlying condition can cure the incontinence. However, if it remains the client should be given help in the management of the condition. There are different types and degrees of incontinence and it should be established which kind the client is experiencing. These require different methods of management. Stress incontinence, for example, is caused by the insufficiency of the pelvic floor muscles. A physiotherapist will advise on an exercise programme to strengthen these muscles. Overflow incontinence, by contrast, is caused by constipation leading to faecal impaction. In this case a dietician will advise on a suitable diet to include more roughage.

Some so-called incontinence may be caused by the client's inability to access the toilet successfully. This may be due to a condition causing a greater urgency of micturition combined with slower mobility, as in the case of Multiple Sclerosis. The home environment can lead to problems; for example, where a client is unable to enter the bathroom with a walking frame, or where too much furniture impedes or slows down access. A home assessment by an occupational therapist will identify these difficulties and modify the environment to overcome them. Equipment is available to improve access to the toilet and thereby eliminate incontinence and improve independence.

The embarrassment caused by incontinence can prevent people coming forward to receive help and the psychological and social effects of it must not be ignored by professionals and carers. Trust will need to be established before a client will seek help of such a personal nature. In many areas continence advisers are available to give practical help on the management of incontinence and stoma care.

Dignity, then, is a practical consideration for society and for individual carers and professionals. It involves the participation of clients in their own treatment through choice and the upholding of basic human rights. It places importance on quality of life rather than mere personal independence and stresses the uniqueness and inherent value of each individual person.

References

1. Hilgard, A. *Introduction to Pyschology*, London: Harcourt, Brace, Jovanovich, 1967.
2. Age Concern, *Old Age Abuse, Lifting the Lid*, England: Age Concern, 1991.
3. McCreadie, C. *Elder Abuse: an exploratory study*, London: Institute of Gerontology, King's College London, 1991.

Further reading

The Law Commission, *Mentally Incapacitated Adults and Decision Making: An Overview*, London: HMSO, 1991.

Age Concern, *The Law and Vulnerable Elderly People*, England: Age Concern, 1986.

McCormack, G.L. Pain management by occupational therapists, *American Journal of Occupational Therapy*, Vol. 42(9), pp. 582–9, 1988.

Mandestam, D. *Understanding Incontinence: a guide to the nature and management of a very common complaint*, London: Chapman & Hall, 1989.

Strong, J. *et al.* The effectiveness of relaxation techniques with patients who have chronic low back pain, *Occupational Therapy Journal of Research*, Vol. 9(3), pp. 184–92, 1989.

Resources

Tissue Viability Society, c/o Wessex Rehabilitation Association, Salisbury District Hospital, Salisbury, Wilts SP2 8BJ. 15-minute video and booklet.

Continence Foundation Helpline: 0191–213–0050.

Chapter 9

Counselling

ELIZABETH CRACKNELL
Head of the Division of Occupational Therapy, School of Health and Life Sciences, Nene College, Northampton

An occupational therapist employed by a a local authority Social Service department received a request from the local hospital to visit a 60-year-old man. Mr B. had just been discharged home following an above-knee amputation and the request for a walking aid had come from the hospital department. The occupational therapist telephoned the hospital to find out a little more about the client and she was told that he had not progressed at all well in hospital – indeed, there was nothing more that could be done for him as he was not making any effort. Mr B. was being sent home to fend for himself as best he could. The occupational therapist was rather concerned at this, so she arranged to see him at home that week. On arrival she found a very distressed person who looked far older than his years, together with a very anxious wife. Both were overwhelmed by the events which had overtaken them. His life had been turned upside down by the unexpected happening. Whereas, prior to surgery, he had been an active, lively confident man he was now an invalid (in-valid) who could not face his family, friends or the future.

The occupational therapist quickly realised that practical help in such circumstances was inappropriate. In the previous year she had under-taken some counselling training and was able to respond to Mr B.'s greatest need. She spent the next one-and-a-half hours listening to the outpourings of grief and anguish through tears as Mr B. expressed all the pent-up emotions that consumed him and which, since the operation, he had had no opportunity to release. In hospital the norm was to put on a brave face as practical difficulties were dealt with. There was no room for emotional adjustments and distress, for there was always 'someone worse off than you'.

This true story of Mr B. illustrates how essential it is for the occupational therapist to be sensitive to all aspects of her client's being. To respond at the level of the presenting practical problems would not have met Mr B.'s most urgent needs. Physical trauma is accompanied by tremendous psychological disturbance both in thought and in feelings and for this man, healing could only begin once the emotional turmoil surrounding his operation and residual disability could be expressed fully. Someone had to give time, a listening ear and understanding. Fortunately in this case the therapist recognised Mr B.'s state of distress, was sensitive to his psychological needs and provided the opportunity that had not previously been available. Within a few weeks, he looked 10 years younger as he walked independently on his pylon and began to plan hopefully for the future. As so often can be the case, the client referred with ostensibly a practical problem of mobility, was in reality a very different requirement. Since the occupational therapist was perceptive and able to respond to the client's state of being she promoted a counselling relationship to respond to his emotional needs.

The concept of counselling

Counselling is an activity which is carried out by many professional people as an integral part of their work, as well as by those who are appointed to designated counselling positions. Clergy, teachers, managers as well as those in the helping professions often find that they are called on to 'counsel' someone even though they may not feel adequately prepared for the task. The demand for such help has led to counselling skills being included in courses for students of occupational therapy so that they can be effective in their work. At this point it must be stressed that basic counselling skills do not make a counsellor, and anyone who wishes to become proficient in this field must seek further training. As a separate discipline counselling has burgeoned in the last 20 years, both in practice and in the numbers of organisations which offer training under the umbrella of the accreditating organisation, the British Association of Counselling.

Most counselling occurs between two individuals, one being in need of help and the other the helper. The term is often used loosely to refer to any help that is given by one person to another, such as advice, but in the counselling milieu information-giving is not considered to come under the term 'counselling'. Counselling is a psychological process whereby one person, the counsellor (for this text, she) helps another person (the client, he) to explore issues of life which are important to him. The exploration is more than a listening process. It is one which accepts the client's view of life and through discussion enables him to learn fresh ways of looking at events and of using his own resources to live a more effective and fulfilling life.

Counselling has been described as treatment;[1] however, this suggests a close link with the medical profession and patient passivity, but this is not so. It is always about active change. Counselling involves the person in his own development and search for wellbeing. Another writer states that counselling aims to help clients who are mainly outside medical settings to help themselves.[2] Note that these definitions are not problem orientated, for many counsellors believe that the basic process has much deeper aims, comprising greater independence, self-responsibility and integration of the individual through growth and development. Carl Rogers (1902–87),[3] to whom the counselling world owes so much, emphasised that the individual is the focus and not the problem. Thus the aim of counselling is not to solve one particular problem but to assist the person to grow, so that he or she can cope with present and future life issues. Rogers assumed that all human beings have internal resources for understanding and changing themselves; that they can remain in control and be responsible for their own lives, and that they do not have to become dependent on others to be helped. If for some reason a person does become dependent upon the counsellor he has lost his autonomy and thereby progress will be impeded.

The British Association for Counselling encapsulates the essence of the process when it says that the task of counselling is 'to give the client an opportunity to explore, discover and clarify ways of living more resourcefully and toward greater well being'.[4]

Counselling has a number of theoretical bases; analytical, behavioural, cognitive and humanistic. It is not possible here to explore them all but it has to be remembered that each perspective provides different parameters and different assumptions upon which the counselling process is based. However, the one thing that all counsellors agree upon is that, just as with occupational therapy, it is the relationship established between the client and therapist which is vital to a successful outcome. In addition both counselling and occupational therapy aim to help people to help themselves towards greater independence of living and life fulfilment.

A holistic model

Human beings are complex creatures who experience the world in a variety of ways. Knowledge of the world comes through the bodily senses which are then interpreted, resulting in experiences, feelings, thoughts and possibly actions. Humanistic psychology, which has its roots in both eastern and western thought, focuses upon the subjective experience of the individual considering it to be the way to understand and help another person. It assumes that people have within them resources for growth which are constructive and creative.[5]

Counselling recognises the complexity and subjectivity of human experience. It encompasses all aspects of a person's being as represented in the concept of self. Self comprises the cognitive processes, such as thinking, memory, willing and learning; affective processes such as feelings and motivations; and behaviour, the way a person relates to the world. This holistic model, familiar to occupational therapists, is based upon the belief that mind and body, psyche and soma, are inextricably linked and each domain effects the other. The depressed person will think, feel and move in a different way from that prior to onset of the depression; similarly, the person who is seriously physically injured will undergo changes in thoughts and feelings about himself, others and the world in general as a result of his trauma. Consequently the view of oneself changes and the regard with which one holds oneself also changes (Fig. 9.1).

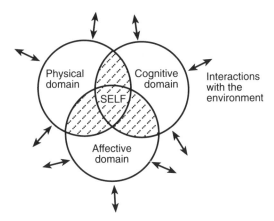

Fig. 9.1 A holistic model of a person

If the above assumptions are correct to treat one aspect of the person, for example, the physical injury, and ignore the psychological aspects will not cater for all the needs of the client and the neglected aspects could interfere with the process of healing. To treat the whole person the therapist must therefore include the psychological, social and physical needs if she is to be truly effective.

Mr B. had experienced a traumatic event which left him with severe disability that seriously impaired his physical functioning. It was a trauma with which he had to come to terms not only in physical functioning but also cognitively and emotionally. Nothing would restore his leg to him; his body would be permanently incomplete and he knew that life for him would never be the same again. Inevitably things would change for he was no longer the man he once was. His feelings about himself and others also changed. He no longer knew how relatives and friends would receive him and was anxious about this. He did not like himself and believed that other people would not like him in this condition either. How could anyone love him now? His thinking became irrational as he felt he could no longer support his wife as he thought he should. Indeed, he felt useless, questioned the purpose of life and could find no reasons for continuing. The occupational therapist found a defeated man. The amputation had changed everything about Mr B. His active life of work and leisure was curtailed and he felt helpless. Worse still, he was so dependent on his wife. His feelings and thoughts were all focused upon his physical state and the changes imposed upon him as a result of surgery. At the time of the visit of the occupational therapist he could see no future for he had no hope.

Humanistic theorists such as Abraham Maslow[6] and Carl Rogers[3] have both contributed to the understanding of the person as a subjective organism. Maslow discussed motivation and the development of the whole person, emphasising the ability human beings have of making choices. Central to Rogers's thinking was that each person has an independent 'self' motivated by positive motivation to enhance one's being. The 'self-concept' comprises all thoughts, feelings and values of the person derived from past experience. Everything that happens to an individual is evaluated in relation to the self-concept. A person with a positive regard for oneself will view the world very differently from someone who esteems themselves low regard. A man like Mr B. may no longer feel good about himself, due to the change in his self-regard resulting from his changed circumstances. By listening to him and allowing him the chance to express his pent-up feelings and find the good things he knew of himself and his life, the therapist was able to help him reconsider who he was and what his choices might be as he faced the future. Only as Mr B. progressed through the transition period of emotional up-heaval was it right for the occupational therapist to offer Mr B. the practical help he needed for mobility, thereby extending his opportunities for action.

The counselling relationship and processes

No two people in a counselling encounter bring to it the same things. Each person has his or her own philosophy of life, personal values, attitudes and beliefs which affect the way events are perceived. Each has his or her own phenomenological view of the world. The humanistic perspective is as much a personal challenge to the therapist as to the client.[7] All events are interpreted in the light of previous experience and responses are made upon these perceptions. Where people are very similar to each other communications tend to run smoothly, but where people differ greatly in their phenom-enology, interactions can give rise to many misunderstandings.

The core characteristics of the helping relationship

Drawing on his extensive work with people in need, Rogers proposed that there are three important ingredients which constitute a helping relationship, irrespective of the theoretical orientation of the therapist. He defined them as *positive regard, empathy* and *congruence*. Rogers was very keen that his work should be validated and these core conditions were tested by researchers,[8] who found they were essential for effective counselling. Without these characteristics the process of counselling is not likely to prove very helpful and at times could be harmful.

Positive regard. The client in distress may behave very oddly to a degree which could be described as bizarre; may have peculiar ideas about himself and prove to be very uncooperative. Even so, it is important that he should be warmly accepted for who he is and be valued unconditionally. Acceptance does not mean approval or agreement with a person's view or life or behaviour, for a person can be accepted without his actions necessarily being condoned. Such a quality is the mark of many friendships, where one can like someone very much but still dislike some of the things that they do. The therapist accepts the views of the other as real for him even when they in no way resemble hers; they are his starting point. The therapist who can accept the client in a non-possessive manner, without judgement and values him for who he is, is more likely to provide the milieu for growth and change.

Empathy. For empathic understanding the therapist has to drop her own view of the world and adopt that of the client. She needs to listen to her client's experiences and feelings as if they were her own, knowing that they are not. To understand the client's story the counsellor has to enter his phenomenal field, perceive events as he does and be in tune with his experiences and feelings. Only then will the counsellor be able to comprehend accurately and reflect what is happening to the client and then together they can explore the possibilities. Rogers writes that it is a way of being with another person where one enters 'the private perceptual world of the other becoming thoroughly at home in it'.[9] It is a very delicate process wherein one is constantly sensitive to the changing emotions of fear, rage, tenderness, confusion or whatever is being experienced.

Congruence. Throughout life human beings play many parts and at times one can be conscious that one is putting on a front, a façade which presents as a mask. Congruence means that the therapist is genuine, sincere and is able to be herself as she really is, without playing a part. Being true to oneself and having the confidence to trust oneself freely requires an authenticity of being. It is the most problematical of these three qualities and depends to a large extent upon one's own personal development. To be congruent the therapist has to know her own boundaries and be aware of her own internal responses. She needs to be comfortable with herself and does not have to pretend to be anything other than she feels herself to be.

Listening and reflecting

Some people are thinkers, some are doers and some are chatterers, but to be an effective counsellor one has to be a good listener. Listening is both an art and a skill which most people have at varying levels of competency, and one which can be developed with practice. It may be defined as concentrating on hearing something and paying full attention to it. In the counselling world empathic listening is a very active process and involves not simply attending to what is being said, but also observing how it is said. Body language conveys the feelings underlying the statements and due regard must be paid to both if one is to hear the messages. It is the kind of listening which allows clients to have the 'psychological space to do their own exploring' facilitated by the therapist.[10] The aim is to help the client to listen to himself, to overcome the blocks which impede his growth to becoming fully himself.

To listen effectively, both therapist and client should sit comfortably in a place where they are not likely to be disturbed. Contrary to the bustle and distractions of an occupational therapy department, it is often easier for the community therapist working in the home to respond to a client who wishes to talk. The therapist listens calmly as the client tells his story which she interprets as far as she is able, from the client's standpoint and not from her own. She will need to attend to the expression of feelings, attitudes and values as he recalls the events which have led him to his current position. Egan[11] calls this the stage of exploration; the period when the therapist is being put in the picture, listening to both verbal and non-verbal messages. While listening the therapist checks with the client so that she knows that she has understood the problem and if confused, she seeks clarification.

A friendly manner, not an inquisitive one, will encourage the client to talk easily. As the therapist listens carefully, more and more of the client's self-concept is revealed. The skill for the counsellor/therapist is in responding to what the client is saying in a way which enables him to open up and expand on particular points which may seem important to the counsellor but not apparent to the client. He may understand for the first time what is happening to him and where he is; through the exploration facilitated by the listener, he may be able to see ways forward.

Questions are useful but should be used with care. In basic listening exercises many students ask so many questions that the 'client' is subjected to an interrogation, which leads to a clamming-up rather than a flow of conversation. Open-ended questions, those which do not have clear-cut answers, are likely to elicit more from a client than those which can be answered by a yes or a no. 'Tell me what happened next' may lead to an unexpected narrative which the client is free to formulate as he wishes. A comment on the listener's observations, such as restlessness when the client mentioned the doctor, may trigger some feelings in him of which he was not wholly aware, and which he is not able to face.

The process of reflection mirrors for the client what he has said and enables him to experience more fully what is going on within him. It shows him that the counsellor is responding sensitively, not from her own frame of reference, but from the client's phenomenal field, for he is the primary reference point.[12] Through the reflections of the counsellor within a relationship of acceptance, unconditional positive regard and empathy, growth and development may occur.

Establishing goals

Sometimes, to listen attentively is all that is required of one person by another in distress. At other times it is necessary to examine ways in which the client can move forward from his current predicament. What does he really want? What actions is he prepared to take to change his position? In his disturbed state he may be blind to what the possibilities are even though at one level he knows there are some. The therapist can make suggestions by drawing upon her own experience and having a much wider knowledge of available resources. Under no circumstances should she impose her own wishes upon the client, for what is right for her may be totally inappropriate for another person. 'If I were you ...' is a phrase which has no place in the counselling world. The consequences of any actions may be thoroughly discussed by both parties, but the decisions as to what goals are set must stay with the client. The aim of counselling is to empower the client, promote his growth so it is essential that he remains in control and takes responsibility for decisions and subsequent actions. However, while in a distressed state he needs the support and guidance of the therapist as he makes his moves.

Making decisions often leads to relief, a reduction of tension and a release of energy. It is an assumption of the person-centred approach of counselling that all people have untapped resources for growth. The decrease in distress results in an increase in personal strength and confidence. He may develop a greater knowledge of himself as he integrates his experience into his self-concept, a process accompanied by a rise in self-esteem. The provision of a relationship which promotes the personal growth of another is rare and precious and those who undertake counselling should themselves be concerned about their own personal development.

The therapist as an agent of change

A fundamental belief which underpins the practice of occupational therapy is that people can change and that one is 'never too old to learn'. Through the learning of new skills or relearning of old skills, treatment is designed to increase all aspects of physical and psychological functioning so that the client can change and lead a fuller life. A therapist must have a strong belief that people can change and if she does not she has little to offer her clients. She must also believe that people are important *as* people and not for the positions they hold in society. Many clients are elderly and no longer command occupational status; they are outside the economic market. Even so, as individuals they need to be valued and respected, each having their own needs, gifts and graces. Therapists are like all other people in that they have their problems, dilemmas, joys and sorrows in life and, like others, will only be partially aware of their own motivations, attitudes and feelings. All human beings have 'blind spots' which are often well known to our nearest and dearest. These unconscious aspects of being can interfere in the relationship with a client and impede the helping process.

Bugental[13] points out that the therapist's own emotions, conflicts and anxieties will inevitably have an effect upon the client's life. Although Bugental was writing from the psychotherapy standpoint this applies equally in the areas of counselling and occupational therapy. The occupational therapist may find herself listening to a client express feelings which he has never before put into words, and she must respect these confidences. It may be that if there is a fear that confidentiality cannot be kept it is better to tell the client and with that information the client can choose whether or not to continue. Another issue is one where the therapist thinks that the client himself should tell another person his story; then it is matter of empowering the client so to do. It is important that trust exists within a helping relationship if personal change is to take place. Wise judgement needs to be exercised as the therapist weighs up the pros and cons of her decision. As already indicated, for a person who is undertaking counselling, the support of a supervisor is invaluable.

Community occupational therapists will work with people of varying ages, occupational experience and backgrounds. People from ethnic minorities may present a meeting of cultures and religions, and the helper has to put aside both her ethnocentricity and her egocentricity. If that cannot be achieved she will appear to be narrow and prejudiced. Clients have different expectations, responsibilities and lifestyles and their varied needs may be associated with any life event. In Holmes and Rahe's Social Adjustment Scale,[14] the death of a spouse is the life event which causes most stress to a person. Divorce is another major event which causes a great deal of stress, when specific counselling may be required. Physical disability may lead to a person suffering grief for the loss of function and problems in one's sexual life. Any event, however small, at whatever period of life, may present a crisis for an individual.

Community occupational therapists operate within different parameters to their colleagues working in organisational departments. Social psychologists recognise that behaviour is strongly influenced by the environment and three important concepts are relevant to community care: territoriality, privacy and personal space.

Territoriality

'The Englishman's home is his castle' is a well-rehearsed maxim. The majority of people live in a house or flat which they feel is their territory. There they are involved in family life and all its activities, eating, sleeping, loving and celebrating. With the medicalisation of birth and death these events often take place elsewhere, but the effects of these happenings are felt powerfully in the home. It is the place where the occupier has full control and where, under normal circumstances, entry is allowed only to those to whom permission has been given. The occupational therapist, like any visitor, is there by privilege which must be respected. A side effect of this is the power that a professional person has when in the hospital or a Social Services department is considerably reduced. As the nature of the counselling relationship is one which requires a more equitable sharing of personal power this changed position of the therapist can be an advantage.

Privacy

While the client is in the counselling role he may share and disclose aspects of himself which he would not do in other circumstances. In hospital, people (in today's language, customers or consumers) have little say in matters regarding privacy. Hospital staff are entitled to ask the most intimate questions which every consumer feels obliged to answer. In the home this situation is reversed. The client is independent of the professional person and he is directing his own life as much as he is able. He is able to determine the extent to which he will allow the occupational therapist and others not only to his home, but also to himself as a private citizen.

Personal space

Edward Hall, an anthropologist, proposed the science of 'proxemics', the way in which space is used in relationships and communication. Each person has a feeling of space around the body which is comfortable and is regarded as personal. Cultural patterns vary, but for most Europeans, if strangers come too near, perhaps within 18 inches (the intimate zone), it feels like an intrusion and can give rise to great discomfort. When customers are treated in hospital, members of the medical team who have no personal relationship with a customer from necessity often violate this feeling of personal space, which for some people causes distress and even anger. In the home the position is different, for the client is the host and the roles of each person demand that the therapist must be more circumspect and sensitive to the communications of the client if she is to be in a position to help him.

People who seek counselling may be experiencing or anticipating changes leading to confusion or distress. They may generally feel unsatisfied with their current place in life and be seeking ways to change their circumstances. Whatever it is that makes someone want to talk to another, the principles of counselling are the same. The helper/counsellor promotes a relationship which is accepting, warm and friendly in which she is genuine in her concern for the other. An opportunity to explore is created and the client is responded to with empathy which enables him to increase his understanding of himself. In this loving relationship (agape) the client may learn to live more resourcefully and creatively and move towards a greater sense of personal autonomy and independence.

References

1. Halmos, P. *The Faith of the Counsellors, 2nd edn*, London: Constable, 1978.
2. Nelson-Jones, R. *Practical Counselling Skills*, London: Holt, Rinehart and Winston, 1983.
3. Rogers, C.R. *Client Centred Therapy*, New York: Houghton Mifflin, 1961.
4. *Counselling: Definition of Terms*, British Association of Counselling, 1985.
5. Mearns, D. and Thorne, B. *Person-Centred Counselling in Action*, London: Sage Publications, 1988.
6. Maslow, A.H. *Motivation and Personality, 2nd edn*, New York: Harper and Row, 1970.
7. Broadbent, F. Counselling: an introduction. *British Journal of Occupational Therapy*, Vol. 48(2), pp. 36–9, 1985.
8. Truax, C.B. and Carkhuff, R.R. *Towards Effective Counselling in Psychotherapy; Training and Practice*, Chicago: Aldine, 1967.
9. Rogers, C.R. Empathic: and unappreciated way of being, *The Counselling Psychologist*, Vol. 3(2), pp. 2–10, 1975.
10. Broadbent, F. op. cit., 1975.
11. Egan, G. *The Skilled Helper, 3rd edn*, California: Brooks Cole, 1986.
12. Mearns, D. and Thorne, B. op. cit., 1986.
13. Bugental, J.F.T. *Psychotherapy and Process: the Fundamentals of an Existential Humanistic Approach*, Reading, Mass: Adison-Wesley, 1978.
14. Holmes, T.H. and Rahe, R.H. The Social Readjustment Rating Scale, *Journal of Psychosomatic Research*, Vol. 14, pp. 391–400, 1970.
15. Hall, E.T. *The Hidden Dimension*, London: Bodley Head, 1966.

Further reading

Atkinson, R.L., Atkinson, R.C., Smith, E.E. and Bem, D.J. *Introduction to Psychology*, Chapter 15, 11th edn, Fort Worth, Philadelphia: Harcourt Brace Jovanovich, 1993.

Dongen-Garrad, J. van, *Invisible Barriers, Pastoral Care with Physically Disabled People*, London: SPCK, 1983.

Etherington, K. The Occupational therapist as a counsellor towards attitude change in disability, *British Journal of Occupational Therapy*, Vol. 52(22), 1990.

Jacobs, M. *Still Small Voice: An Introduction to Pastoral Counselling*, London: SPCK, 1982.

Jacobs, M. *Swift to Hear. Facilitating Skills in Listening and Responding*, London: SPCK, 1985.

Kroll, U. *Sexual Counselling*, London: SPCK, 1980.

Nelson-Jones, R. *The Theory and Practice of Counselling Psychology*, London: Holt, Rinehart and Winston, 1982.

Nichols, K.A. *Psychological Care in Physical Illness*, London: Croom Helm, 1987.

Rogers, C. *On Becoming a Person*, London: Constable, 1967.

Rogers, C. *A Way of Being*, Boston: Houghton Mifflin, 1980.

Speck, P. and Ainsworth-Smith, I. *Letting Go: Caring for the Dying and Bereaved*, London: SPCK, 1983.

Books of the Series *Counselling in Action*, ed. Windy Dryden, London: Sage
  Publication.

Resources

Tapes, literature and a list of approved courses are available from the British Associ-
  ation of Counselling. BAC publishes a monthly journal for members. Regent Place,
  Rugby, Warwickshire, CV21 2PJ.
Relate, previously known as The Marriage Guidance Council, Herbert Gray College,
  Rugby, Warwickshire.
Cruse. An organisation which aims to relieve distress among the widowed. There are
  local branches in most areas.

Chapter 10

Equipment – help or hindrance?

ANN MOY
Head Occupational Therapist, Learning Disability Services, Norwich Community Health Partnership NHS Trust

Equipment is by definition a set of tools or a device designed for a specific purpose to aid or assist an activity: hence the now out-moded term 'aid'.

Everyone, whether able-bodied or incapacitated with some form of handicap, either short- or long-term, regularly use equipment to facilitate their daily lives. The well-known Nelson knife and Wellington boot no doubt resulted from the needs of their famous namesakes. Even today, many items are designed by one person for their own particular needs and it is not until they are marketed that a wider application is appreciated. The last 30 years have, however, witnessed dramatic developments in equipment for disabled people as medical knowledge has increased life expectancy, and the recognition of people's rights and potential has resulted in those with a disability leading fuller and more integrated lifestyles than ever before.

Designers and manufacturers quickly realised the potential for commercial development and equipment for a wide range of needs poured onto the market. This continued deluge has meant an increasing responsibility for professionals involved in the assessment and recommendation of equipment, and up to date knowledge and information regarding new items is essential if the service is to be effective and responsive. In addition to this multiplicity, there is a growing trend away from equipment designed specifically for disability towards that designed for a particular need, irrespective of whether a person is designated able-bodied or disabled. In the long term this trend can only prove positive and encourage high quality design and realistic pricing, as well as encouraging disabled people to feel accepted within the community. For example, an elderly person who would resent being termed disabled may welcome a handle on the bath, a non-slip surface and a tap which could be easily gripped and turned. To term such items 'special equipment' would result in rejection by many. Even people with quite difficult-to-manage needs can, because of the improvement in design, use attractive standard equipment instead of the basic and utilitarian items previously designed specifically for them and thus identifying them as disabled.

Everyone appreciates equipment that helps with a particular task and it is often selected for its cost, appearance, recommendation or advertised effectiveness. Items that do not assist become a hindrance and are eventually rejected. In fact, studies[1,2] have shown that significant amounts of equipment supplied to elderly and disabled people were never actually used, due mainly to initial inappropriate recommendation, poor design and quality, or inadequate training and reassessment.

In many situations a new technique in achieving a required activity is far more appropriate than the provision of more equipment and may provide a quick solution to the presenting problem. An adjustment to an existing piece of equipment or furniture may also be a simpler and more acceptable solution. For example, someone unable to exert sufficient pressure to cut up their food might find it easier if the table and chair were repositioned. There will, however, always be those people for whom no alternative technique or standard piece of equipment is available and who require a specially designed item. In these situations professional advice and training in their use are essential as incorrect choice can prove an expensive mistake and possibly detrimental to their condition.

Reassessment of the suitability of equipment supplied should be carried out, particularly where a person's condition improves or deteriorates. Equipment no longer required should be removed, as it may take up valuable space, and in the case of deterioration become a sad reminder of previous achievements.

Criteria for selection

Once it has been established that equipment is required, four aspects should initially be considered:

- the needs of the user;
- the needs of the relatives/carers;
- the objectives to be achieved;
- possible improvisation.

The needs of the user

Equipment can only be of benefit to the user when it is recognised by them as being needed. At first it may only be the physical aspect that is consciously recognised, but unless social and psychological needs are also satisfied, the item may be quickly rejected. In fact, there is a tendency by some to strive for physical achievement if the equipment is psychologically and socially acceptable to them. The occupational therapist must therefore include social, psychological and physical needs in the assessment.

The needs of the relatives/carers

At times throughout a week more than one relative or carer may be involved in the use of a piece of equipment, for example a hoist, and consequently all their needs and viewpoints must be considered. Discussion and training are essential to ensure that all involved recognise the benefits and know how to use the equipment safely.

The objectives to be achieved

As well as satisfying personal needs and wants, equipment must achieve the clearly defined objective for which it is issued. For example, the main objective for issuing a special seating system and wheelchair for a person with a severe multiple handicap may be to enable that person to sit comfortably and be transported safely. The therapist may wish to achieve a posturally acceptable position to prevent further deformity and pressure areas as well as ensuring safety and comfort. However, the user may simply want to be comfortable, achieve certain activities and receive the least amount of handling. The carer, on the other hand, may want a system that they can safely transfer the user to and from, possibly alone or by means of a hoist. They also may need to transport the chair in a car; therefore the seat will need to be easily removable and lightweight. Finally, the overall appearance must be aesthetically acceptable to all.

Often complex needs have to be considered and resolved, otherwise equipment will be rejected, resulting in distress and complications with a considerable waste of time and money.

Possible improvisation

Improvisation may sometimes be possible, particularly for an urgent short-term need or deteriorating condition, where the speed of achieving a solution is essential. Improvisation can also provide a temporary answer while waiting for other equipment to be delivered. For example, a piece of foam with a cut-out area may not be perfect but could prevent a spinal pressure area deteriorating into an actual sore while waiting for a more appropriate cushion to arrive.

Choice of equipment

Choice varies considerably depending on the activity to be achieved. For some, only one or two items are available, such as small polypropylene or bone spoons for feeding someone with severe athetoid cerebral palsy, while for others there is a bewildering selection. A systematic approach to the consideration of any of the following aspects relevant to the equipment required will prevent unnecessary confusion and ensure a more informed decision.

Design

Good design is vital if the item is to be aesthetically acceptable to the user and carer otherwise it is far less likely to achieve its objective and be regularly used.

Method of control

Some equipment is mechanically or electrically controlled. Where there is a choice of mechanism, such as in self-rise chairs or food whisks, the ability of the user must be carefully assessed to ensure that the item selected can be used safely and efficiently. The actual choice will depend on three equally important factors: the degree of disability of the user, their personal preference and finance.

Mechanically operated equipment usually requires considerable hand and upper limb movements, the degree of necessary muscle power depending on the design. Electrically or electronically operated equipment is easier and can sometimes be controlled by various parts of the body if suitable adaptations are available; for example by the forehead, chin, elbow or knee. The position and type of switch must ensure safety with minimal muscle power and movement.

Comfort

(a) Pressure. The user and carer must be aware of any potential pressure points likely to be caused by the use of an item. Pressure can result from the:

- size and shape of the equipment;
- type of material in actual contact with the body;
- the composition of the support beneath the surface;
- physical condition of the user such as bony prominences, sensitive skin, excess perspiration;
- degree of muscle power required to operate the equipment.

(b) Position and posture. Correct positioning will ensure the effective use of equipment. Considerations should include:

- support of deformities;
- elimination of spasticity;
- frequency of use;
- required quality of performance.

Safety

(a) Stability. Any type of support equipment, for example chairs, standing frames or hoists, must be stable enough to enable the user to be left

unattended for short periods of time. Back and front extensions, while assisting stability, can if badly designed, create obstacles for others. Equipment and furniture attached to the wall, floor or ceiling must be firmly secured to withstand any amount of pressure or weight that is anticipated to be exerted on it while in use. It is important that both user and carer have confidence in the equipment's stability or the item will be rejected.

(b) Potential hazards. Anticipating hazards can be difficult as the most unlikely situations may suddenly occur, thus causing an accident. General considerations to be aware of, however, include:

- sharp edges;
- small apertures which may trap fingers;
- insecure, collapsible or adjustable parts;
- easily removable parts that may be dropped;
- exposed rods or poles;
- required movements that are detrimental to the user or carer, thereby causing pain or damage, for example a lever that would prove difficult for a rheumatoid arthritic hand or a low chair that could cause damage to a carer's back during a transfer procedure;
- inappropriate materials that might break while in use (Photo. 10.1).

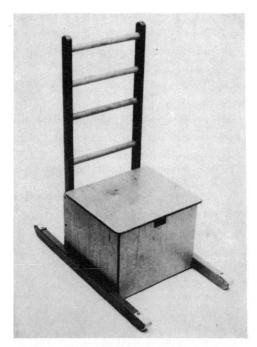

Photo. 10.1 Example of a child's chair with extensions to increase stability

Durability

Good design cannot hide inferior materials or workmanship and similarly unstable, shabby and badly designed equipment cannot be disguised by attractive materials and good workmanship over time.

Access

Ease of access to and from all equipment should be uncomplicated, bearing in mind emergencies such as choking, fits, bleeding or fire. Difficulties may be caused by:

- the height and position of the item;
- the type of straps or other method of fastenings;
- fixed or removable trays and tables;
- methods of postural support or restraint other than straps, for example abduction blocks or angled seats;
- the physical deformity or weight of the user and the number of carers required to assist, or the non-availability of a hoist (see Chapter 11).

Adjustments

(a) Method. Equipment can be adjusted by a variety of means. When an option is available consideration should be given to:

- how frequently the adjustments need to be made;
- where the equipment is to be used and by whom;
- how difficult the adjustment is to carry out and whether tools or assistance are required and if so whether they are accessible;
- whether the user can remain in position while the adjustment is made; and
- the cost, for example between an hydraulically adjustable table and a manually operated cantilever model.

(b) Range. The range of adjustment should be sufficient to accommodate all the required needs for a realistic period of time. For example, a correctly selected chair could 'grow' with a child for 2 or 3 years.

(c) Security. It is very important to ensure that:

- the method of adjustment is secure in all positions;
- the equipment is stable at all times and in particular at the top of the range;
- the method of maintaining the adjustment is secure. Some switches, pegs or wingnuts, for example, can be easily removed especially by

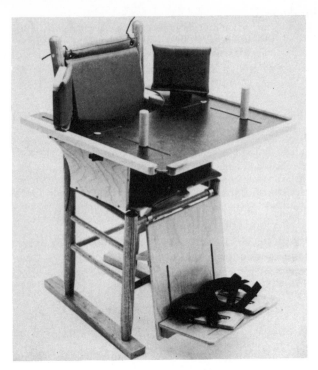

Photo. 10.2 Velcro straps and a quick-release mechanism on the tray allow a child to be quickly removed from this specially designed chair

some children, or accidentally knocked, thus causing an accident (Photo. 10.2).

Weight

This is a vital consideration if the equipment is to be transported regularly. A correctly positioned handle will make lifting easier but if one is not present a non-movable part, that affords a secure grip, should be identified.

Bearing in mind the manual handling regulations, any item that is too heavy or awkward to lift should be transported on a trolley or have castors attached (see Chapter 11). Some items are permanently fixed but have moving parts, for example an electric hoist or stair-lift. The weight of these, therefore, becomes less important to the user or carer. However, it is essential that the supporting structure, such as wall or ceiling, must be able to withstand the combined weight of the equipment and user (see Chapter 13).

Dimensions

Equipment can be referred to as standard or adjustable within the following specifications.

- Standard equipment is non-adjustable and designed to suit the average person and their needs. However, some equipment, particularly children's, is produced in more than one size, with growth being accommodated by a new item rather than by an adjustable variety.
- Adjustable equipment may be designed to satisfy variations such as height, ability, strength, angle of vision or hearing. The degree of adjustment must always be sufficient for the required need.

Transportation and storage

For those items that needs to be transported, either regularly or occasionally, and stored for periods of time, the following points need to be considered.

(a) Foldability. The ease of folding or dismantling an item and how frequently this needs to be done.

(b) Weight. This aspect has been considered in detail in the section 'Weight'.

(c) Design. The shape, dimensions, type of construction and materials used especially in relation to transportation and storage and in particular including:

- extensions and irregular shapes;
- overall height, length and width of item when folded and where it is to be assembled;
- type of material used;
- movable and removable parts (care must be taken to avoid loss or damage);
- carrying handles in the correct position.

Cleaning

Smooth, rounded or continuous surfaces help to facilitate cleaning while inaccessible cracks and corners collect dust and dirt, thus becoming a health hazard. Equipment used by a number of people will require more frequent and harder cleaning than if used by only one careful owner. Fabric covers and padding should be removable, respond to frequent cleaning and preferably be able to dry quickly. Equipment used for eating and drinking must be able to withstand a dishwasher when required[3] and should be checked for suitability.

Maintenance and repairs

Equipment must be checked regularly to ensure it remains functionally correct and safe, as well as continuing to satisfy the required needs.

Some firms provide their own maintenance service for large items such as hoists and responsibility for the contract must be identified when the equipment is purchased. When the need for repair occurs too frequently the cause may be due to an inappropriate item, or an incorrect size having been issued or purchased.

Availability

Delay between identifying a piece of equipment and actually receiving it can prove a source of much anxiety and frustration as well as prolonging pain and discomfort. Delivery times vary and are often unreliable; therefore, every effort should be made by the therapist to hasten delivery and find a temporary solution for the interim period. Equipment resource centres can, if efficiently organised, provide a valuable service both for assessment and temporary provision. Certain equipment may only be manufactured to order, for example an extra-large chair, and may take 2–3 months to arrive. If the need is urgent it may be preferable to compromise and adapt an available item rather than prolong suffering.

Price

As with all equipment prices can vary between one shop or catalogue and another. Therapists should be aware of these variations and be able to recommend value for money. Disabled people can be exempt from VAT[4] and the appropriate forms should be completed at the time of purchase.

Factors influencing acceptance of equipment

Even after assessment and careful consideration of the above aspects there are still some areas relative to the actual use that need to be considered.

Suitability for use

This can be difficult to assess unless the equipment is available for a trial period in the intended situation with all involved present. The aspects to consider are whether or not the equipment is:

(a)   *Functional.* It must achieve one or more of the following:
  - enable the user to carry out a previously impossible activity or a previously difficult one more easily;
  - allow more enjoyment or sense of achievement;
  - increase independence and/or of lesser dependence;
  - reduce pain or discomfort;
  - improve quality of life;
  - improve the life of the carer/s.

(b) *Efficient*. Equipment should enable the activity to be carried out with ease, within the required period of time and to an agreed or acceptable standard.

(c) *Reliable*. It should be capable of regular use and consistently achieve the required result. Unreliability results in frustration, lack of confidence and rejection as well as possible injury.

Training

However basic and straightforward equipment may appear to the therapist, it is important that verbal and written instructions are given relating to the correct assembly, use and care. A training session for user and carer/s is essential in identifying the equipment's purpose and potential, and should take place in the intended area of use or one that is realistically related. Points to cover are as follows.

(a) *Preparation*.
- correct assembly such as position of slings on a hoist;
- correct adjustment of height and angle;
- secure adjustments;
- secure attachments.

(b) *Use*.
- routine for access, e.g. bed to chair to toilet;
- routine for required activity using equipment.

Convenience for others within the same environment

Wherever the situation occurs, all involved should understand the reason for the equipment being provided but at the same time not be inconvenienced by it. Therefore, to ensure that it is acceptable to other people as well it should not be:

- disliked, e.g. a fixed toilet seat may not be welcomed by other members of the family;
- a disturbance, e.g. a particularly noisy piece of electrical equipment;
- a hazard, e.g. a child could easily cause damage or be hurt if allowed to 'play' with an electric wheelchair belonging to someone else.

The therapist should always try to anticipate potential inconvenience, damage and hazards that might occur and recommend basic guidelines for use.

Factors influencing rejection of equipment

Personality. Like any household furniture or equipment an item may be rejected for many reasons, especially personal preference. A brightly coloured drinking mug may be very acceptable to a young person but rejected by someone older.

Family influence and lack of perception. Equipment disliked by the family will not, or very rarely, be used especially if the use is not valued by them. The reason for using equipment must be recognised by user, carer, family and friends if the benefits are to be appreciated. For example, the use of a particular knife and fork might enable a couple to eat together and visit friends for a meal, whereas previously they ate at home with the husband feeding his wife.

A learning disability. A user with a learning disability may lack concentration or ability to persevere with equipment unless the training is appropriate and continuous. The co-operation of family or carers is essential in this and a special training programme which recognises achievement essential.

Time lapse. If the period of time between the referral, or onset of the disability, and the commencement of intervention by the therapist is too long, the person may reject all equipment, having in the meantime become too dependent on the family or carer.

Inadequate assessment. This is perhaps the most important factor. All information relative to the intended activity or required objective must be considered thoroughly during the assessment and prior to the recommendation of equipment (see Chapter 7).

Lack of training. As indicated above, lack of training is a common cause of rejection.

Lack of follow-up and/or reassessment. Few situations remain constant for any length of time and therefore it is crucial to review the situation at appropriate intervals to ensure that the equipment still satisfies the requirements. Equipment has been defined as something that 'assists' or helps to achieve an objective. If an item fails to assist it is no longer a help and may quickly become a physical, social or psychological hindrance.

Legislation

Apart from the British Standard Institute requirements legislation is now in place to ensure safety of all medical equipment and that required by disabled people. This includes the following.

Medical Devices Directorate. A government organisation with responsibility for medical devices and products used by the NHS and other health care sectors. It exists to ensure that these items meet acceptable standards of safety, quality and effectiveness by:

- operating the Manufacturers Registration Scheme (MRS);
- co-ordinating adverse incident reports and investigations (via NATRIC);
- undertaking equipment evaluations;
- participating in the development of standards;
- playing a major role in the development and implementation of the EC Directives on medical devices.

National Reporting and Investigation Centre (NATRIC). NATRIC was established in 1987 to co-ordinate reports concerning accidents involving medical equipment, devices and materials. It aims to improve the standard of reporting, issue hazard and safety bulletins and liaise with manufacturers and suppliers regarding product specification.

CE mark. This mark means that a manufacturer claims his product satisfies the requirements essential for it to be considered safe and fit for its intended purpose. Its aim is to harmonise and regulate the safety and marketing of products throughout the European Community, instead of the present situation where each member state has a different criteria that manufacturers have to satisfy.

Disability equipment assessment (DEA). The Medical Devices Directorate publishes reports (DEA reports) on a wide range of devices used in the NHS. Particular areas of interest to therapists are the disability and mobility equipment. The reports are issued free to the NHS.

References

1. Page, M. et al. *The Use of Technology in the Care of the Elderly and Disabled: Tools for Living,* London: Pinter, 1980.
2. Barrow, S. and Derbyshire, M.E. *Survey on the Usefulness of Aids: Lancashire County Social Service Department,* 1975.
3. Temperatures for Mechanical Washing and Double Wash Hand Washing, recommended by the British Institution of Environmental Health Officers.
4. *VAT leaflet 701/7/86,* HM Customs and Excise, local branches.

Resources

DEA Reports, Ordering Department, Room 222, 14 Russell Square, London WC1B 5EP.

Medical Devices Directorate, Department of Health, 14 Russell Square, London WC1B 5EP.

Disabled Living Foundation (DLF), 380/384 Harrow Road, London W9 2HU.

Local Independent Living Centre: details available from DLF, above.

Chapter 11

Lifting and manual handling in the community

JOYCE CHENEY
Manual Handling Adviser, Norwich Community Health Partnership NHS Trust

The aim of this chapter is to look at manual handling, all that is involved in its safe practice and how this may be applied to the community setting. Much has been written on manual handling and reference may need to be made to these documents in order to gain a wider view of the whole issue.

Manual handling injuries account for 55 per cent of all staffing injuries reported annually to the Health and Safety Executive (HSE) from the health care sector.[1] Patient handling is the most common source of reported injuries in nurses and carers, accounting for 70 per cent of the total. Back injuries account for 45 per cent of all musculoskeletal problems but the rest of the body is also vulnerable. Each year 60 million working days are lost because of back pain and NHS treatment for sufferers is estimated at a cost of £350 million.[2] The cost is considerable to the employers and to the victims who may never actually recover. Back pain is a major occupational hazard for nurses and other NHS patient handlers. However, informal carers who look after friends/relatives at home are also very much at risk of back injury since a high proportion will have had little or no training in handling techniques and may be poorly informed as to the availability of equipment.

The Manual Handling Operations Regulations 1992 (MHOR) came into force on 1 January 1993 under the Health and Safety at Work Act 1974. These regulations give a hierarchy of measures (Fig. 11.1) that employers should take in order to ensure that the risk of injury to employees from manual handling is reduced to the lowest level that is reasonably practicable.

Avoiding hazardous manual handling operations may be achieved by using mechanical lifting equipment such as hoists, trolleys, forklift trucks or by changing the system of work. The *assessments* should have an ergonomic overview and as such should have regard for the task, load, working environment and individual capability; and as a result of the assessments, *actions* are recommended to reduce the risk of injury.

The community within the context of health and social care is a workplace

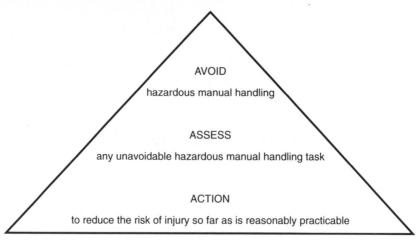

Fig. 11.1 The measures for manual handling

and as such the employer is required to do all that is reasonably practicable to make it safe. The overall responsibility for safety largely rests with management but the specific responsibility for each handling task lies with the individual practitioner or carer. It is essential that assessments are made to determine the most appropriate approach to the movement of loads and if at all possible these should be made prior to manual handling intervention. Relevant training is needed to provide a level of competence for all in order to decide the safest and most appropriate way to carry out the task, using assistance and equipment as necessary. The employee should conform to the systems set up as a result of the assessments.

What is manual handling?

The phrase is defined within the MHOR as 'any transporting or supporting of a load (including the lifting, putting down, pushing, pulling, carrying or moving thereof) by hand or by bodily force'. The MHOR states that the load is a discrete moveable object and includes any person or animal.

What does safer manual handling involve?

It is suggested within the MHOR guidance that training should be more than simply teaching techniques since such sessions make little difference to the numbers of injuries caused by handling. In order to make manual handling as safe as possible there needs to be consideration of the whole work system and where the risks might lie. By having an ergonomic approach to the moving and handling of loads, the ultimate aim is to 'fit the task to the man'.

The work system is made up of the *task*, the *working environment*, the *load* and the *individual*. Consideration of each of these areas in a handling situation can go a long way to reduce the risk to the handlers. It is obvious that even with a good technique, if the working environment is unsafe the handler could still be injured. A checklist of factors to consider when going into a handling situation is important and structures the thoughts of the handler. See the checklist example in Fig. 11.2.

If individuals are in a situation that offers a high risk of injury they should be assertive enough to refuse to undertake the task and to consult with management in order to examine how the risks might be minimised. Within the home the provision of hoists and other handling equipment can at times be traumatic for patients and carers because it may be seen as a way of losing independence and being identified as 'disabled'. However, the introduction of equipment, the need to move loose rugs or suggesting repositioning of furniture may be the only way of reducing risk and can take some considerable negotiation.

Many musculoskeletal problems are cumulative resulting from poor posture, excessive repetition of load-bearing movement and continually working in an unsafe environment, rather than being attributed to any single manual handling incident. Consequently, it is important to be aware of what the body is going through 24 hours a day and not only for the specific handling period.

Adequate, correct and specific moving and handling training should be complementary to eliminating and reducing manual handling hazards and subsequently reduce injuries if used alongside other methods of risk reduction, such as safe systems of work and a safe handling environment. However, in considering the individual capability it is true that to teach handling techniques as well as the ability to assess, is a further way to reduce the risk of injury.

Principles of safe load handling

It is not within the scope of this chapter to look at anatomy and biomechanical features of the spine and other potential areas of risk, but obviously some of the principles for safe handling are based on the acquisition of such knowledge.

There are general principles for the movement of all loads as well as other factors to be considered when these are applied to the safe handling of disabled people. The handling task will vary considerably, such as putting a wheelchair into the boot of the car; fitting a raised toilet seat; transferring the patient in/out of the car; aiding dressing; undertaking a bathing assessment; and so on. The following general principles apply to all situations.

The load

1. Never lift manually unless it is absolutely essential. Consider alternatives such as sliding, use of a trolley or hoist.

WORK SYSTEM AREA	ASSESSMENT CONSIDERATIONS	RISK REDUCING ACTIONS
Individual capabilities (all handlers)	Is the task within the handler's limits?	Handlers to know their limits
		Ensure help is available
	Are health problems going to compromise safety?	Health problems reported to manager
	Are the handler's clothing, footwear, jewellery appropriate?	Ensure roomy clothing, flat supportive footwear, minimal jewellery
	Does the handler have the skills required to perform the task safely?	Consider training needs
		Communication essential
Working environment	Is there adequate space?	Create access/space
	Is the area cluttered?	Clear the area for handling
	Is appropriate equipment available?	Know the equipment and how to use it
	Is the floor suitable?	Remove loose rugs, mop up spills
	Is the lifting/handling between hip height and shoulder height?	Change lifting heights
		Plan stages
	Is the noise level satisfactory?	Reduce the noise level
Task	The posture of the spine	Avoid twisting/bending
	The height/reach distance	Raise/lower work surfaces
	Frequency	Reorganise the task to allow more rests
	Distances carried/pushed	Consider equipment
Load	Is it too heavy, bulky?	Can the load be split?
	Is the shape awkward?	Can it be repacked or given handles?
	Is it unstable?	
	Does it have sharp edges?	Can you use equipment?
	Is it hot, cold, slippery?	Is the weight marked on it?
	Is it unpredictable?	Is the heaviest side shown?
The disabled person	The ability of the client to help and understand	Encourage the disabled person to help as much as possible
	Are they unpredictable?	Communication between handlers essential
	Their weight, shape	Get help/equipment if needed
	Their: medical condition	Reassure, communicate
	attitude	Ensure privacy but adjust hazardous clothing
	clothing	
	age, sex, cultural and religious background	Respect these and get appropriate help if needed

Fig. 11.2 Checklist for manual handling

2.   (a)   Assess the load – its weight and centre of gravity; whether or not it is slippery; difficult to grasp.

         (b)   Assess the patient – how much help is needed, does he understand, can he co-operate, what is his medical condition, and so on.

The environment

1.   Assess and prepare the handling area by moving obstacles and making more room to manoeuvre.
2.   Ensure that all equipment used is appropriate and near to hand.

The task

Assess and decide on the handling method to use, i.e. the task.

Individual capability

1.   The handler should be aware of their own limits.
2.   The handler's clothing should allow free movement and footwear must be suitable, i.e. flat shoes.
3.   The handler's posture is crucial in order to reduce the risk of injury.

         (a)   Place the feet apart, with one foot pointing in the direction of the move, the handler's weight balanced between them (Fig. 11.3).

unstable   stable

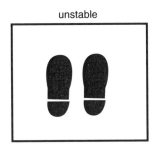
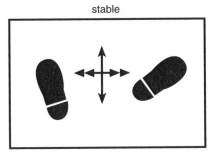

Fig. 11.3 Position of feet for lifting

         (b)   Knees and hips should do the bending, not the back (Fig. 11.4).

         (c)   Maintain the three natural curves so keeping the spine in the least stressful position (Fig. 11.5).

         (d)   Do not twist and bend the back (Fig. 11.6).

         (e)   Use the whole of the hand in a firm, comfortable grasp.

         (f)   Lead with the head to maintain good spinal posture.

         (g)   Keep elbows and abdominal muscles tucked in.

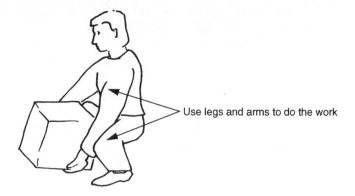

Fig. 11.4

(h)   Hold the load as close as possible in order to minimise the strain on the back.
4.   The load should always be moved towards the handler.
5.   Use rhythm, timing, a smooth movement and clear instructions.
6.   Communication with the patient and handlers is essential for safe practice.

All patient handling involves the facilitation of normal movement within the limitations of the individual and there needs to be allowance made for such incapacities as the reduction in joint range and acquired movements. There may also be a tendency for patients to forget how to move easily and efficiently, to which the handler acts as a reminder. Bearing in mind the basic principles it is possible to move all loads safely.

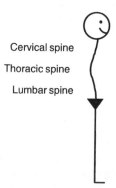

Fig. 11.5 Natural curves of the spine

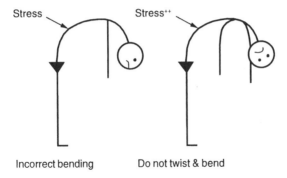

Stress

Stress++

Incorrect bending   Do not twist & bend

Fig. 11.6 Incorrect bending positions

Sitting to standing

It is considered to be bad practice to lever a patient from the chair or along the bed with the handler's arm hooked under the patients axilla (usually from the front) – the 'draglift'.[2] It is not only painful for them, but dangerous and inefficient for the staff who rely on this technique.

Helping the patient to the front of the chair

In order to help the patient to stand more easily the following steps should be taken.

1. Check the starting position. There is a need for the patient to be at the front of the seat, which can be done by encouraging him to hitch his bottom forwards.
2. The handler needs to place their hands on the patient's hips to encourage a rocking movement from one hip to the other in order to bring the patient forwards (Fig. 11.7a).
3. The patient then places his hands on the arms of the chair, brings his feet back to the chair base, slightly apart and with one foot slightly in front of the other, and then leans forward, 'nose over toes' to prepare for standing.
4. Continue to lean forward and push on hands and feet to stand up. If the patient needs some assistance it may be appropriate to stand at the side facing the same direction as him (Fig. 11.7b).
5. The outside foot of the handler should be forward with the nearside foot level with the centre of the seat just behind the patient's hips. The handler's nearside arm goes around the patient's waist, or just lower, and the outside hand is used to support the arm.

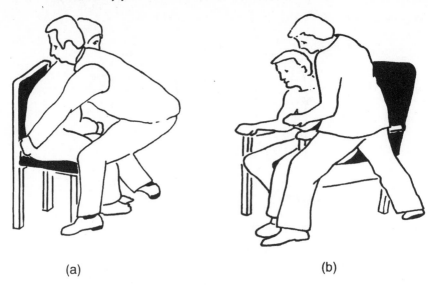

| (a) | (b) |

Fig. 11.7a and b Helping patient to rise from chair

6.   Both handler and patient lead with their heads and the movement can be helped by using momentum and rocking prior to standing.

Communication and timing is very important. This manoeuvre could be done with one or two handlers, depending on the patient's needs.

Standing to sitting

The recommended method is as follows.

1.   The patient walks up to the seat and turns round, feels for the surface of the chair with the back of the legs then, bending at the hips and knees, reaches for the arms of the chair.
2.   He lowers his body down and pushes his bottom to the back of the chair.

It is essential to move with the patient. If all the items of furniture involved in transfers are of compatible optimum height the task will be easier.

Car transfers

For wheelchair users the car needs to be far enough from the kerb so that the patient can place his feet on the road. When getting into the car the wheelchair should be placed on the road alongside the car, the patient is brought to the standing position in the chosen method and then encouraged to turn with his back to the seat of the car, sits down, hitches his bottom backwards, followed by his legs and feet. The use of a transfer board or turntable, depending on the

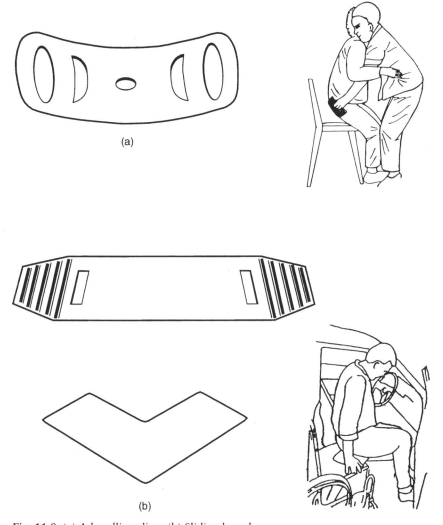

Fig. 11.8 (a) A handling sling. (b) Sliding boards

needs of the disabled person, could make the transfer easier. In all situations the handler should be aware of their spinal posture.

When getting out of the car, the legs are brought out first, then the bottom hitched forwards to make standing up easier. It may be easier to use a sliding sheet to help turn the patient in the seat and move to the edge more easily, so making it less effort for both patient and handler. Sitting to standing may be aided by a handling sling (Fig. 11.8a), but if the patient is unable to stand then a sliding board (Fig. 11.8b) may be necessary to transfer to a wheelchair. All these techniques require some training and practice and assessment of the situation. See Chapter 12 for further information.

If a walking aid is to be used it should be close to hand. Above all, encourage the patient to help and plan the manoeuvre beforehand. It is essential the handler is aware of the position of their back to maintain the natural curves to make the tasks less stressful to their spine.

Fallen/falling client

While supporting the patient the handler may find that she is taking too much of the patient's weight. In these situations it is often safer to lower the patient to the floor in a controlled manner by being at the side and slightly behind the patient, so that she can hold him securely and slide him down her body while at the same time ensuring she keeps her back in a reasonable position.

If, however, the handler is some distance from the patient, the best that can be done is to break the fall by getting behind the patient if time allows. It is a high risk situation to attempt to hold a patient up if he is falling.

Finding a patient on the floor is a potentially hazardous situation and assessment is crucial, giving consideration to the safety of both the patient and handler. First it is important to establish if the patient can be moved or needs medical attention. If in doubt make the patient comfortable and seek advice. Once the decision has been made to move the patient thought needs to be given to the task, the environment, the load and the abilities of the handler.

For the less dependent patient who is prone to falling, or greatly at risk of falling, then they may already have been taught how to get up from the floor with minimal help. This involves getting onto their knees and then to the half-kneeling position with one foot on the floor in preparation for pushing up onto an adjacent chair. Perhaps the use of a belt round the patient's waist will help the handler to grasp the patient and guide the movement. This should not put stress on the handler.

For the dependent patient, and when the lift is from the floor, the only safe method is by hoist. When working on one's own in the community, and no hoist is available, no attempt should be made to lift the patient but help must be sought. Any help summoned will depend upon the circumstances but there is a need to ensure they are capable of helping. In some situations calling in one of the emergency services for help is the only option and several districts have local agreements for this. The therapist should be conversant with any local arrangements for dealing with such situations.

With other activities that may involve handling such as going up/down the stairs, or helping the patient in/out of the bath, then all the principles should be applied. Equipment may be available to help with handling, such as sliding boards, sliding sheets, handling belts and slings or trolleys, and seeking advice from a manual handling adviser or appropriate personnel may be very valuable.

If the load is not a person the same principles apply; thus, when putting equipment into the boot of a car an assessment is made considering all the areas described earlier and then, by bracing the knees against the boot, the arms rather than the back can do the work. It is important to remember when putting a load into the boot to slide it into position. A blanket is very useful for this. Before taking it out of the boot, the object should be slid as close to the handler as possible.

Manual handling involves more than simply lifting. It is very important to take time and make the effort to do it in the safest way possible. Do not take the body for granted but assess the situation, consider the task, the load, the working environment and the individual's capability for safe practice. Always consider whether it is necessary to lift. If not, consider other possibilities, such as sliding the load. All handling tasks involve an element of risk and handlers should remember this and assess accordingly.

References

1. Health and Safety Executive, *Manual Handling Operations Regulations*, London: HMSO, 1992.
2. National Back Pain Association, *The Guide to the Handling of Patients*, 3rd edn, London: National Back Pain Association in conjunction with the Royal College of Nursing, 1992.

Further reading

Disabled Living Foundation, *Handling people (equipment, advice and information)*, London, Disabled Living Foundation, 1994.

Grandjean, E. *Fitting the Task to the Man*, London: Taylor and Francis, 1988.

Health and Safety Executive, *Manual Handling Operations Regulations*, London: HMSO, 1992.

Health and Safety Commission, *Guidance on the Manual Handling of Loads in the Health Services*, London: HMSO, 1992.

Hutchinson, M. and Rodgers, R. *Moving and Lifting for Carers*, Hemel Hempstead: Woodhead Faulkner, 1991.

Royal College of Nursing and National Back Pain Association, *A Guide to the Handling of Patients*, London: Royal College of Nursing, 1992.

Pheasant, S. and Stubbs, D. *Lifting and Handling: an ergonomic approach*, Middlesex: National Back Pain Association with Thorn EMI UK Rental, 1991.

Chapter 12

Out and about – solving problems of mobility

(i) General mobility

BARBARA RICHARDSON
Lecturer in Physiotherapy, School of Occupational Therapy and Physiotherapy, University of East Anglia

Central to client autonomy within the ethos of the new National Health and Community Care Act of 1993 and the concept of promoting independence within rehabilitation programmes is the development, maintenance and promotion of an optimal level of physical mobility. A perceived sense of independence is firmly based on the interrelationship between psychological, sociological and physical functions and the ability to be able to choose when and how to move to interact with the environment and with others. The goal of a 'seamless service' draws on the assumption that the client is not so much concerned with issues of multidisciplinary demarcation as in receiving a service that is both effective and efficient.[1] The therapist may take the role of facilitator or educator or use interdisciplinary teamwork to promote mobility of the client. The needs of the client may be best met by taking advice from a range of professionals in the health care team including occupational therapists, physiotherapists, dieticians and social workers. This may occur during assessment or in coming to a final consensus on the most appropriate programme of care for the client and the most appropriate person to carry it out.

What is mobility?

Mobility results from a change of position or movement in individual joints, limbs or body parts. The ability to move all or part of the body in order to achieve self-directed goals is fundamental to the concept of self as an independent entity. It provides a means of interacting with the environment and expressing feelings and is the basis from which we interact with others as equal human beings. Mobility requires some level of intact and co-ordinated function of the musculoskeletal, cardiovascular and nervous systems. Anatomy, physiology, psychology, biomechanics and sociocultural awareness are all involved with initiating and controlling movement. Effective mobility is that which achieves a purposeful endpoint.

The age at which pathology occurs is important. For example, the infant with neurological damage from cardiovascular accident, trauma will lack a background knowledge on which to base movement and learn skills of mobility which are fundamental to developing social and interpersonal skills. However, the adult with neurological damage has already experienced normal movement and may have retained a memory and drive for movement, although this may be complicated by the loss of ability to modulate muscle tone and the resulting excessively decreased or increased tone. In contrast, rehabilitation of a person with musculoskeletal injury, loss of a limb or degenerative arthritis may be hindered by individual psychosocial factors despite a physical potential for attaining a functional level of mobility.

Any mobility is better than none at all and for each individual the more time and vigour put into mobilising, the greater the improvements and benefits which will ensue. Studies have shown that regular episodes of brisk walking result in an increase in general wellbeing. Aerobic exercise, that is activity which increases the rate and depth of respiration, is associated with decreases in systolic and diastolic blood pressure, and maintaining mobility prevents the stiffening of joints and the atrophy of muscles.[2,3] Further, it is thought that short periods of skeletal stress may increase bone density. Although it has not yet been determined what the minimum daily requirement of skeletal stress may be, recent studies indicate that even a few seconds of grip exercise each day may stress the forearm sufficiently to stimulate a local gain in bone mineral content.[4] Mobility also promotes mental activity and helps to prevent withdrawal of interest in, and attention to, the environment. Mobility thus confers not only physical and physiological benefits but also psychological and social benefits on an individual and together these can promote physical and mental wellbeing.

General principles of mobility for people at home

It is important that the aim of mobility be towards some independent movement, at whatever level, for the client. Possible future changes in the ability of the client to move, whether engendered by physiological or psychological factors, should be kept in mind. Within a potential situation of increasing dependence there is a need to try to preserve some perception of independence for the client for as long as possible. Equal attention must also be paid to potential increasing demands on the carers both now and in the future. Social and family support in physical care is of key importance in caring for clients in their own home. Careful collaboration, sensitive assessment and good planning must be carried out to determine how much mobility can be encouraged and promoted in the client, and how much should be borne by the carers at any one time (Photo 12.1). While initially carers may need to be encouraged to hold back or give minimal help so that the client can

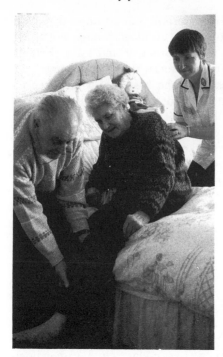

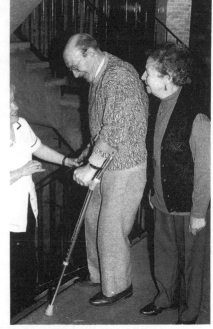

Photo. 12.1 Mr K finding a way to help his wife

Photo. 12.2 The goal to be achieved is discussed with a patient and his wife

Source: *The East Anglian Group of Chartered Physiotherapists with special interest in elderly people.*

persist in attempting an activity (Photo. 12.2), it should be understood that these very activities may be those that may demand more help as time goes by.

Aids to mobility

Much independent mobility can be preserved and promoted through taking an ergonomic approach and attempting to 'fit the task to the person', as Grandjean expressed it.[5] Using this approach, both the person and the environment are kept in focus. Optimal conditions for creating, encouraging and maintaining client mobility can be achieved by the selection and positioning of furniture and equipment; the general arrangement of the physical environment and through the attitude of carers. Design characteristics and position for use of the bed, chair and toilet are of particular importance in encouraging independent mobility.

The bed

It is easier to move around on a firm mattress and this may be afforded by simply inserting a plywood board between the mattress and the bedframe. It is important that the wood is wide enough to rest on the bedframe and to extend at least from the hips to the shoulders of the client in order to prevent mattress-sagging which can hinder mobility. Synthetic sheets can promote mobility from one side of the bed to the other, although it must be remembered that they may cause overheating. A rope attached to the bed end or a 'monkey pole' may assist independent movement up and down the bed for those with some strength in the upper limbs.

The bed height is critical. It should allow the client to reach the floor comfortably for easy transfers or if attempting to walk. The height of a divan bed which is approximately 550mm may be suitable for many clients.[6] However, for continual nursing the bed will need to be higher to suit the height of the carers, if it is to minimise the musculoskeletal stress of caring activities. Wooden blocks may therefore be needed to raise the bed or, on occasions, it may be necessary to shorten the bed legs.

The chair

Attention should be given to selection and use of dining and easy chairs. The aim should be to provide not only an appropriate height but seat dimensions and quality such as to provide firm support for the length of the thighs without cutting into the back of the knees, as well as support for the whole length of the spine. Lumbar support cushions are a matter of personal comfort related to spinal mobility and the normal posture of the individual and therefore are better provided separately to match individual needs. The covering fabric also needs careful selection, since plastic/PVC may be hot and sweaty, whereas silky material can encourage slipping.

Chairs should offer independent access and egress for the client and must be stabilised in some way, either by being braked or placed against a wall. It is essential that the client has a good view of their surroundings and can actively participate in their chosen activities. For example, there may be an opportunity to seat the hemiplegic patient in a way which encourages looking towards the direction of the weak side, so helping to reduce unilateral neglect. On the other hand, if it is obvious that unilateral neglect is irrevocably established it is punitive to sit him in such a position when he could enjoy many stimuli with his good eye.

The toilet

A wide range of toilet seats and frames is available to promote independent use of the toilet. The final choice is often determined by the dimensions of the toilet area and the ability of the disabled person. Standing and turning to use a toilet, or at least a commode chair, preserves mobility and provides stimuli to proprioception and balance mechanisms as well as a measure of personal independence and dignity. The client should be encouraged to persevere rather than to use a bedpan and initially it may be helpful to set aside areas in other rooms for this purpose if it is not possible to use the bathroom. Toilet/grab rails set in strategic positions may be essential to assist this independence, not only for access and egress, but also for support while adjusting clothes.

Soft furnishings

Rugs and soft furnishings must be appraised according to individual need. Mobile clients need floors which are free from small obstacles and hazards presented by rugs. Loved rugs could be hung on a wall or placed to one side of the room away from the walking thoroughfare. Soft furnishings can present a hazard to someone who needs to grasp the arms of chairs for extra help in getting up and sitting down. However, for others who must be lifted from one place to another, they may be a source of pleasure for their colour, texture or appearance.

Walking aids

Walking aids help to provide increased stability for those who have reduced balance, muscle weakness or loss of confidence. They widen the supporting base of the individual and thus keep the centre of gravity of the individual within it. Walking aids, including frames, crutches, sticks and quadrupeds, should not be introduced without weighing the benefits of increasing the stability of mobilisation against the costs of any loss of independence or limitations to walking. The client and carers need clear information on their purpose and whether it is expected that the walking aid will be required permanently or temporarily. It is often a matter of negotiation between the client and therapist over which walking aid is selected. Each has advantages and disadvantages according to individual need. Sticks are lighter and more easily used on stairs and steps, but they do not provide the stability of a walking frame. On the other hand, frames encourage a less than natural gait pattern; do not leave any hand free to open doors or hold a bag; and steps and stairs are difficult, if not impossible, to negotiate. To counteract this within a house, it may be necessary to have one walking frame for use upstairs and another downstairs.

Only crutches and walking frames, which allow the body weight to be taken entirely through the arms, can be considered to provide partial or non-weight-bearing mobility. The theory underpinning some recent approaches to rehabilitation of clients with neurological damage[7,8] makes use of quadruped frames a contentious issue. Sensible decisions on their use need to be made, taking into account the stage and type of disability, and the needs and wishes of the client. In these instances it may be appropriate to consult a physiotherapist or other expert in the field.

Assessment for the height of the handgrip of walking aids is achieved customarily by measuring from the proximal wrist crease (the level of the ulnar styloid) vertically to the floor when the client is standing and wearing appropriate footwear. This accommodates the few degrees of elbow flexion required to allow for arm extension during walking and avoids the shoulder girdle being stressed. Handgrips need to be comfortable and are best achieved by selection for shape or by repositioning the angle of the grip, rather than indulging in padding which can loosen quickly and become a hazard.

The walking pattern naturally adopted by the client using a walking aid is the one most likely to persist. Careful explanations are needed to persuade clients of the benefits of the wider base of support afforded through the use of the stick in the hand opposite the weak limb, or the more normal gait movement achieved through use of a four-point gait.[9] With older people an easy functional movement using minimal effort may be more acceptable than an awkward strenuous attempt at biomechanical perfection. It must be remembered that crutches and sticks will widen the base of support and stability only in the direction in which they are placed. Stability may therefore only be improved in a lateral direction unless clients are encouraged to keep the walking aids in front of them, particularly when pausing between taking steps (Fig. 12.1). Walking frames provide a wider base and some support to the body in front, but not behind, and consequently clients will become unstable if they lean backwards.

Walking involves moving body components in an orderly manner, requiring an ability to adapt to a variety of surfaces and space dimensions and an ability to perceive hazards. The whole sensory input is involved and a disorder of any part of the sensory system will affect gait. When issuing

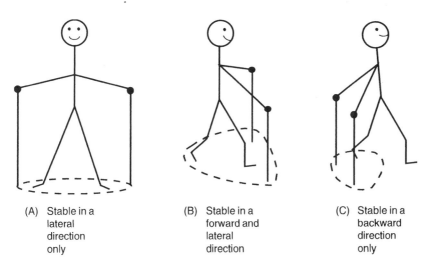

(A) Stable in a lateral direction only

(B) Stable in a forward and lateral direction

(C) Stable in a backward direction only

Fig. 12.1 Increasing stability through use of walking aids

walking aids the health care professional should satisfy themselves that the client, with the help of carers where necessary, can use the aid safely to get out of a chair; walk forwards and backwards; negotiate steps; turn around and sit down. If this is not the case then clear warnings must be given to the client (and carers) on the limitations of their use. Care of walking aids should be taught, e.g. rubber ferrules must be renewed at the first signs of smoothness and hence reduction in grip; screws, nuts and bolts on metal aids must be kept tight and clean.

Maintaining and improving mobility

While it may be necessary, on occasion, for the client to follow a programme of specific strengthening or mobilising exercises recommended by a physio-therapist, increasing general mobility is often a matter of providing encouraging opportunities which help to promote an increase in confidence. In negotiation with the client, the establishment of daily routines and patterns of activity which promote mobility play an important part in this.

Clients who are able to carry out self-care activities of daily living around the home and be independent in the garden may, with encouragement from

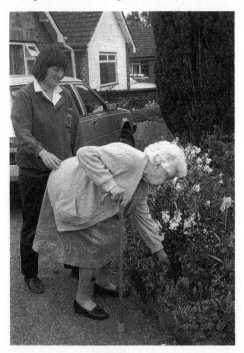

Photo. 12.3 Testing her ability to balance

Source: *The East Anglian Group of Chartered Physiotherapists with special interest in elderly people*

others and initial accompanied visits, be enabled to become confident to go to the shops or to make visits to friends, relatives or social groups. Clients who are unable to endure long periods of physical activity away from home may be encouraged to become more mobile between the house and the garden (Photo. 12.3). The ability to simply step outside the door and walk a few steps in the garden or sit on a chair the other side of the doorstep opens up realms of possibilities for communication with neighbours and passers-by, and for observing the passage of time by events such as people going to and from work and school or the milkmen, postmen or builders carrying out their jobs.

For those whose mobility is confined to the home, all attempts need to be made to identify a range of possible areas in which to pass some time. This will allow choices to be made and habits to be set up which give some variety to life; for example, breakfast in the kitchen followed by moving to another room to watch activities in the street or to carry out a hobby, followed by taking a short rest in the bedroom after lunch, and then from another window to watching the sunset or the birds fly over in the afternoon. Despite the physical effort required, if this kind of movement pattern can be achieved it should be encouraged and all provision made to facilitate it. This is far more preferable physically, psychologically and emotionally than merely transferring from bed to one chair and back again each day.

The same principles can be applied to the person who is confined to one room. A number of positions affording a variety of views can be identified for passing the day and then a variety of seats provided to stimulate the postural and balance mechanisms of the nervous system. These might entail moving from bed to hard chair to a softer chair for a short period of time and back again. If it is possible for the client to stand for a short while each day this should be encouraged for the particular benefits it provides to the musculo-skeletal, cardiovascular and renal systems.

Similarly, the person confined to bed needs to be encouraged and shown how they might make full use of it during the day by moving from supine to alternate-side lying positions to sitting upright, or into different reclining positions to carry out various activities. The ability to sit unsupported for a few minutes on the edge of the bed should also be explored.

With some thought and ingenuity, any environment is capable of providing a range of experiences for all individuals. Needless to say, the attitudes of carers and relatives are crucial to any endeavour to maintain and promote mobility. A good understanding of the long-term benefits and hazards of certain lifestyles and patterns of behaviour will help them to appreciate the importance of their own role in reinforcing or discouraging client behaviours.

Mobility and sexual activity

The ability to express oneself through sexual activity is natural and a fundamental right and any discussion and plan to maintain physical mobility is not complete unless the sexual needs of the client have been considered. For many clients whose problems stem from stiff joints, weak muscles and loss of range of movement, suggestions of alternative positions or use of pillows for support may be all that is required.[10] Others may be better helped by being put in contact with a support group, such as Sexual Problems of the Disabled (SPOD).

Mobility and hobbies

Hobbies can provide an enjoyable means of maintaining and promoting mobility as well as fulfilling psychological and social needs of the client. The natural inclinations of the client should be followed, as often these encourage social interaction. An interest in gardening may be the vehicle to joining a local gardening group, or a love of cricket or football may be encouraged by a local supporter who will arrange visits to games held in the area. Swimming can be carried out at one's own speed and encourages general physical exercise and breathing exercises. Many local swimming pools hold regular sessions dedicated to a particular age range and some have special hoists to assist the disabled swimmer.

For those clients confined to their homes there may be opportunities to carry out handcrafts which can be donated to local charities and relationships may be built up around these. An increasing number of people confined to their homes like to take part in radio or TV shows via letter or telephone.

A variety of interactions with people, experience of a range of environments and good use of local facilities, the media and audio-visual aids should all be recognised and exploited as a means of providing stimulus to enjoy life and encourage mobility, whether of individual limbs or of the client's whole body. The goal of mobility may be achieved through utilising direct and indirect intervention; the philosophy of client-focused care challenges health professionals to adapt and modify traditional skills and approaches to care to that end.

References

1. Biggs, S. User participation and interprofessional collaboration in community care, *Journal of Interprofessional Care*, Vol. 7(2), pp. 151–9, 1993.
2. Astrand, P. Exercise physiology and its role in disease prevention and in rehabilitation, *Archives of Physical Medicine Rehabilitation*, Vol. 68, pp. 305–9, 1987.
3. Davison, R.C. and Grant, S. Is walking sufficient exercise for health? *Sports Medicine*, Vol. 16(6), pp. 369–73, 1993.
4. Beverley, M.C., Rider, T.A., Evans, M.J. and Smith, R. Local bone mineral response to brief exercise that stresses the skeleton, *British Medical Journal*, Vol. 299, pp. 233–5, 1989.
5. Grandjean, E. *Fitting the Task to the Man*, London: Taylor and Francis, 1988.

6. Pheasant, S. *Bodyspace – Anthropometry, Ergonomics and Design*, London: Taylor and Francis, 1986.

7. Ada, L. and Canning, C. *Key Issues in Neurological Physiotherapy*, Oxford: Butterworth-Heinemann, 1990.

8. Davies, P.M. *Steps to follow: A guide to the treatment of adult hemiplegia*, Berlin: Springer Verlag, 1985.

9. Hollis, M. Re-education of walking, in *Practical Exercise Therapy, 3rd edn* (ed. Hollis, M.), Oxford: Blackwell Scientific Publications, 1989.

10. Grieve, G. *Common Vertebral Joint Problems*, Edinburgh: Churchill Livingstone, 1981.

Further reading

Burns, R.B. *Essential Psychology for Students and Professionals in the Health and Social Services*, Lancaster: MTP Press Ltd, 1991.

Compton, A. and Ashwin, M. *Community Care for Health Professionals*, Oxford: Butterworth-Heinemann, 1992.

Galley, P.M. and Forster, A.L. *Human Movement – an Introduction Text for Physiotherapy, 2nd edn*, Edinburgh: Churchill Livingstone, 1987.

Golding, R. and Goldsmith, L. *The Caring Person's Guide to Handling the Severely Multiply Handicapped*, London: MacMillan Education, 1987.

(ii)   Wheelchairs – assessment and availability

Wheelchair and Seating Occupational Therapist, South West Thames Region with Roehampton Rehabilitation Unit

Though frequently classified as a mobility aid, a wheelchair is much more than a device to deliver a person from one place to another; for many it is an aid to independence. Good assessment and prescription, together with training in the use of the wheelchair, can enhance the life of the user and increase their mobility both inside and outside the home, whereas poor assessment can have an adverse effect on morale and restrict the activities of both the user and the family or carer.

There are more than 500 000 wheelchair users in the United Kingdom, the majority of whom are aged 65 years or over. Many of them are dependent on a carer who also may be elderly, while others, given the right equipment, can lead full, active and independent lives. Approximately 15 per cent of wheelchair users are children with varying degrees of disability. Wheelchair selection therefore must take into account their changing needs and general development and enable each individual to reach their full potential, whether at home or in the school environment.

Occupational therapists, with their training in assessment of functional skills in relation to environmental and social needs, have an important part to play in assessing and advising in wheelchair matters, providing they have a good understanding of the biomechanics of a wheelchair and the models currently available.

Recent years have seen an increase in the number of both wheelchairs and accessories but, in spite of this, a wheelchair is still a compromise and unlikely to satisfy all the needs of an individual.

Obtaining a wheelchair

A wheelchair may be acquired in one of three ways.

Temporary loan

1.   For use following an accident or operation resulting in short-term difficulty with walking.
2.   Social needs, e.g. holiday, wedding, day centre outing.
3.   Rehabilitation, during specific period of short-term rehabilitation. Prior to prescription of appropriate permanent wheelchair.

NHS wheelchair centres do not generally provide wheelchairs for short-term loan, although it is advisable to check with them. Other sources for loan include:

- joint medical loan stores;
- British Red Cross – local branch;
- wheelchair repair firm;
- commercial wheelchair supplier; and
- voluntary groups, e.g. Scope, Multiple Sclerosis Group.

Most loan services provide standard non-powered wheelchairs. A few may supply recliners or heavy duty and powered chairs. There will normally be a hire fee which can be any amount from £5–40 per week with delivery and collection extra. 'Shopmobility' is available in some areas. This is a local initiative which allows individuals to hire a wheelchair while shopping in their locality. A wide range of chairs is generally available and the attendant is trained to assess for choice and instruct the user.

Permanent loan

Anyone with a disability that results in making walking permanently difficult or impossible will be provided with a wheelchair through the NHS. This will be on permanent loan, free of charge. Prescription will be made following an assessment. The form this takes will vary depending on local guidelines and the user's requirements. Information about the NHS wheelchair service is given below.

Privately funded

In some cases people prefer to purchase their own wheelchair as this gives them a wider range of choice in both performance and appearance of the chair. Certain charities may be willing to help with funding. Those purchasing privately should be made aware of the additional costs of maintenance, repair and replacement of parts, particularly batteries, which they will need to meet from their own funds.

Placement, Assessment and Counselling Team

The Placing Assessing Counselling Team (PACT) is a government-funded organisation which provides funds for equipment including wheelchairs and pavement vehicles and in some cases alterations, to enable people with disabilities to return to work. Contact the local Job Centre for information (see Chapter 14).

The NHS wheelchair service

Wheelchairs are available, free of charge and on permanent loan, to anyone who has a mobility problem that permanently restricts or prevents walking. Most district health authorities have a wheelchair centre although in some areas two or three districts run a joint service. The level of service provided and the range of equipment available will vary as each district has its own guidelines. Some centres provide a full range of services while others refer those with complex postural or mobility needs to a regional or supra-district clinic for assessment by a specialist team. It is important that all occupational therapists are familiar with local procedures and policies before assessing any client for a wheelchair. The local district wheelchair service should be the first point of contact for any wheelchair query. Staffing levels and services available at each centre will reflect local need as well as budget level, but most centres will provide all or some of the following.

- Identified wheelchair therapist able to assess, prescribe, review, provide information and training in use of wheelchair equipment to all users of the service.
- Co-ordinator clerk or helper to support clinical staff; deal with clients' queries; arrange appointments; organise clinics and domiciliary visits; take responsibility for administrative duties including ordering and equipment information.
- Rehabilitation engineer to provide technical information relating to clients' needs, modifications, safety matters and new equipment. To oversee quality control of repairs, modification, reconditioning and other services undertaken by the contract repairer.

All referrals and requests for wheelchair assessment or equipment should be sent to the service which is local to the client's home address. If this is in another district, a letter or a telephone call to the appropriate centre will inform them of the involvement of a therapist and they can then provide details about local policies and requirements.

Types of wheelchairs

Wheelchairs can be broadly categorised as follows.

Non-powered wheelchairs

1. Transit. Attendant controlled.
2. Self-propelled:
    (a) standard;
    (b) specials, e.g. reclining, one-arm drive, heavy duty;

(c)   high performance, central folding or rigid frame;
(d)   sports wheelchairs.

Powered wheelchairs

1.   Indoor use only.
2.   Indoor and outdoor use.
3.   Clip-on pack to convert non-powered chair to powered chair.

It is also possible to convert a powered chair from user to attendant control by means of a special control or switch.

Special wheelchairs

These may be self-propelled or powered wheelchairs which have a specific function over and above mobility, such as tilt-in-space; elevating seat, stand-up wheelchairs.

Additional equipment

Pressure care cushions

Many wheelchair users may be at risk from pressure sores. A large number of pressure cushions are available either through the NHS or by private purchase to help prevent these. Full assessment of risk is essential before any prescription is made as much time and money can be wasted on inappropriate provision. The wheelchair therapist, district nurse or tissue viability adviser at the local hospital should be consulted as pressure care information is a multidisciplinary responsibility.

Accessories

A wide range of accessories is available, such as trays, harnesses, footrest extensions and head supports, which can be supplied from the wheelchair centre, to clip-on cupholders; rain covers; shopping bags; camera fittings and others which can be purchased privately.

Careful assessment is essential as supplying an inappropriate accessory can affect mobility and may not be required, e.g. provision of a tray will inhibit self-propulsion, restrict forward movement such as opening doors and prevent transfers, unless the user is able to remove and replace it independently. It may also be more beneficial for them to sit at a table with others and therefore the provision of desk arms would be a better option. On the other hand, desk arms could be contraindicated if full-length arms are required for independent transfers.

Any additions or alterations to a wheelchair can adversely affect another aspect of use, so careful thought must be given to all aspects. The wheelchair service therapist or rehabilitation engineer can offer advice.

Special seating

For those with postural problems and spinal deformities, special seating can be provided by the wheelchair service. Assessment for this seating is generally undertaken by a multidisciplinary team which includes a consultant, bio-engineer and specialist therapist. Depending on the complexity of the problem, the postural support provided can be divided as follows:

(a)   inserts;
(b)   modular seats; and
(c)   custom-made seat.

Further information about these can be obtained from the district wheelchair service.

Principles of assessment

All too often a negative attitude is adopted by both medical and lay people to the provision of a wheelchair, but good selection can improve quality of life. It is therefore important that the occupational therapist adopts a positive, realistic, yet sensitive approach when advising and assessing a client for the first time.

Experienced users quickly learn to identify their own needs and unless their condition has deteriorated, will require the occupational therapist only to keep them informed of new equipment or policy changes. District wheelchair centres provide their own criteria for prescribing. Some accept prescriptions from any qualified therapist and will only reassess if inadequate information is provided, whereas others have a list of 'accredited' therapists who have undergone local training and can prescribe to an agreed level. There is no national accreditation scheme but many districts run local awareness or wheelchair training courses. For community therapists with clients from other district health authorities, it may seem confusing to have different guidelines but it is essential to follow local procedures and to liaise closely with the wheelchair service therapist in order to ensure a good service for all clients.

Assessment for a wheelchair should not be treated in isolation but be part of an overall assessment for total rehabilitation needs. It is essential that occupational therapists, when assessing and prescribing for wheelchairs, are not only knowledgeable and well informed about disability and the range of equipment available, but should actively involve the user, family or carer when establishing priorities relevant to the choice of chair. Comprehensive assessment should address three main areas.

The user

Clinical and functional factors.

(a)   *Diagnosis and prognosis* to establish the anticipated course of the disability. This may be improving, static or progressive.

(b)   *Ability*. Range of movement, muscle power and tone, deformity of spine, trunk stability and sitting balance. Upper limb power. These factors will indicate the type of wheelchair required, e.g. self-propelling, transit, powered chair.

(c)   *Other medical factors* include poor circulation, pain, incontinence, sensory disturbance, visual limitations. These are relevant in choice of chair and accessories such as elevating leg rests, shaped joy sticks, practical covers for washing.

(d)   *Pressure care*. Time spent in the wheelchair may increase the risk of pressure sores. Ability to change position, method of transfer and general condition, will all influence the choice of a pressure cushion. This should preferably be selected at the time of wheelchair prescription as change in depth of the cushion will alter the height of the seat and other support surfaces.

(e)   *Attitude*. Motivation and individual expectations will affect attitude to using a wheelchair and the success of provision.

(f)   *Physical size and weight*. Most chairs have set seat sizes and a specified weight limit. An ill-fitting chair can create problems and discomfort for the user. Exceeding the weight limit will put the user at risk, particularly if being used up and down pavements, causing additional stress to the frame.

(g)   *Postural support*. People with postural problems may require additional support in their wheelchair, whereas for others minimal support will allow greater freedom to function.

Carer

Many carers are elderly or also have health problems. Assessing and actively addressing their needs, providing appropriate training in the use of a wheelchair together with clearly printed information, will improve the quality of life for both user and carer. The following will need to be considered during assessment.

(a)   State of health.
(b)   Ability.
(c)   Expectation.
(d)   Additional help and information required.

Environment and social factors

Where will the chair be used? The answer to this will influence choice of size and features such as type of castors, folding mechanism and many other details. Factors to be considered include:

(a)   width of doors;

(b)   turning spaces;
(c)   surfaces – smooth, gravel, thick carpets all affect performance and power required;
(d)   height for transfer and work surfaces; and
(e)   space for access, turning, transfer in specific situations, e.g. bathroom. Can furniture be rearranged? Is it acceptable to carry out major alterations?
(Remember, changes in a home environment may affect other members of a family or community.);
(f)   external access – ramps, steps;
(g)   social activities – day centre, sports club, shopping;
(h)   transport requirements.

Work, school and social requirements should also be considered, although if these conflict with home needs it may be preferable to provide separate equipment rather than compromise on one piece of equipment. Access in public places cannot always be altered to suit the individual but local councils need to be made aware of any environmental problems which may restrict a wheelchair user.

Technical requirements

A wheelchair is basically a seat on wheels and should fulfil the following criteria.

(a)   Provide comfort
                stability
                support, yet freedom for function
(b)   It should be easy to use
                easy to maintain
                durable
                cost effective
                attractive
                appropriate for the individual need
                conform to safety regulations
(c)   An additional requirement for mobility is ease of propulsion. This is affected by the weight of the user; the design of the chair; the size position and width of the wheels and castors; and types of tyres, e.g. pneumatic tyres provide a comfortable ride but solid tyres reduce energy for propulsion on smooth surfaces.

As can be seen, there will be many conflicting requirements and compromises will have to be made. Where this is the case, the user's preferences should be respected whenever possible.

Prescription

Following assessment, the relevant prescription form should be completed and sent to the wheelchair centre. Failure to complete all sections of the form can result in a delay in receiving the wheelchair. Once final selection has been agreed, all concerned should be aware of the model chosen and the reason for this choice. There will always be limitations, but some of these can be reduced or overcome by good training in handling the wheelchair.

Training in using a wheelchair

Unless alternative arrangements are made, the wheelchair will be delivered to the client's home by the contract repairer, who will explain the basic principles of opening and closing the wheelchair. A more detailed training, preferably in the home environment, should be carried out either by the occupational therapist, rehabilitation engineer or a trained helper. Many therapists do not have the necessary skills to instruct a new user with a high performance wheelchair, in which case an experienced user or mobility adviser from an appropriate voluntary organisation should be contacted. The Spinal Injuries Association and Association for Spina Bifida and Hydrocephalus (ASBAH) are two groups who provide information and practical advice. For school children, the Royal Society for Prevention of Accidents (ROSPA) have a proficiency scheme, which encourages children to get the best from their wheelchairs.

Maintenance and repairs

Each district has a contract with a repairer to repair and maintain NHS chairs, free of charge. They also recondition and store chairs for the district. The conditions of the contract vary in different districts, but in general the contract repairer collects and delivers chairs, demonstrates their use and gives information on handling and caring for it to new users. The free repair service covers all wheelchair users with an NHS chair within a district even if they are resident from elsewhere for a limited period of time. However, in the case of temporary residents, they should call on the local contract repairer for emergency problems only.

In order to obtain a speedy and efficient repair service users should, when requiring repair or maintenance, make direct contact with the repairer themselves. All users are issued with a reference number and model of wheelchair when the chair is issued. Users should be encouraged to keep these details to hand although they can be obtained from the local wheelchair centre should they be mislaid. Any details of the problem will also help the repairer to provide a speedy response.

Repairs to private wheelchairs may be carried out by the contract repairer but the full cost must be met by the user or owner of the wheelchair. A private agreement must be made, as this is not the responsibility of the NHS wheel-chair service.

Community occupational therapists can play a major part in helping users to get the best from their wheelchair by encouraging clients to keep their chair clean and in good working order. Regular checking of tyre pressures, tightening loose nuts and cleaning all parts will increase efficiency and performance and reduce the number of calls to the repairer. Occupational therapists should actively carry out minor maintenance, such as pumping up tyres, adjusting footrests and checking batteries while on a routine visit.

It should, however, be remembered that work affecting safety or stability of a chair should not be attempted by a therapist but reported immediately to the contract repairer.

Further reading

Cochrane, G.M. (ed.) *Wheelchairs, 7th edn, Equipment for Disabled People*, Oxford: The Disability Information Trust, 1993.

Green, E.M., Mulcahy, C.M. and Pountney, T.E. *Postural Management Theory and Practice*, Witton: Active Design Ltd, 1992.

Jay, P. *Getting the Best from your Wheelchair*, London: Radar, 1992.

Male, J. and Massie, B. *Choosing a Wheelchair*, London: The Royal Association for Disability and Rehabilitation (RADAR), 1990.

Mandlestam, M. *How to get Equipment for Disability, 3rd. edn*, London: Jessica Kingsley and Kogan Page for the Disabled Living Foundation, 1993.

Pope, P.M. A study of instability in relation to posture in a wheelchair, *Physiotherapy*, Vol. 71, pp. 124–9, 1985.

Tuttiett, S. *Wheelchair Cushions Summary Report, 2nd edn*, Department of Health Disability Equipment Assessment Programme, 1990.

Societies and useful addresses

National Posture & Mobility Group, Membership Secretary, Dr A. Turner-Smith, Senior Lecturer in Rehabilitation Engineering, Centre of Rehabilitation Engineering, Bowley Close, Farquahar Road, Crystal Palace, London SE19 1SS.

Special Interest Group in Orthotics and Prosthetics (including Wheelchairs) (SIGOP), College of Occupational Therapists, 6//8 Marshalsea Road, Southwark, London SE1 1HL.

Resources

Department of Health Wheelchair Training Resource Pack (1991), Includes range of tapes, slides, videos, booklets and bibliography. From local District Wheelchair Services.

Wheelchair Information Pack, Disabled Living Foundation, 380–384 Harrow Road, London W9 2HU.

(iii)   Car drivers, passengers and powered vehicle users

MORIGUE CORNWELL
Director, Banstead Mobility Centre, Surrey

In the first two sections of this chapter, indoor and short-range mobility have been considered but in order to complete the mobility chain and to enable a person to gain optimum independence, long-range mobility must also be included. Mobility in this area may be as a car driver, a passenger or, in some cases, as a powered vehicle user. Public transport may be a further option for some people but is beyond the scope of this publication.[1]

Almost everyone with a disability is either a driver or a passenger and many of the considerations are common to both, such as access, seating, egress and for some people, wheelchair loading. In addition, disabled drivers need to consider their ability and suitability for the driving task together with any control modifications which may be required. A few more disabled people may need to consider the various special vehicle options which would enable them to drive or be a passenger while seated in their wheelchair.

Vehicle choice, access and egress

The community therapist may be called upon to give information and advice concerning car choice to disabled people and their families. Most clients can be helped by talking through a list of options together with their various merits and disadvantages, while mobility centres can provide more detailed information (see Further resources). However, as in many cases, the outcome usually involves compromise. A useful publication is *Ins and Outs of Car Choice*.[2]

The two-door saloon or three-door hatchback

Each side door of these cars is wider than in four-door versions, thus allowing more leg room. However, in some parking situations there may be insufficient space to open the door fully, although this should not apply in designated

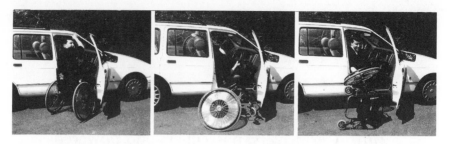

Photos 12.4a–c Paraplegic driver transfers and loads his own rigid framed wheelchair on the front passenger seat

disability spaces marked out in accordance with Part M of the Building Regulations. The second disadvantage is that a large door is heavier to open and close. Some full-time wheelchair users are able to load their own folding wheelchairs behind the front seats through the wider doors or a rigid framed wheelchair onto the passenger seat (Photo. 12.4a,b,c). It is worth noting that currently there is no two-door estate car available in the United Kingdom with level rear loading, which would be a first option for some disabled people.

The four-door saloon or five-door hatch and estate car

These cars give easier access to the back seats. The smaller doors are lighter to open and close and less space is required at the side of the car to open them fully. However, a narrower space between the door pillars makes entry and exit with stiff, awkward legs more difficult. It is almost impossible to load a folded wheelchair into the space behind the front seats unless the user can stand, and there is less space to lift a rigid framed wheelchair onto the front passenger seat.

Choosing between a saloon, hatchback or estate car

If a wheelchair user or carer is going to load a wheelchair into the rear loading space of the car, the height between the sill or floor of the car and the ground is relevant. While the flat floor of an estate is easiest, the angle of slope of the hatchback rear window will dictate whether the wheelchair can be loaded vertically. Often it necessitates the removal of the parcel shelf. A rear seat which splits may help the loading of larger wheelchairs. All wheelchairs should be secured because a loose one could be dangerous if the vehicle was involved in an accident.

An estate car is definitely an advantage when loading a powered scooter or wheelchair, as this offers the option of ramping which is cheaper than powered wheelchair winches (Photo. 12.5a, b). If the tailgate cannot be reached, a webbing strap may facilitate closure.

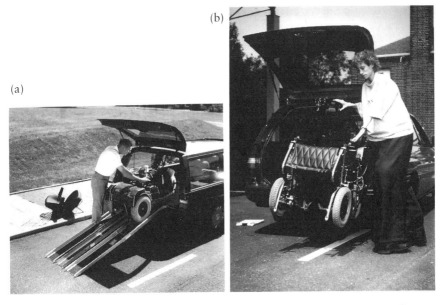

Photo. 12.5a Using 3 portable ramps to load a powered scooter. **5b** An electric winch to load a powered wheelchair

Features and aids to facilitate access of people and wheelchairs

Cars with adjustable seat height and low door sills are helpful. The removal of the door pocket gives more leg room. A window wound down will give the hand a suitable grab point to assist standing up and an extra 'ceiling' grab rail on the driver's door may help. Sliding boards, especially the shaped variety, may assist a wheelchair user over the gap between the car and the wheelchair seat. A plastic bag or purpose-made swivel cushion may facilitate the turn through 90° into the car, Special swivel and sliding/swivelling car seats are available but *these must always be tried first*. Leg lifters may ease a foot over the door sill or a polythene bag may provide a cheap, immediate alternative. A powered fore and aft seat slide can be useful if someone is unable to operate the manual seat slide mechanism.

One of the most useful inputs that a therapist can give is to assess the present and future needs and abilities of the carer/s. In some instances, careful tuition of lifting principles and techniques will suffice and prevent injuries (see Chapter 11). In other instances, more expensive wheelchair and passenger-lifting equipment is needed. This may mean referral to a mobility centre for assessment and practical demonstration.

Seating

Correct seating is vital to car drivers to provide adequate, safe vision, good ergonomic position to operate car controls and provide comfort and stability.

The last two points also apply to passengers. Some car seats are notoriously bad at providing suitable lumbar support and so additional support may have to be added. Many people require the seat raised to improve vision. One method of achieving this is to wedge the back of the seat up, tapering the raise to nothing at the front. This retains sufficient thigh space below the wheel; reduces the flexion required at the hip and knee and, combined with bringing the back of the seat forwards, provides a better upper limb position to ease steering for drivers with restricted shoulder and elbow movement and for those with reduced sitting height (Photo. 12.6).

Feet should be supported and, if necessary, a false floor inserted in the well of the car to achieve this. Lateral stability can be increased with arm supports or devices such as a webbing belt but these must always be in addition to, not instead of, the safety restraint (Photo. 12.7). Seat belts can almost always be modified to suit individual users. This is preferable to the option of a seat belt exemption.

Special vehicles for wheelchair passengers and drivers

In addition to the larger minibuses, which offer tail-lift access to passengers in wheelchairs, there are smaller vehicles for family use, usually modified small vans. Access may be via a rear or side tail-lift or it may be possible to use ramps, assisted by a powered winch on steep gradients.

Wheelchair drivers have a more restricted choice of vehicle because they need a level floor to access the driving position and sufficient headroom with adequate vision. Specialist help should always be sought from a mobility centre.

Accessible vehicles are used by full-time wheelchair users, especially powered ones which give the individual independent mobility once they reach

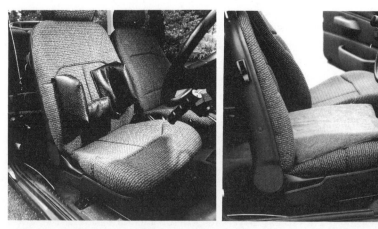

Photos. 12.6, 12.7 Seat wedge used to reduce hip flexion and/or increase visibility

their destination. The therapist involved in wheelchair prescription should consider additional items such as a higher back rest and head restraint, to provide support during the journey and a degree of protection should there be an impact. It is important that the wheelchair is secured to the vehicle structure by at least two clamps or preferably a four-point webbing tie-down. The user should be separately secured to the vehicle, preferably by a three-point lap and diagonal belt, as for other car users.

Car driving

Driver licensing regulations

Many drivers are unaware of the wording on their licence which states:

> You are required by law to inform DVLA, Swansea at once if you have any disability which is, or may become likely to affect your fitness as a driver, unless you do not expect it to last for more than three months.

Therapists treating patients or visiting clients who they know are driving should enquire as to whether they have notified DVLA of their disability. The groups who are most at risk of slipping through the information net are those with a gradual onset disability, such as rheumatoid arthritis and Multiple Sclerosis. Once they have written, they will be sent an enquiry form asking for details of their disability and permission to seek medical information from their doctor. On some occasions, DVLA may ask the driver to undergo an independent medical examination. Contrary to popular opinion, drivers are very rarely asked to take another driving test and licences are only revoked if they do not meet certain requirements, such as levels of vision and control of epilepsy. If the driver has a progressive condition, the licence expiry date may not be their 70th birthday. A 'restrictive licence' may be issued, renewal being at 1, 2 or 3-year intervals. If the driver requires control modifications, the wording may include 'Entitled to drive ... with controls adapted to suit disability'. The driver should also notify his insurance company of his disability.

A person in receipt of Higher Rate Mobility Component of Disability Living Allowance can apply for a provisional licence at 16 years of age.

Driver assessment

People with disabilities can be divided into two groups when driver assessment is considered.

1.   Those whose disability arises as a result of organic brain damage, whether congenital or acquired. This group includes people who have had a stroke or sustained head injuries and those born with cerebral palsy, spina bifida or hydrocephalus. They need to consider their fitness to drive as well as physical control requirements.

2.   People with physical limb disabilities, such as arthritis, spinal injuries or myopathies. They only require assessment of their car control requirements. Booklets are available for people who have had an amputation or a stroke and for professionals involved with people from these disability groups.[3-6]

All drivers require information and help with choice of car, access and seating, as described previously. This help is available from all members of the UK Forum of Mobility Centres (see Further resources). Precise assessment procedures vary according to the centre visited but for drivers with brain damage, consideration will be given to medical fitness to hold a licence; visual testing; psychological testing to include perception; speed of reaction; concentration; memory; and risk awareness. Physical ability will be assessed including overall mobility; use of wheelchair as appropriate; which limbs will operate the major controls (steering, accelerator and brake) and how secondary controls will be operated. While measurements of steering strength, brake pressure and reaction times will be taken in a static rig, the most important consideration is in-car assessment. This allows the safe operation of the car controls to be checked, as well as the residual driving ability in people with previous driving experience (Photo. 12.8).

Modifications

Many drivers with a disability require automatic transmission and benefit from factory-fitted power assisted steering. Approximately 80 per cent of the more severely disabled drivers only require simple modifications such as right hand 'single combined lever' to accelerate and brake, or a left foot accelerator (Photo. 12.9). This will, however, be an additional cost to the vehicle. One-handed drivers should use an infra-red device to operate the secondary functions such as horn, indicator, lights, washers and wipers. A small percentage (perhaps 2 per cent) of the most severely disabled drivers need high technology solutions such as very light power assisted steering; joystick steering; powered accelerator and brake and, in some cases, to drive from their wheelchair. As these are extremely expensive vehicles, with the total cost being as high as £30,000, these drivers definitely require specialist help. It is essential that the vehicle is chosen in conjunction with the modification company, who should check the fitting with the driver as the conversion progresses.

Tuition

Careful tuition with an experienced driving instructor, who must be Department of Transport Approved, is essential. A National Disability Tuition Register of approved driving instructors is available from Banstead Mobility Centre (see Further resources). Severely disabled drivers with high technology

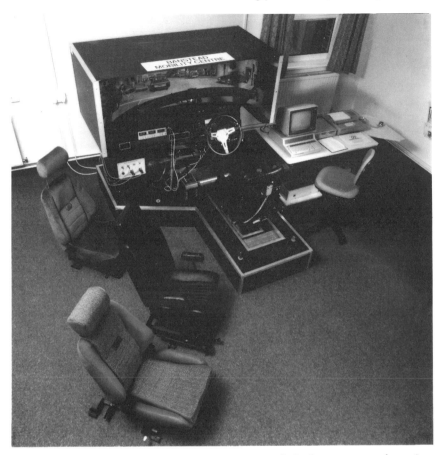

Photo. 12.8 Static rig used to measure steering strength, brake pressure and reaction times

controls are likely to take tuition on their own tailor-made vehicle, but other drivers who only require items such as power-assisted steering, automatic transmission, hand controls or a left foot accelerator may be lucky and find a local driving school car. The British School of Motoring (BSM) have recently equipped 150 school cars for disabled pupils. It is important that lessons are frequent (at least one a week) and uninterrupted. It is worth noting that the national average is said to be one-and-a-half hours of tuition for each year of your life.

Funding

For many disabled people, whether drivers or passengers, funding is the biggest problem. Those who are unable, or virtually unable, to walk are eligible to receive the Higher Rate Mobility Component of Disability Living

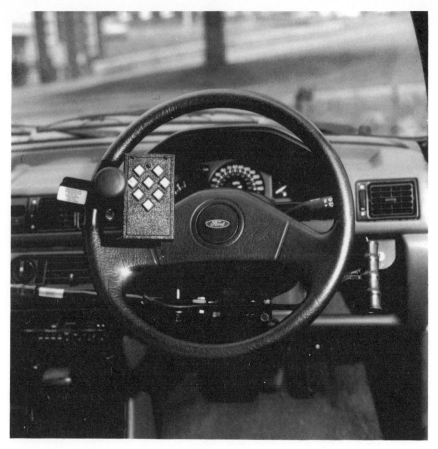

Photo. 12.9 Right hand single combined lever to accelerate and brake. Infra-red secondary controls and steering aid for left hand steering. (The bar on the left is an extension bar to allow the driving instructor to brake in an emergency.)

Allowance (Mobility Allowance). They are exempted from paying Vehicle Excise Duty. These people can apply to Motability, an independent charity, set up to enable 'Mobility Allowance' recipients to convert their allowance into a vehicle. The most favoured scheme is a contract hire scheme which provides a car, insurance and maintenance in return for the 'Mobility Allowance'. Smaller, manual transmission cars do not require additional money but larger cars do need an initial sum of money which is non-returnable. People who are unable to afford this or the cost of conversions or tuition can apply to the Grants section of Motability for financial help. There are two additional funds who may be able to help – the Mobility Equipment Fund, set up to help the more severely disabled people, and a Drivers' Fund to assist those who need to use a wheelchair accessible vehicle and drive from their wheelchair seat.

Insurance can be expensive although, in theory, premiums should not be loaded because the driver has a disability. There are specialist brokers who are keen to assist and information on this and many other aspects can be found in *Motoring and Mobility for Disabled People*.[7]

Parking

Anyone who is entitled to the Higher Rate Mobility Component of Disability Living Allowance, or those who would be if they had not been over the age of 65 years at the onset of disability, are eligible to apply to their local Social Services Department for an *Orange Badge*. This allows certain privileges and concessions, including free parking in meter bays and some car parks, entitlement to use designated parking bays and free use of certain toll roads. The Orange Badge is recognised almost nationwide although sadly, there are a few places which have designed their own parking schemes.[8]

Breakdown and recovery

The AA, RAC Response and National Breakdown Recovery Service all offer special schemes for the disabled motorist. There are pennants and illuminated signs to alert people that they have broken down. Details are available in *Motoring and Mobility*.[7]

Powered vehicles

In the 1988 No. 2268 Statutory Instrument – *The Use of Invalid Carriages on Highways Regulations*,[9] vehicles were divided into:

> *Class I:* An invalid carriage which is not mechanically propelled.
> *Class 2:* Mechanically propelled invalid carriage incapable of exceeding 4 mph.
> *Class 3:* Mechanically propelled invalid carriage capable of exceeding 4 mph but incapable of exceeding 8 mph.

Class 1 has been covered in the previous section.

Class 2 vehicles

These can be divided into indoor/outdoor; outdoor/indoor and outdoor electric wheelchairs; three- and four-wheeled scooters and a few four-wheeled buggies.

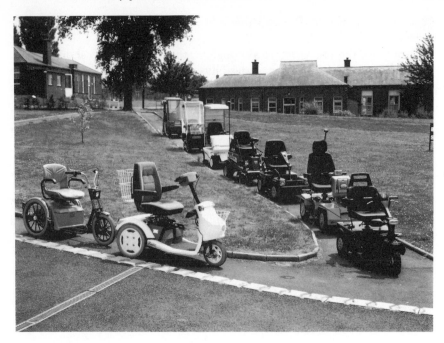

Photo. 12.10 A range of Class 3 vehicles

Class 3 vehicles

These can be divided into outdoor wheelchairs, scooters (usually four-wheeled) and buggies (Photo. 12.10). Although users do not require a driving licence nor is insurance obligatory, it is very highly recommended and members of the British Association of Wheelchair Distributors will not sell a Class 3 vehicle without insurance.

Assessment for powered vehicles

In many ways assessment for these vehicles is similar to assessing someone for any other wheelchair but there is a different emphasis on the importance of the topics considered. These vehicles are used on pavements and sometimes on the road and, therefore, safety of the user and other members of the public must come first. Minimum visual recommendations should be considered as indicated in *Which One Should They Buy? A Powered Vehicle Prescription Guide for Therapists.*[10] Balance will be extremely important because the vehicle may be used on uneven terrain and to mount and descend kerbs. Pain and fatigue may be exacerbated because of the terrain and the length of the journey. Joint restrictions in the neck and trunk may make manoeuvring in busy or restricted areas more hazardous. Everyone *must* try a selection of vehicles extensively before committing themselves to a purchase, for it can be an expensive mistake.

Training

ROSPA run a training scheme for Class 2 and 3 vehicle users and details are available in *Adviser Care for Class 3 Invalid Carriages*.[11] Users need to have a thorough knowledge of the Highway Code and road behaviour.

Linking powered vehicles in the mobility chain

Some powered vehicles, especially the Class 2 vehicles, are carried in the backs of appropriate cars but another growing facility is 'Shopmobility'. These schemes offer the loan of powered and non-powered wheelchairs and scooters to shoppers. Many of the users are elderly people who have reduced walking ability as part of the ageing process. This increased usage is helping to heighten public awareness and to reduce the stigma of using a mobility product.

References

1. Department of Transport, *Door to Door. A guide to Transport for People with Disabilities*, London: Department of Transport, HMSO, 1992.
2. Department of Transport, *Ins and Outs of Car Choice, A Guide for Elderly and Disabled People*, London Department of Transport, 1985 (available from MA-VIS, address below).
3. *How to Get Behind the Wheel, Information for Amputees Wishing to Drive a Car*, compiled by the UK Forum of Mobility Centres, 2nd edn, April 1992 (available from Forum members).
4. *Driving after Amputation, Information for Professionals*, compiled by the UK Forum of Mobility Centres, January, 1991 (available from Forum members).
5. The Stroke Association, *Driving After a Stroke. How to get back behind the wheel if you have had a stroke or transient ischaemic attack*, the Stroke Association in co-operation with UK Forum (available from CHSA House, Whitecross Street, London, EC1Y 8JJ).
6. The Stroke Association, *Driving after a Stroke or Transient Ischaemic Attack, a leaflet for general practitioners and other medical professionals*, the Stroke Association in co-operation with UK Forum (available from CHSA House, Whitecross Street, London, EC1Y 8JJ).
7. Darnborough, A. and Kinrade, D. *Motoring and Mobility for Disabled People*, London: Radar, 1991.
8. The Orange Badge Scheme, Department of Transport, T/INF/222, London: HMSO, 1991.
9. 1988 Statutory Instrument No. 2268, *The Use of Invalid Carriages on Highways*, London: HMSO, 1988.

10. *Which One Should They Buy? A Powered Vehicle Prescription Guide for Therapists*, Medical Devices Directorate Report No. MDD/M93/01, London: Department of Health Store (free to NHS and Social Services).
11. *Adviser Care for Class 3 Invalid Carriages. A Code of Practice for those advising the users of 4mph/8mph Vehicles*, Department of Transport (available from MAVIS, address below).

Further resources

Banstead Mobility Centre, Damson Way, Orchard Hill, Queen Mary's Avenue, Carshalton, Surrey SM5 4NR.

Mobility Advice and Vehicle Information Service (MAVIS), Department of Transport, TRL, Crowthorne, Berks RG11 6AU.

UK Forum of Mobility Centres: a full list is available from Banstead or MAVIS.

BSM, Mobility Advice Unit, 81/87 Hartfield Road, London SW19 3TJ.

Department of Transport Mobility Unit, Room S10/21., 2 Marsham Street, London SW1P 3EB.

Motability, Gate House, West Gate, Harlow, Essex CM20 1HR.

National Federation of Shopmobility, c/o Helmsdale, 80 Hilton Street, Aberdeen AB2 3QS.

National Disability Tuition Register is available from Banstead Mobility Centre (address above).

Chapter 13

Home assessment and housing adaptations

VALERIE DUDMAN
Senior Occupational Therapist and Care Manager Physical Disability Team, Oxfordshire Social Services Department

The ability to live as normal a life as possible within the home environment is the right of every disabled person. This philosophy is supported by the White Paper *Caring for People*.[1] Suitable housing is an important part of community care and, wherever possible, elderly and disabled people should be enabled to remain in their own homes. Population censuses and surveys in England have identified more than four million people of all ages as having one or more physical disability or sensory impairment, ranging from slight to severe of whom more than one million are aged between 16–64 years; more than 400 000 of these having a severe or very severe disability.[2]

The Health of the Nation[3] identified poor housing and environmental amenities as some of the main causes of ill health, along with low income and unhealthy behaviour. The aim of the government's housing policy is to 'put decent housing within reach of all people'. This supports the World Health Organisation's[4] 'Health for All 2000' Target No. 24, which states: 'By the year 2000, all people of the region should have a better opportunity of living in houses and settlements which provide a healthy and safe environment'. Between 1985–8 around one-and-a-half million disabled people in Great Britain had some form of home adaptation.[5]

A disabled person is not by definition a handicapped person, but this may follow if they are unable to function independently within the confines of their own home or the environment in which they live. Poor housing can result in increased family stress or incidence of illness such as asthma or other chest complaints, while inappropriate housing for the physically disabled person can cause accidents. Elderly and disabled people are all likely to spend a greater proportion of their time within the home compared to fitter people of a similar age, and will need to spend a larger amount of their limited income on keeping warm.

Familiar surroundings, family and possible employment prospects are all important factors which may encourage both client and the statutory local services to consider adaptation of their present home as the most viable solution, rather than considering alternative housing. It may be possible to achieve independence by the provision of small items of equipment, such as grab rails; however, for some it may be necessary to consider adapting, altering or even extending the existing dwelling. Many ambulant disabled people are able to use standard facilities even with minimal adaptation, whereas everyday activities may appear insurmountable to one who is confined to an unsuitable house with steps, stairs and inaccessible facilities. For those who are wheelchair-dependent special considerations will need to be made, including the option of moving to a purpose-built dwelling in order to become totally independent.

Layout and general design within the home is an important factor in determining the degree of handicap associated with a disabled person. The decision to adapt the home should be taken only after consideration of the total physical problems; the nature and prognosis of the medical condition; the client's view of his disability; level of handicap; and the family situation.

This chapter is mainly concerned with structural work to the dwelling in order to facilitate independence. Major alterations may include building work or the provision of fixed items such as stair-lifts and through-floor lifts. In some cases the existing structure of the house need not be altered at all, merely added to or altered internally while maintaining external proportions. Utilising existing space or changing the use of rooms may well be a more acceptable solution than extending the fabric of the home.

Legislation

It is essential that occupational therapists working in the community should have a clear understanding of the relevant, current legislation relating to the provision of services for disabled in their area. Although housing adaptations are mentioned in numerous acts and circulars, the provision for adaptation comes under the broad responsibilities outlined in the Chronically Sick and Disabled Person's Act 1970 (CSDPA),[6] Disabled Person's Act 1986 and 1989[7] and the Local Government and Housing Acts 1985, 89, 92 (England, Wales and Northern Ireland) and Housing (Scotland) Act 1987.[8] It should be noted that the method of execution of these responsibilities may vary in different areas of the country. Occupational therapists should ensure that they keep abreast of all new legislation, its implications for their work, and local interpretations. For further information see Appendix I.

Identifying the housing needs of the disabled person and his family

In most cases these people requesting adaptations who apply directly to either their local housing department or Social Services (social work department in

Scotland) will be referred to the community occupational therapist, who acts as an adviser not only to the disabled person but also the statutory authorities.

It is important that the needs of the disabled person are recognised early, whether this is by the individual himself, his family, carers, members of the primary health care team or others. There is a fine balance between becoming dependent or achieving and maintaining independence.

During assessment the occupational therapist may be aware that the disabled person or their family have ideas on how they see the solution to the problem. However, this may sometimes be based on a lack of knowledge and understanding of the disabled person's abilities, or as a result of poor or misinformation. Therefore, an objective assessment is essential.[9] This requires the full co-operation of all parties involved so that the solution that best meets the needs of the client is found. It is also important for the occupational therapist to identify the framework of the assessment clearly and work in partnership with the client, their family and carers in enabling them to identify the issues and make informed decisions.

The following points should be considered when identifying the problem. *What is the need*:

1.   as expressed by the client related to his perception of his disability and role within the family?
2.   as identified by family or carers involved with the client?
3.   as the objective view of the occupational therapist related to medical knowledge, prognosis and nature of the disability?

The assessment may identify that there are activities which the disabled person values more than others; for example, being independent in showering may be considered more important than cooking a meal. Also, there may be many different options to resolving the identified needs and an adaptation may not be the answer: for example, a different method of climbing stairs may negate the need for a stair-lift, or a mobility problem is resolved by waiting for further recovery or by advising a treatment regime. Conflicts can arise when the client's perceptions and ideas are questioned, such as the client who may request a ground floor extension because of difficulty managing the stairs, while the occupational therapist may identify that a stair-lift would be a more cost-effective solution, at the same time still meeting the client's needs of easy access to the toilet and bedroom. It is part of the occupational therapist's skill and responsibility to identify to the client all the possible options, discuss their suitability and help the client and their family to consider the alternatives to enable them to make an informed decision. Reference to the following points need to be made in these discussions.

(a)   Does it meet all the perceived and actual needs (functional, emotional and cultural) and what affect would it have on the client and carers?

(b)   Is it feasible, taking into account the length of time from inception to completion and costs?

(c)   Will it continue to be suitable in the future?

Conflict of ideas may well occur but must be resolved and agreement made by all parties otherwise dissatisfaction and non-use of the adaptations may result. While some options may be eligible for financial assistance, others may not and this may affect the client's choice and final decision. Assistance given is dependent on departmental policies and criteria, which vary considerably countrywide.

Adapting present accommodation

It is often possible to improve the use of existing living areas in the home or create more space for the disabled person by very simple measures, such as partitioning larger rooms, moving doorways or changing the use of a room. Other common home adaptations are:

- additional grab rails;
- temporary or permanent ramps or step-lifts;
- automatic garage doors;
- storage for wheelchairs;
- special doors and windows;
- door-answering intercom and emergency call facilities or warning system;
- special kitchen units and lever taps;
- special baths and shower units;
- special toilets;
- hoists, stair lifts and through-floor lifts;
- ground floor extensions to provide bathroom and/or bedroom.

Lifts. In some instances a lift will be the solution to the problem of access to existing facilities, e.g. bathroom or bedroom. There are two main types of lift – stair-lift and through-floor lift.

Stair lifts are fixed to the stair treads and there are many different manufacturers and models. The track can be straight, curved or even spiral. The seat on which the disabled person can sit or perch can be fixed or swivel, facing either forward or sideways; or there is a platform on which they can stand and can be large enough to accommodate a wheelchair. The usual weight limit of these is 20 stone but some manufacturers have heavy duty models, or will look at methods of adapting these to suit the individual if at all practical, although there will be a cost implication to this.

Stair lifts are not suitable for very narrow stairways. Room is needed at both the top and the bottom of the stairs and consideration of headroom must be made for standing models. It is possible to use a straight lift on a curved flight by using a dropped manual or motorised platform that bridges across the landing. This is dependent on the client's abilities and safety in transfers.

Through-floor lifts go up through the ceiling from one room to another and when on the ground floor the top of the lift forms the floor of the room above. There are some types suitable for the wheelchair user, and others simply for people to stand or use a seat. Space is needed on both floors and the track must be fixed to a load-bearing wall, preferably an outside one, as this reduces the noise disturbance to neighbours.

All the lifts are fitted with key switches to enable them to be turned off to prevent children playing with them. Lifts also have microsensitive pads on the base of the through-floor lift and the foot plate of the stair lift, which will trigger a safety mechanism the moment it touches or lands on an object. It is important to ensure that any lift installed complies with the current safety standards set by the British Standards Institute.

Extensions to the property. Where there is insufficient space within the dwelling to adapt the property an extension may be the only alternative. Most extensions are built either to the back or side of the house owing to building line regulations. Factors which will affect this are the position of existing drains, soil pipes, manholes or boundary walls. An extension to the side of a semi-detached house may reduce access to the back garden, driveway or garage, whereas if built onto the back of a terraced house there may be the loss of existing windows, which will therefore mean additional lighting being required.

Rehousing

Some disabled people living in the private sector on low income, with low-valued houses or negative equity will find that moving to a more suitable property may not be a viable proposition. This may be because the type of accommodation required may not be readily available within their financial resources, the cost of moving prohibitive or a suitable dwelling is not available in the area. Even the opportunity to move into purpose-built council or Housing Association property is not always possible because of insufficient resources and high demand. However, those living in the public sector do appear to have more opportunities for moving to more suitable accommodation than those in the private sector. Many housing departments give high priority to tenants who need to transfer because of medical reasons and require partially adapted or purpose-built dwellings.[10] Most new projects now include a few homes suitable for disabled people.

Financial help available for adaptations

The Home Improvement Grants (Housing Act 1985) has been replaced. Since 1990 the major source of financial help now available is through Disabled Facilities Grants (England, Wales and Northern Ireland) administered by local environmental health departments of boroughs or districts.[11] A maximum expense limit of £20,000 for eligible work was introduced in January 1994.

These grants, available to disabled people for adaptations which improve access to essential facilities in the home, require support from the local authority (Social Services) as being 'necessary and appropriate'. They apply to both private and public sectors, and although financed differently are mandatory or discretionary.

A mandatory Disabled Facilities Grant cannot be given unless it is for enabling or improving the disabled person's access. For example:

- entry to and from the property; to rooms used to sleep in or the main family room;
- provision or use of basic facilities such as a toilet, bath, shower or wash-hand basin;
- enabling the preparation and cooking of food;
- improving or providing a suitable heating system so that the disabled occupant can control power, light or heat; and
- to enable a disabled person to look after someone in their care.

Discretionary Disabled Facilities Grants cannot be given unless it is to make a dwelling or building suitable for the disabled person's welfare, accommodation or employment. For example:

- a safe play area for a disabled child; or
- adapting or providing a room which might be used as a workplace by someone housebound but still able to work from home.

The property should be in reasonable repair to obtain a grant but, if it is not, help may be available to assist via a Renovation Grant. Other works may be eligible, but grants for these may be offered at the discretion of the housing authority.

The Environmental Health Officer (EHO) will carry out a financial test of resources (means test) which is similar to the housing benefit resource test. This is to determine the applicant's ability to contribute (notional loan) towards the cost of the proposed work. The amount assessed is based on their income and savings and ability to take out a loan, such as a second mortgage. This amount is then deducted from the cost of the work and a grant is given to cover the remaining cost, if any. In the case of owner-occupiers, the applicant is tested; where there are couples (married or not), the test covers both of their incomes and savings. Joint owners or tenants living in a property are tested individually, whether or not they all applied for the grant. For Disabled

Facilities Grants, the disabled person is also tested, whether or not a applicant. If the client feels that by taking out a loan it would cause financial hardship they can apply to their local Social Services department, which in certain circumstances may offer help (see Fig 13.1 and section on 'Topping up').

Minor Works Assistance (England, Wales and Northern Ireland)

'Staying Put' and 'Elderly Resident' discretionary grants are available to people over the age of 60 years. Assistance is only available to owner-occupiers and private sector (including Housing Association) tenants on income-related benefit. They are aimed at enabling an elderly person to remain in their own home in greater comfort or to make it more suitable for them. The therapist needs to be conversant with current arrangements, as the grant system is continually revised.[12]

Improvement Grants (Scotland)

These are available to disabled people both in the private and public sectors. They are mandatory or discretionary, dependent on the assessed purpose of the adaptation.

District Council

Housing authorities can adapt their own housing as part of 'duties' to their own stock, free of charge to tenants. This is usually decided by the housing liaison officer and needs support from an occupational therapist or other authorised person. Many councils have specific budgets (CSDP) to do this work which is usually for minor adaptations and with set limits. Alternatively, for some work the district council or housing authority will expect tenants to apply for a Disabled Facilities Grant. This can vary countrywide, and even neighbouring authorities can be considerably different. For example, in Oxfordshire one district council has a £50 limit for minor works, while another has a £1,500 limit. Some housing authorities will make up the difference between the grant awarded and the total cost of the works by paying the client's assessed contribution, or may undertake to fund the work completely.

Housing Associations

Tenants can also apply for grant assistance, or the association can apply on their tenant's behalf. In some circumstances the Housing Association may fund the work themselves but will ask for recommendations from the therapist.

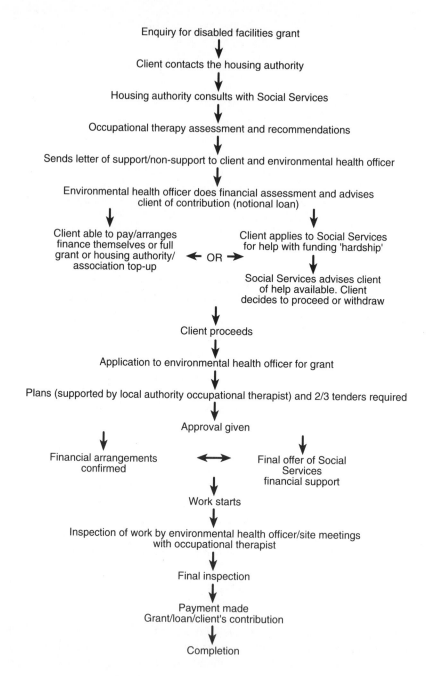

Fig. 13.1 Flow chart of a grant enquiry

Privately rented property

Tenants can also apply for grant assistance after gaining agreement from their landlord, or the landlord can apply on their behalf. Social Services may help towards the cost.

Valued Added Tax. VAT is chargeable on all building work. However, the VAT (Handicapped Persons) Order exempts specific items such as ramps, widening of doorways and the installation of a WC and bathroom on the ground floor. This only applies to first time installations and not to existing facilities.

Stair lifts and through-floor lifts. These are often provided in a variety of ways depending on local policies.[13] Some Social Services departments may provide lifts in 'emergency' situations for clients whose prognosis is poor, e.g. motor neurone disease or terminal cancer, to eliminate the stress of making a grant application. In other areas, Social Services departments offer help with servicing and maintenance to clients who have purchased these privately with the assistance of a disabled facilities, improvement or minor works grant. In return they may claim ownership of the lift when no longer required. Occasionally a housing authority may choose to install a lift on the client's behalf as an alternative to rehousing.

'Topping up'. In certain circumstances financial help may be available from Social Services or the housing authority to those who have been assessed within a grant process to pay towards the cost of any work identified.[14] This involves meeting some or all of the difference in cost of the work and the amount of grant and may be given as a grant or repayable loan. It is usually dependent on a financial assessment.

Charitable funding. This may be considered as an alternative method of paying a percentage of the costs not covered by grant aid. However, the sums of money available from this source are usually nominal and consequently it is difficult to raise large amounts from charities.

Designing for the disabled

Many books give general standard measurements; however, it cannot be emphasised too strongly that each person has individual needs and the effect that illness or handicap will have is determined by their abilities, motivation and the environment in which they live. Any structural alteration must therefore be tailored to meet the individual's requirements based on an accurate assessment.

Anthropometric drawings

Using anthropometric measurements will enable the therapist to determine the design needs of the client (see Fig. 13.2a, b). For example, they are particularly useful when planning the layout of kitchen facilities, especially in relation to positioning of shelves and depths of cupboards.

Scaled plans

An architect will produce drawings of the proposed adaptations using the scales of 1:20, 1:50 and 1:100. In order to check that these plans are correct a proper scale rule must be used, so that door widths, sizes of rooms and turning spaces are verified. The position of facilities can be determined by positioning scale models of wheelchairs, baths, WCs and showers on the drawings until the most appropriate design is found. This is a more effective method of identifying design options than producing numerous scaled plans (see Fig. 13.3a, b).

Checklists

Checklists are helpful when undertaking complex adaptations to ensure that nothing has been forgotten, and the therapist should go through this with the architect to determine the specific measurements and equipment necessary and record agreed details. The checklist might include any of the following:

> Access requirements (carport, ramps, rails or shallow steps).
> Kitchen layout (safety and ease of use).
> Bedroom layout (room for transfers).
> Bathroom layout (wash basin, bath/shower, toilet position and heights).
> Floor finishes (non-slip).
> Doors and door furniture (sliding, bi-fold, hinged and lever handles).
> Windows (safety glass, security/operation).
> Refuse systems.
> Heating (flexibility, type and position of controls and time switches).
> Electrics (numbers of plugs, position and height).
> Alarms and communication equipment (intercoms, door-openers, flashing lights, or vibrating).
> Storage (internal/external).
> Leisure facilities (raised flower-beds).
> Other specific equipment needs (reinforcement of joists for electric ceiling-mounted hoist).
> Rails (for transfers, guiding, colour contrasted, wall-mounted, floor-fixed or folding).
> Living/workroom.
> Garage.

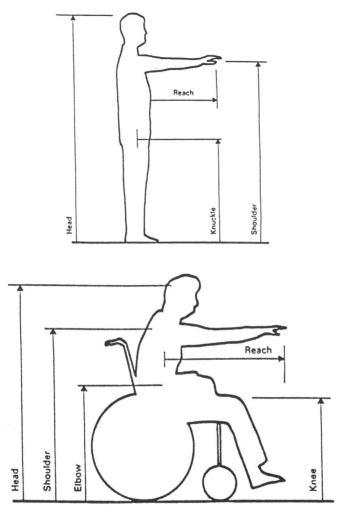

Fig. 13.2a Anthropometric drawings for ambulant and wheelchair adult

Planning and execution of the scheme

Once the scheme has been identified, the work involved in planning and execution is similar in both public and private sectors, however, the procedures regarding finance and general administration will vary widely.

Briefing the architect

The architect involved with the project may be independently employed by the client, from an 'in-house' team of the housing authority or from an

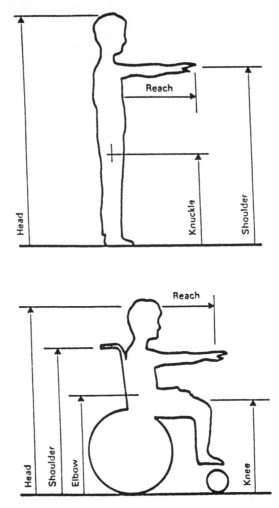

Fig. 13.2b Anthropometric drawings for ambulant and wheelchair child

agency. As he may have little or no specific knowledge of such adaptation work, it is essential that the therapist is very clear in her briefing and gives as much information as possible within the bounds of confidentiality to enable the architect to produce the required plans. It is helpful if the therapist has already had discussions with the client on what information and disclosures would be acceptable to them as being essential to the project. Ideally, the following points should be included in these discussions.

1.   The client's disability and needs.
2.   Present home circumstances, e.g. number of people in the household and their ages.

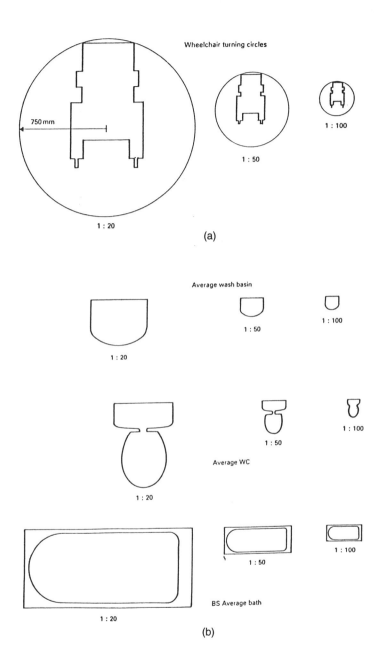

Fig. 13.3 (a) Wheelchair turning circles. (b) Scaled plans

3.   Details of the proposed work.
4.   Additional equipment/aids to be incorporated in the scheme.

An initial site meeting should follow this discussion, when the architect will undertake a survey of the existing layout and examine the feasibility of the proposed scheme. A preliminary sketch will then be produced for discussion with the client and therapist. Sometimes a visit by therapist, client, architect and builder to a similar completed project is helpful, so that everyone has the same understanding of what is being proposed. A final, mutually agreed plan can then be produced. It is advisable to gain a written agreement from the client indicating their acceptance to the final scheme, as this can avoid possible misunderstandings at a later date. In some instances, the client may wish for additional work to be done at the same time. This can be arranged. However, the architect would need to specifically identify this and cost it separately as expenses of any additional work, including the related proportion of the architect's fees, would have to be borne by the client.

Detailed plans and documentation

Detailed plans should indicate the layout of the property to be adapted, and the proposed scheme. The plans may include both ground plans and elevations of the property showing present drainage, electrical points and details of the house construction. Details of the work required will be added to these plans. The types of material to be used, the quality and quantities and method of construction will be prepared separately as a specification for the builder. The working drawings are then used when an application is made for planning permission and building regulations.

For complex work a project sheet (Fig. 13.4) may help the therapist and architect to keep track of the progress of the work, especially if there are delays or long time-lapses between the various stages.

Rules and regulations related to building work

The present building regulations are aimed at ensuring the health and safety of the inhabitants of buildings. Any work which involves structural alterations, or extensions to domestic property, needs the approval of the building inspector. Examples of this would be the provision of a WC and drainage; installing a beam when making two rooms into one; or changing the use of a building, such as making a garage into a habitable room. There are local authority bylaws which govern changes to existing plumbing systems. Apart from fire regulations, the local authority can relax regulations for special cases. The building inspector will visit the site at various stages during the work to ensure compliance.

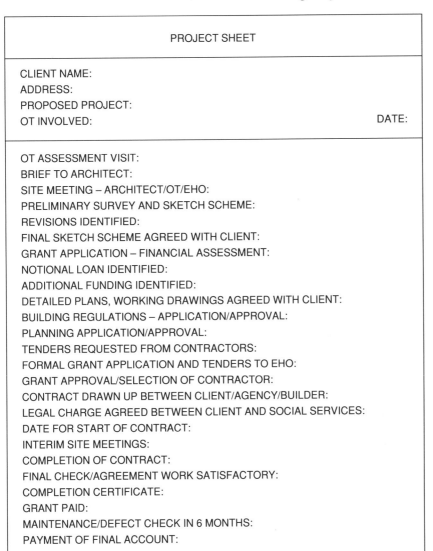

Fig. 13.4 Example of a project sheet for monitoring stages of an adaptation

Planning permission. Internal work is not normally subject to planning permission unless it is a change in use, such as dividing a house into flats. However, this may still require building regulations approval. Permission, however, is always required for listed buildings and usually also needed in designated conservation areas. As these regulations can change quite frequently it is always best to check first.

Estimates and selection of contractor

Where adaptations are funded by Social Services under the Chronically Sick and Disabled Persons Act (CSDP) 1970 either in-house technicians (for rails) or local builders are used to do the work. Some Social Services departments offer advice on the 'feasibility' of a major adaptation proposal through their planning and property services, many of which are now contracted out, but may not provide architectural support in following the project through. Minor works within the district or borough council are usually undertaken in-house by their direct labour force. For complex adaptations councils may use their own technical services or an agency to draw up plans. It is likely that the technical services or planning department will hold a list of builders from which they can invite estimates or tenders, as all work now has to be offered for competitive tendering, in which their own department can participate. Costs are based on the final plan and specifications produced by the architect. Where a disabled person is applying independently for a grant without help from other sources, he or she is normally expected to obtain these estimates, which could be done by an employed architect. There are several ways of drawing up a list of possible architects or builders; for example:

- contacting local planning departments for advice;
- personal recommendations;
- trade associations; or
- local advertisements.

In some areas of Britain agencies have been set up to help applicants through the grant system: for example, 'Staying Put' and 'Care and Repair'.[15]

Grant application

The Environmental Health Officer (EHO) will visit the client to determine which grant is most applicable and to explain the procedure for its application (see section on funding). For the grant application to be processed, plans (if appropriate) and at least two sets of tenders will be required. Work can only be started on the project after formal approval from the housing authority or district council has been received, although in exceptional circumstances permission may be given to commence before this. The EHO will visit the site during the work to ensure that the scheme is progressing satisfactorily. Once the building or alteration is completed the therapist may be requested to visit and confirm that the work meets the needs of the client before the grant is paid. In some situations it is, however, possible for the grant to be paid in instalments.

The contract

Some architects have a standard contract for use in building adaptations. However, for those who intend to work independently the following points will indicate the most important items which need to be included.

1. The commencement date of the scheme.
2. The completion date with clauses for non-completion or variations in completion date; reference to compensation and agreement by the builder to proceed with work on a regular basis.
3. Who will be responsible for obtaining building regulations and planning permission (if appropriate).
4. How alterations to the contract will be agreed.
5. Confirmation that the builder is suitably insured to cover any losses or damages incurred to persons or property during the course of the contract (repair of any defects should be at the builder's own expense).
6. A clear statement of the conditions under which the contract can be terminated by either the client or the builder.

Working with the builder

It is important that all parties have the same well-drawn scale plans and that the builder has clear, written specifications. It is in the client's best interest to have a formal contract with the builder setting out terms and conditions as a safeguard against possible difficulties. The builder must be aware of the problems of the disabled person so that they have daily access to basic services such as WC, cooking facilities and water and periodic rests. If this is not going to be possible, it must be identified at an early stage in the planning so that alternative accommodation can be arranged.

The builder may request interim payments during the course of the project, but this should always be agreed prior to the commencement of work and set out in the terms of the contract. Advance payments may also be requested but this is not recommended practice. The contract may, however, state that the client has the right to withhold a percentage of the builder's final account for a period of 6 months to ensure that the contractor will return to put right any defects which may have occurred during that time. The actual position of fitments such as wash-hand basins, rails and shower controls, although shown on detailed plans, are often best arranged on site. It is important to keep an accurate record of such meetings and discussions in case of dispute. The builder is usually responsible for arranging the inspection of the site by the building control officer at various stages during the project.

Completion of the scheme

A final assessment of the work should be made to satisfy the client, occupational therapist, architect and funding authority to ensure that the project meets the needs of the client and is to a good standard of workmanship. This may be necessary before finance for the scheme is released.

References

1. *National Health Service and Community Care Act 1990*, London: HMSO, 1990.
2. *Health Services for Physically Disabled People Aged 16–64*, National Audit Office, London: HMSO, 1992.
3. *The Health of the Nation – Health Survey for England*, London: HMSO, 1991, 1992.
4. *Health for all targets: the health policy for Europe* (Health For All series, No. 4) Copenhagen: World Health Organisation, 1993.
5. *OPCS surveys of disability in Great Britain. Report No. 4*, London: HMSO, 1989.
6. *Chronically Sick and Disabled Persons Act 1970*, London: HMSO, 1970.
7. *Disabled Persons (Service, Consultation and Representation) Act 1986*, London: HMSO, 1986. *Disabled Persons (N. Ireland) Act 1989*, London: HMSO, 1989.
8. *Local Government and Housing Act 1989*, London: HMSO, 1989.
9. Centre on Environment for the Handicapped (CEH), *Assessment criteria for house adaptations*, London: CEH, 1987.
10. DOE Joint Circular 92/75, *Wheelchair and Mobility Housing, Standards and Costs*, London: HMSO, 1975.
11. DOE Joint Circular 10/90, LAC(90)7, *House Adaptations for Disabled People*, London: HMSO, 1990.
12. PIEDA (1993) *Monitoring the new renovation grant system: final report*, London: DOE, 1993.
13. Centre for Accessible Environments (CAE), *The disabled facilities grant: stairlifts*, London: CAE, 1991.
14. Centre for Accessible Environments (CAE), *Policies and practice on 'topping up'*, London: CAE, 1991.
15. Centre for Accessible Environments (CAE), *The local authority agency services*, London: CAE, 1991.

Further reading

House adaptations for people with a physical disability, London: HMSO, 1990.
Cheshire County Council, Department of Architecture, *Made to Measure*.
Domestic Extensions and Adaptations for Physically Handicapped People, 1980.
London Boroughs Occupational Therapists Managers Groups (LBOTMG), *Occupational therapists' criteria for the provision of adaptations in the homes of people with disabilities*, London: LBOTMG, 1988.
Mandelstam, M. *How to get Equipment for Disability*, 3rd edn, London: Disabled Living Foundation.

Edgington, A. Survey of major adaptations, *British Journal of Occupational Therapists*, Vol. 47(II), p. 46, 1984.
Penton, J. Access for all, *The Architects' Journal*, 16 February, 1983.

Further resources

Care and Repair, Castle House, Kirtley Drive, Nottingham NG7 1LD.
Centre for Accessible Environments, 35 Great Smith Street, London SW1P 3BJ.

Chapter 14

Employment opportunities

RHODA BAXTER

Head Occupational Therapist, Coleraine Hospital, Coleraine, Northern Ireland

There are many reasons why people work. Some would say that it is a means to an end – *they work to live*. Others, who put much value on the nature of their work, might claim that basically *they live to work*. These are contrasting attitudes; it is worth considering them both.

Working to live. People who have this attitude work for extrinsic motivations and rewards – usually money. Work is an unavoidable necessity – something that has to be done in order to acquire the resources for survival and material wants or for 'real living', which begins as work ends. A slogan seen on the back of a lorry, sums it up (Fig. 14.1)!

Some would say they have no choice but to work; they see it as a curse or drudgery – a necessary evil to 'put up with'. Slogans and posters around a workplace may be indicative of true tales (Fig. 14.2).

Another motivation may be success – work can make one successful - upwardly socially mobile.

Living to work. With this attitude people work for intrinsic motivations and rewards. Work is viewed as having the potential to develop a person's abilities and exercise his creativity. It also answers a deep-seated need to be useful, promoting self-esteem and identity.

Some see work as their duty: a service to humanity; it can be a demonstration of their philosophy of living or religious faith.

Both approaches to work can, however, be exploited. In many cases factories have alienated the worker from his work by treating him as a human machine repetitively making a small part, the purpose of which he knows nothing about. Labour can also be physically and mentally incapacitating through repetitive strain. It can even be used as a punishment.

On the other hand, some people who gain much fulfilment from work can become 'addicted' to the point where it completely takes over their lives.

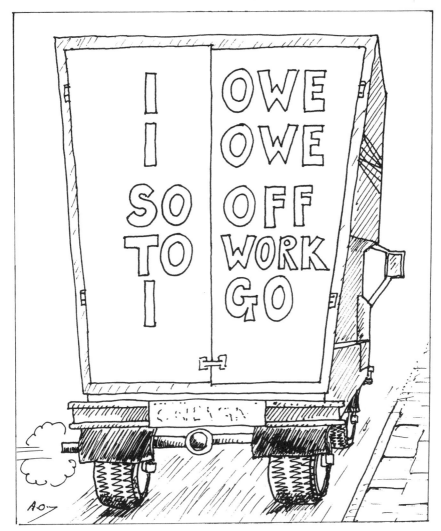

Fig. 14.1

Again, this can be detrimental to their physical and mental health, compromising social relationships.

The effects of unemployment

Since 1980 unemployment in Great Britain has risen from 4.3 per cent to 9.4 per cent of the estimated work force (from 8.4 per cent to 13.3 per cent in Northern Ireland).[1] No matter the attitude to work, remove it from people's lives and in many cases there are serious consequences. According to Grint[2] employment generates the structures of time, routine, status and social

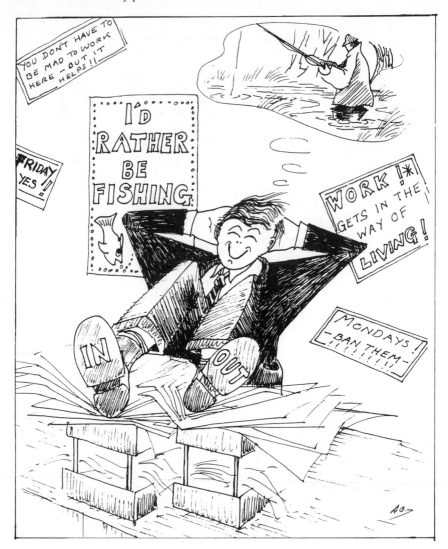

Fig. 14.2

networks; unemployment destroys these. Redundancy may lead to financial difficulties and a drop in living standards. Emotional depression and loss of hope for the future may also result, even leading to suicide.

Employment, health and disability

Kahn[3] defines work as 'a human *activity* that *produces something of acknowledged value*'. He suggests that all three elements in the definition are important for health – the activity, the experience of producing something (abstract or concrete) and the recognition of value. He believes that 'providing work is paramount for individual and social well-being' but also that 'the adequacy of jobs is almost as important as their availability'.

Government figures indicate that people with disabilities are three times more likely to be unemployed than able-bodied people.[4] Unemployment is therefore a major problem in the disabled population.

In promoting employment for people with disabilities, occupational therapists need to be proactive in the community so that specific jobs that can be undertaken by disabled people are identified, thus making work more available. The disabled person will then have the opportunity to 'work to live', or in other words have the resources to lead a full life, enjoying the quality of living desired.

However, 'any job' will not do; it has to be *adequate* for the person so that he can 'live to work', that is to enjoy, as much as possible, fulfilling employment with the psychological and social benefits this brings. Assessment and preparation by occupational therapists may help to fit the right job to the person and encourage a balanced lifestyle. This may be an idealistic approach in today's situation of high unemployment but it is important that people with disabilities have the same opportunities as their peers.

Legislation related to work and disability

The relevant legislation is to be found in *The Disabled Persons (Employment) Acts 1944 and 1958 (1945 and 1960 Northern Ireland) and the Companies Act 1985* (see Appendix I).

According to the Royal Association for Disability and Rehabilitation (RADAR)[4] the effectiveness of these Acts is limited as follows:

- Only approximately 1 per cent of the workforce is currently registered as disabled. This may be because many disabled people have not heard of the scheme; do not regard it as worthwhile or do not like being labelled 'disabled'. The register is therefore not a true indication of the numbers of disabled people in the workforce.
- In 1992 only 20 per cent of employers (with more than 20 staff) met their quota, yet those who failed were not prosecuted. In fact, only 10 prosecutions have ever been brought about under the Acts and none since 1975! It can, however, work for in 1986 the London Borough of Lambeth decided to implement the quota, and within 5 months had increased the proportion of disabled employees from 1 per cent to 4 per cent of its workforce.
- The law against unfair dismissal gives some protection but this only applies to those employees who have been with their employer for at least 2 years and it is unclear about what action is legally required of employers.

Discrimination in employment on grounds of gender and marital status, religion and race is now illegal through the equal opportunities, fair employment and race relations legislation.

Statutory organisations related to employment

The main statutory body in Great Britain concerned with employment and disability is the Employment Service: Disability Services Branch. This organisation overseas 'Placing, Assessment and Counselling Teams' (PACTs) located throughout Job Centres and nine Ability Development Centres (ADCs) throughout Scotland, England and Wales.

Placement, Assessment and Counselling Team (PACT)

PACT is a team of disability specialists giving advice and support 'to help the disabled person assess his abilities and plan his next steps back to work'.[5] It brings together the former work of the Disablement Resettlement Officers, the Disablement Advisory Service and parts of the Employment Rehabilitation Service.

A person's first link with PACT is the Disability Employment Adviser based at the Job Centre. He or she can give advice about:

- suitable jobs;
- assessment;
- useful equipment;
- employment rehabilitation;
- training;
- back to work schemes;
- homeworking; and
- sheltered workshops.

In addition, the PACT team can offer to employers:

- advice on the Code of Good Practice on the Employment of Disabled People; and
- advice on using the disability symbol to show that an organisation is 'positive about disabled people' (Fig. 14.3).

Ability Development Centre (ADC)

These aim 'to promote the *ability* of disabled people by working

- for more and better employment opportunities;
- to create chances for disabled individuals to realise their own potential'.[6]

The ADC's role includes:

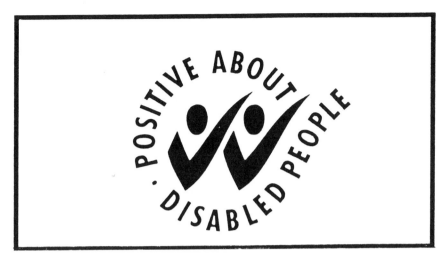

Fig. 14.3

- training for Employment Service (ES) personnel, and others, so that they can best facilitate people with disabilities into jobs;
- assessing and preparing people with disabilities for employment, referred by the PACTs; and
- liaising with employers and other organisations to minimise the effects of disability in employment and maximise ability.

In Northern Ireland the equivalent statutory body is the Training and Employment Agency (TEA): Disablement Advisory Service. This organisation oversees Disablement Employment Advisers (DEAs) based in local TEA offices, and a Mobile Employment Assessment Unit that will bring employment assessment facilities to a local centre on request. Apart from this difference in structure, the services offered are similar to those in Great Britain.

Employment assessment

The conventional approach to employment assessment and preparation for clients who have physical disabilities or mental health problems is one of assessing functioning followed by training and the securing of a job; that is, *assessment–training–job*. An alternative model will be presented later in relation to people with learning difficulties.

Assessment may be carried out in various settings and the professionals involved will largely depend on the place and the client group. Traditionally occupational therapists have always been committed to helping people return to work but the 1980s brought a revival of interest in this area of practice, particularly in the United States, where much literature has been published. In

1992 the College of Occupational Therapists produced a document entitled *Employment Assessment and Preparation in Occupational Therapy.*[7] This outlines what an occupational therapy service may offer; defines current terminology and gives practical advice on how assessment and preparation of clients for employment may be undertaken.

The person who is being assessed for employment is in one of three situations. Either he is being assessed for return to his previous employment or for new employment, or he has never been employed.

Assessing for return to previous employment

It will be necessary to obtain the following information about the client:

- medical information;
- level of performance: physical, psychological and social;
- self-maintenance abilities needed for the job and to get to the location;
- level of work skills related to the demands of the job;
- standard of work behaviours; and
- level of work tolerance.

Medical information should be obtained and following the assessment of performance and self-maintenance abilities, the client's job should be simulated through a programme of practical tasks as similar as possible to those that the job demands. Relevant pencil and paper tests may also be used. The occupational therapist, together with the client, will then be able to identify whether the required skills, behaviours and tolerance to return to his previous job are achievable with or without modifications to the tasks, equipment, environment or hours worked. Supervisors and colleagues will need to have some understanding of his condition. If modifications have financial implications the DEA should help with these, such as paying for specialised equipment; returning part time, or on a reduced output basis (refer to section on 'Back to work' schemes).

If the client is not able to meet the demands of his previous job perhaps he may need more treatment to improve his general condition or more employment preparation. If he is still unsuccessful, it may be concluded that his previous job is unsuitable. The client should therefore be assessed for new work opportunities.

Assessing for new employment

It will be necessary to obtain further information about the client from that mentioned above, to include:

- background information – educational level and attainments,

employment history, leisure pursuits, ideas about future employment;
- financial viability of employment and social situation; and
- job aptitudes.

Because the client is now approaching the 'world of work' and not just one job, drawing on past achievements and experiences may be helpful as a starting point. Any new employment must be considered in the light of his present income. Many clients find themselves in a 'benefit trap'; they want to work but would be at a financial loss by accepting a job which receives less remuneration. The Disability Working Allowance is an attempt to resolve this problem.

To evaluate properly job aptitudes, specialised assessment material will be required such as the following.

(a)   *Standardised material*
This includes commercially produced vocational questionnaires; pencil and paper tests, practical tests and standardised work sample tests.

(b)   *Non-standardised material*
    (i)   Non-standardised work sampling by which a client may try out components of a job off site in the occupational therapy department. Samples may be obtained from local firms who are usually helpful in donating or lending samples, or from Training Centres.
    (ii) Non-standardised tests and tasks, devised by the occupational therapy department.

In many instances non-standardised materials are used as adjuncts to standardised ones, as they allow more time to observe work skills, behaviours and tolerance which may not be apparent during standardised testing.

Both the College of Occupational Therapists' (COT) document[7] and Jacobs[8] give details of the specific tests available. Some occupational therapists may be restricted in using certain psychomotor tests, so liaising with the local PACT team and occupational psychologists can be advantageous.

Assessment locations

The client may be assessed in various locations, such as:

(a)   an occupational therapy department: where pencil and paper tests, practical tests and tasks may be used;

(b)   a 'placement situation': such as a hospital or Social Service canteen, office or supplies department where a specific job may be tried with support and supervision;

(c)   a work site: where the client's skills, behaviours and tolerance for a specific job may be assessed in the competitive employment situation. This could also include the home if home-based work is being considered.

In either situation, close co-operation with the supervisor is essential in order to make any special arrangements, insurance coverage and links with unions if required. Feedback from the employer and other employees on the client's functioning will help to determine the client's employment prospects.

Employment preparation

Employment preparation may be needed when assessment shows that the client is not yet ready for the demands and commitments of his previous job or a new one. If the client has been unemployed for a long time or never been employed, preparation may commence prior to assessment.

The aim of employment preparation is to increase the client's employment potential.[7] This may be defined as:

> the ability of the individual which if realised, will result in his maintaining a paid job. The client's employment potential will depend on his:
> * level of work skills,
> * standard of work behaviours,
> * level of work tolerance.
>
> Level of functioning in one or more of these factors may have to be improved in order to improve the client's overall employment potential.[7]

Work skills

Work skills may be defined as 'the psychomotor and social skills related to the demands of employment'.[7] According to Jacobs[8] they are 'the capabilities that an individual has learned or has the potential to learn, for example, typing, cooking, sewing, welding. They have been frequently called vocational skills'. Occupational therapists can aid clients to develop these skills and a knowledge of the skill acquisition theory can help in the choice of teaching/learning methods.

When a skill requires extensive education or training the client should be referred to the appropriate agency. This may include a general course offering experience in a number of activities as a further assessment of job aptitudes, or a specific course related to one subject or skill. The PACT team (or equivalent) can help to arrange this.

Work behaviours

Work behaviours may be defined as the 'conduct of a person in the work situation'.[7] They can be subdivided into:

> *Work attitudes:* the expression of the person's thoughts and feelings towards work, such as values related to work ethics; motivation.

Work habits: the regular tendencies of the person in a working environment, such as attendance, punctuality.
Work traits: the characteristics of the person required to perform a job
or component of it, such as reliability, responsibility[7]

People who have been unemployed for long periods or who have never had
jobs may find initially that they need to improve work behaviours. For
example, a person who has a poor self-perception as a worker may think his
work skills are limited and is afraid of failing. Someone else who is out of the
habit of a daily routine may find punctuality difficult; others lack job-seeking
skills and an ability to self-motivate. Behaviour modification techniques
through a programme of work-related tasks should be used to improve work
behaviours. Group sessions, where clients share their attitudes to work and
discuss work habits and traits necessary for certain jobs, can be beneficial.

In certain settings 'job clinics' are formed to develop job-seeking skills such
as:

- finding advertisements;
- making contact with employers: in writing and/or by telephone;
- preparing a CV;
- completing an application form;
- preparing for an interview, e.g. interpreting a job specification and
  job description, anticipating questions and preparing answers;
- interview skills:
  - (a) verbal, e.g. manner, clarity, amount and content of speech,
         listening and requesting further explanation;
  - (b) non-verbal, e.g. punctuality, appearance, eye contact, posture
         and facial expression.

  Ways of being courteous and coping with nervousness can be
  handled by verbal and non-verbal means;
- self-appraisal following interview.

Within these sessions learning may take place through talks; information
gathering; pencil and paper exercises; and video role play.

A programme of leisure activities may be a useful starting point to develop
work behaviours, as this may have an immediate appeal to certain clients.
Skills such as reliability, responsibility, initiative and perseverance can be
developed through these and later transferred to a work setting.

Work tolerance

Work tolerance may be defined as 'the ability of the person to endure the
requirements of the job without performing in an unsatisfactory manner,
such as stopping work activity'.[7]

It can be that a person has the work skills and behaviours necessary for a
job but not the physical or mental stamina to tolerate a full day or week at

work. However, he may be able to tolerate a certain number of hours before symptoms develop which subside with rest and he is then able to return the next day.

'Work hardening' is an idea that has developed in the United States since the 1980s.[8] Programmes are run from 2-12 weeks to develop a client's work tolerance. Often these are multidisciplinary in nature and consist of stress and pain management, cardiovascular conditioning, work simulation activities and vocational counselling. They are usually held in a group setting as 'this structure can be a powerful force in motivating injured employees to improve their physical and emotional status and ultimately return to work'.[8]

On a smaller scale, the occupational therapist working with the individual client can enhance his work tolerance through a graded programme of work samples and tasks. The client will aim to achieve an increased level of output as the daily length of programme increases.

Special techniques related to employment of people with learning difficulties

The conventional approach to employment assessment and preparation can also be used with people who have learning difficulties, and certain assessments have been designed specifically for this client group, e.g. 'Jacobs' Prevocational Skills Assessment'.[8]

Assessment and training usually occurs within Adult Training Centres (ATC) run by Social Services or voluntary agencies. Although work preparation and training does take place, the facilities offered can generally be termed *sheltered employment*. Schemes range from co-operatives (involved in a certain activity, e.g. horticulture), training cafes, training workshops (selling goods to the public), to more 'segregated' workshops where contracts are undertaken. A small wage is usually paid to the workers. While some workers do progress to open employment, others remain in the centres for many years.

During the late 1970s another approach to helping this client group find employment was developed by Marc Gold[9] in the USA. At that time he termed his approach 'Try Another Way'. Instead of the traditional *assessment–training–job* model, he developed the *job–training–assessment* model.

Assessment–training–job versus job–training–assessment

Gold asserted that in traditional work assessment, people are tested to discover the amount of skills they have; but he believed that what should be tested is the amount of training power it takes to teach a skill. He devised a system of teaching a skill by meticulously analysing a task: breaking it down into its smallest steps and then slowly and patiently teaching it in small 'chunks'. This system is now called *systematic instruction*.

Gold's model 'turns things around' by first securing a job for the worker then instructing him (through a job coach) to do specific tasks on site and assessing performance afterwards. Employment tasks or 'routines' are categorised into the following.

1. *Core work routines:* routines that are regularly repeated without significant interruption, e.g. in laundry work: sorting items to be washed, loading the washer.
2. *Episodic work routines:* routines that occur infrequently (two or three times per shift), e.g. in restaurant work: cleaning the dishwasher at the end of a shift, taking out the rubbish.
3. *Job-related routines:* routines involving tasks that are not explicitly required for the job, e.g. in factory work: using the drinks machine in the workers' lounge, getting back from break on time.
4. *Accommodations to the work site 'culture':* acceptable and unacceptable behaviour while at work, e.g. in grocery work: touching customers walking by the aisle, opening and eating a packet of biscuits while stocking the shelves, would both be unacceptable.

Each routine is learnt separately by breaking it down into steps and when learnt thoroughly, it is then linked with the next routine.

Learning on site with a job coach instead of 'simulation learning' means that there does not need to be transference of skills. This process is now called *supported employment.*

Exponents of Gold's theory believe that many people with severe learning difficulties are in sheltered (segregated) employment.

> Their placement is not a function of their inability to learn the skills necessary to obtain and maintain employment in integrated environments. Rather, it is a function of our inability to design systems that are responsive to their learning needs.[9]

Supported employment and *systematic instruction* methods are explained in *Getting Employed and Staying Employed* by Mcloughlin, Garner and Callahan.[9] In this text the methods of job analysis, training and assessment are clearly covered together with strategies for obtaining job opportunities. Many centres are now using this method to achieve entry into work for people with learning difficulties. 'Pathway' a division of Mencap, is an example of a supported employment service. Training in Systematic Instruction (TSI) is an organisation which runs courses in this method.

Third level education and training

Many disabled people are able to prepare for open employment by undertaking further study, or participating in various schemes now available to the unemployed.

Educational establishments

Colleges of higher and further education have many vocational courses but do need adequate facilities for access. Some universities and colleges have advisers particularly for disabled students and may offer extra support. A few run special courses for people with disabilities.

Distance learning is a facility provided by some colleges and organisations, which allows students to study away from the base and communicate by correspondence and telecommunications. Some colleges have outlying centres where elements of a course may be taken (see Resources section).

In a sense, *open learning* is a form of distance learning but differs in that minimal entrance qualifications are required and the student is largely permitted to study where and when it suits him best. Though study at home is the basis of this approach there are opportunities for tuition and group discussion at local centres. The Open University and Open College provide courses using this type of learning.

Training schemes related to the Department of Employment

Local enterprise companies (LECs) in Scotland, Training and Enterprise Councils (TECs) in England and Wales or Local Training Agencies (LTCs) in Northern Ireland can provide a range of training opportunities such as 'Training For Work' ('Job Training' Northern Ireland) or 'Youth Training'. Each Job Centre (or equivalent) will have directories of educational courses, open learning and training facilities in the United Kingdom.

Specialist facilities

Residential Colleges. Some people with disabilities find that it is more profitable to attend a residential college, or a training facility, particularly suited to their needs as a preparation for open employment. The residential aspect may also help to overcome difficulties in obtaining suitable accommodation and transport (see Resources section).

Training in information technology. Recent advances in information technology have opened up employment opportunities to people with limited physical functioning but whose cognitive functioning is fully intact. Certain organisations exist to help people with disabilities acquire knowledge and skill in this area, such as the following.

1.   *The National Federation of Access Centres* is a national network of centres in further and higher education seeking to help people with disabilities make choices about a range of microtechnologies, low-tech aids and study methods.

2.   *The Computability Centre* offers education and training about the

opportunities that computers give to people with disabilities, particularly at work, and information and advice on choosing the right equipment.

3. *British Computer Society Disabled Specialist Group* offers information on electronic equipment for people with disabilities, employment opportunities in computing, training facilities for people with disabilities and assistance to employers.

4. *The National Bureau for Students with Disabilities*, entitled 'SKILL', exists to develop opportunities for young people and adults with special needs in third level education, training and employment. It is based in London, and has branches throughout the United Kingdom.

'Back to work' schemes

The occupational therapist needs to be aware of current government schemes and benefits that are available to disabled people, as these change from time to time.

Disability Working Allowance. Currently this is designed to solve the problems of the 'benefit trap' by topping up a low wage to make it higher than the total of a person's benefits.

Therapeutic earnings. If a person can do some work but not as much as 16 hours per week, he may apply to the department of Social Security (DHSS in Northern Ireland) for permission to make therapeutic earnings in addition to his benefits. A medical officer's letter, supporting the value of such earnings in this person's rehabilitation, must accompany the application. The DEA will advise on the current earnings limit.

Sheltered Placement scheme

This is a scheme designed for those who can work full time but whose output is reduced. A Sheltered Placement is an agreement between a 'sponsor company' and a 'host' company whereby the person is employed by the sponsor company to work on a 'placement basis' for the host.

The disabled worker is assessed on his output. If, for example, it is 50 per cent of standard output expected for the job, the host company will pay half his wage with the sponsor paying the other half. Sponsorship can be up to 70 per cent of the person's wage.

A Sheltered Placement may extend from a minimum period of 6 months to an unspecified number of years. It is arranged and monitored by the DEA. If necessary a person on a Sheltered Placement scheme can also receive Disability Working Allowance.

Job Introduction scheme

This scheme exists to encourage employers to employ people with disabilities for a trial period. In this way any serious doubts about their ability to cope with the proposed job or place of work can be resolved. From the disabled worker's point of view it is also a suitable scheme for those who are keen to work full time but are afraid of not being successful.

Under this scheme a grant is paid to the employer towards the person's wages. The trial period is normally 3 months.

Access to Work services

Access to Work is an initiative to provide people with disabilities and their employers with advice and practical support so that successful entry to employment is achieved. The following are examples of the sorts of help that Access to Work will provide:

- a communicator for someone with a hearing impairment;
- a part-time reader or assistance at work for someone with a visual impairment;
- a support worker if someone needs practical help either at work or getting to work;
- equipment (or adaptations to existing equipment) to suit individual needs;
- adaptations to a car, or taxi fares or other transport costs, if someone cannot use public transport to get to work; and
- alterations to premises or the working environment.

Access to Work is flexible to suit each person's needs in his particular job.

In Northern Ireland the above amenities are available but are part of the general facilities provided by the Disability Advisory Service.

Voluntary organisations related to employment

There are many voluntary bodies (national and local) concerned with employment and disability. Some offer a *general resource* service such as the provision of literature and guidelines on employment issues, information and advice. Others offer a *particular* service to an individual including assessment, training, job securement with a job coach (i.e. supported employment), job securement (i.e. unsupported employment but with guidance and follow-up), sheltered placement sponsorship, sheltered work, design of specialist equipment and loan of specialist equipment (see Resources section).

Working from home

Home working may be a consideration, if a person has mobility or transport problems or is unable to work away from home because of disability or family commitments. The occupational therapist can play an important role in this.[8] Modern technology now makes it possible for people with many kinds of disability to work from home in a variety of ways.

There are four main options for home employment, as follows:

1.	Computer work:	data entry and analysis, software applications, word processing and programming.
2.	Telemarketing:	information gathering, direct sales, product marketing and public relations.
3.	Service functions:	clerical responsibilities, small business and professional assistance.
4.	Manufacturing:	light construction of parts for industry (in accordance with appropriate legislation).

A number of organisations run homeworking schemes for disabled people, such as the *Blind Home Workers'* scheme which caters for people with different types of disability, not only those with visual impairment. The *Working at Home with Technology* scheme provides computer equipment and other assistive devices related to employment free of charge as well as essential adaptations to the home. *Teleworking* is a form of employment where an employee, through using a microcomputer, works at a distant base from the location of the firm. Some large firms, such as British Telecom, Rank Xerox and Shell, employ people in this way. The DEA will advise on how to apply for home-based employment.

Employment protection. An employee working from home may qualify for protection depending on the number of hours worked and the length of time he has been in the job. Free advice on legislation related to employment protection may be obtained from the Advisory, Conciliation and Arbitration Service (ACAS).

Starting a small business

Government finance is available to assist those who wish to start their own business. Further information is available from the Department of Trade and Industry (LEDU in Northern Ireland).

The *Guild of Disabled Homeworkers* exists to foster self-employment. It is the only free sales outlet in the United Kingdom for goods made by people with disabilities and who must work at home. As a national organisation, it will receive products from anyone in the United Kingdom.

Voluntary work

Voluntary work differs from employment in that there are less constraints. The agency does not have to pay the volunteer; the volunteer is under no obligation to carry out the tasks and usually no contract is signed.

However, it is not leisure; it is still work and if Kahn's definition of work is used as a 'yardstick' there still must be *productive activity* which is of *value*. Because there is no financial remuneration – one of the principal ways of attributing value to work – the volunteer will have to be rewarded in another way; that is, by receiving what he perceives to be a worthwhile experience. In return his work skills, behaviours and tolerance must be of a satisfactory standard otherwise he will be a liability to the agency, rather than an asset. Local volunteer bureaux and local charitable organisations will provide information on available work in the volunteer's neighbourhood.

Assessing for voluntary work

Voluntary work *can* offer:

- a change of status/reversal of roles;
- an awareness of other's difficulties and an opportunity to help oneself through giving;
- the chance to make a commitment/take responsibility;
- an opportunity for personal development, i.e. confidence building; increasing awareness of abilities;
- involvement in the community; and
- an up to date reference.

Voluntary work can *not* offer:

- a job or the promise of one;
- the sole answer to someone's problems;
- clinical therapy;
- a considerable amount of long-term supervision/support;
- security; or
- money.[10]

It is presumed that the client being assessed for voluntary work is in this situation because an appropriate paid job is not available at the present time. He should, however, have already passed through the employment assessment process or screening process. It must be stressed that it is just as important to thoroughly assess and prepare a person for voluntary work as it is for employment, for an unsuccessful placement will be upsetting for the volunteer, difficult for the agency and disappointing for the referrer.

As with the assessment and preparation for a paid job it is imperative to be realistic about the client's abilities in these situations, so that attainable goals can be achieved. The amount of supervision needed must be gauged and a decision taken on whether the agency can provide this, as most prefer that volunteers work with little supervision after initial support.

When a particular area of voluntary work has been chosen, the agency should list the demands of the tasks and number of hours required. The client's work skills, behaviours and tolerance should then be assessed in relation to these demands, including self-maintenance abilities. Only when a satisfactory level in all these tasks is achieved should the placement commence. Transport may also need to be arranged and financed.

A consequence of the lack of financial incentive may be that the person's work behaviours may deteriorate, especially for those tasks which are less attractive. It is therefore important that the client's attitude is appropriate to the work and that he is well motivated giving the commitment it requires. Work habits, such as punctuality and attendance, should be maintained and work traits, including reliability and flexibility, consistent.

Planning the placement

Success may be facilitated if the client is personally introduced to the agency, place of work and has a 'link person' who will oversee him. This may or may not be his supervisor. He should know to whom he should report and from whom he will receive instructions. In some cases adaptations to the working environment or provision of specialist equipment may be necessary. The occupational therapist may give advice on these and may liaise with other bodies to acquire funding.

It is encouraging that in the mid-1990s there appears to be a revival of interest in people with disabilities obtaining employment. 'Day care' is realised to be no longer adequate and the increasing awareness that people have a need to be productive is leading to discussions about employment rights and the tapping of a valuable workforce. The Occupational Therapy Service can bridge the gap between health, Social Services and employment agencies. Let us hope it is given the resources to do so.

References

1. Department of Employment and Department of Economic Development (Northern Ireland), Labour Market Monthly Reports, 1994.
2. Grant, K. *Sociology of Work*, Oxford: Polity Press, 1991.
3. Kahn, R.L. *Work and Health*, Chichester: J. Wiley & Sons, 1981.
4. Royal Association for Disability and Rehabilitation (RADAR) Statement on Civil Rights Bill, 1994 and Document on Disability and Discrimination in Employment, 1993.
5. Employment Service, *Make it work – employment advice for people with disabilities*, 1993.
6. Employment Service, *Ability Development Centre*, 1993.
7. College of Occupational Therapists, *Employment Assessment and Preparation in Occupational Therapy*, London: College of Occupational Therapists, 1992.

8. Jacobs, K. *Occupational Therapy. Work-Related Programs and Assessments*, 2nd edn, Boston: Little, Brown and Company, 1991.
9. Gold, M. Quoted by Mcloughlin, C.S., Garner, J.B. and Callahan, M. *Getting Employed and Staying Employed*, Baltimore: Paul H. Brookes Publishing Company, 1987.
10. Edinburgh Volunteer Exchange, *Guidelines for those referring patients/clients for voluntary work*, Edinburgh: Edinburgh Volunteer Exchange, 1990.

Further reading

Ryken, L. *Work and Leisure in Christian Perspective*, Portland, OR: Inter-Varsity Press, 1987.

Royal Association for Disability and Rehabilitation (RADAR),
Employment Rights, 1992.
Disability and Discrimination in Employment, 1993.
Employment Factsheet 1 – Guidelines for Policies on the Employment of Disabled People, 1991.
Employment Factsheet 4. Training for Disabled People, 1994.
Factsheet 2. Working from Home, 1992.

Cromwell, F.A. (ed.) *Work-Related Programs in Occupational Therapy*, New York: Haworth Press, 1985.

Fletcher, J. *How to Get that Job*, 3rd edn, Plymouth: How to Books Ltd, 1993.

Dyche, R. *Get Yourself a Job*, London: Longman Group, 1989.

Beyer, S. Employment and People with a Mental Handicap, in *Changing Approaches to Mental Handicap* (ed. Jenkins, R.), Swansea: University College of Swansea School of Social Studies, Occasional paper No. 23, 1994.

Lister, T., Ellis, L., Phillips, T. *Survey of Supported Employment Services in England, Scotland and Wales*, NDT, St. Petersport, 8 Trumpet St., Manchester M1 5LW, 1992.

Lowe, K., Byer, S., Kilsby, M. and Felce, D. Activities and engagement in day services for people with a mental handicap: a pilot study, *Journal of Intellectual Disability Research*, Vol. 36, pp. 489–503, 1992.

Floyd, M. (ed.) *Information Technology Training for People with Disabilities*, Jessica Kingsley Publishers, 1993.

Hawkridge, D. and Vincent, T. *Learning Difficulties and Computers*, Jessica Kingsley Publishers, 1992.

National Council for Voluntary Organisations, *Voluntary Agencies Directory*, London: NCVO, 1995.

Scottish Council on Disability, *Directory of Voluntary Organisations on Disability in Scotland*, Edinburgh: Disability Scotland, 1995.

Northern Ireland Council for Voluntary Action, *Directory of Voluntary Organisations in Northern Ireland*, 1995

Underwood, L., Consumers Association, *Earning money at home*, London: Penguin, 1994.

McClean, S. and Turner, K. *Physically Disabled Volunteers and Voluntary Work*, Belfast: Voluntary Service, 1990.

Darnborough, A. and Kinrade, D. *Directory for People with Disabilities*, London: Royal Association for Disability and Rehabilitation, 1994.

British Association of Occupational Therapists, *Reference Book*, London: British Association of Occupational Therapists, 1992.

Useful addresses

ACAS, Head Office, 27 Witton Street, London SW1 7AZ.

British Computer Society Disabled Specialist Group, c/o BCS Information Officer, 13 Mansfield Street, London W1M 0BP.

Computability Centre, PO Box 94, Warwick, Warwickshire CV34 5WS.

Guild of Disabled Homeworkers, Enterprise Aid Centre, Stag House, Woodchester GL5 5E2.

National Federation of Access Centres, Banstead Place, Park Road, Banstead, Surrey SW17 3EE.

Pathway, 5A Gravel Lane, New Market Square, Blackwood, Gwent NP2 1AG.

SKILL: National Bureau for Students with Disabilities, 336 Brixton Road, London SW9 7AA.

Training in Systematic Instruction, Unit 62, Euroline Business Centre, 49 Effra Road, London SW2 1BZ.

Resources

Residential colleges for people with disabilities – details available from RADAR (below).

Royal Association for Disability and Rehabilitation (RADAR), 12 City Forum, 250 City Road, London EC1V 8AF.

Rehabilitation Resource Centre, City University, Northampton Square, London EC1V 0HB.

Remploy Ltd, 415 Edgware Road, Cricklewood, London NW2 6LR.

Employment Opportunities for People with Disabilities, 1 Bank Buildings, Princess Street, London EC2R 8EU.

Association of Disabled Professionals, 170 Benton Hill, Wakefield Road, Horbury, West Yorkshire WF4 5HW.

British Institute for Industrial Therapy, 63 South Street, Bishops Stortford, Herts CM23 3AL.

ITO (Ulster) Ltd, Unit 5, Duncrue Place, Duncrue Industrial Estate, Belfast.

The Volunteer Centre UK (information service will supply a printout of literature related to disabled volunteers), Carriage Row, 183 Eversholt Street, London NW1 1BU.

Video: *Talking jobs – Interview skills for candidates*, Jumpcut, Bank Chambers, 2 Lidget Hill, Pudsey, N. Yorks LS28 7DP.

Chapter 15

The child with special needs

JANET LEESON
Head Occupational Therapist, Children's Services, Norwich Community Health Partnership NHS Trust

The role of the occupational therapist working with children and young people is to develop their optimum level of independent function, physically, psychologically and socially, bearing in mind their age, their needs, the environment in which they live, and the lifestyle and culture of the family. There are many excellent sources of information for therapists working with children and therefore the aim of this chapter is to act as an introduction to this extensive field; to give the inexperienced therapist an understanding of what working with children and their families involves, and a base from which to develop her skills.

Working with children and their families is exciting and challenging. The therapist, however, has to be flexible, open to new ideas, accept change and be willing to accept that, on some occasions, she may be wrong or not know the answer and will have to try again. Both children and their carers will be a constant source of information which the therapist will need to use skilfully to develop the child's potential. This information will need disseminating so that it can be used by other parents of children with similar needs.

A child cannot be seen in isolation. Not only are they an individual in their own right, but each is part of a family which will have its own particular characteristics and dynamics. These need to be understood and respected. The needs of both the child and the family must be integrated into the therapist's plan of intervention.

The therapist can be one of a long list of professionals involved with each child; therefore, liaison is essential. Parents may become confused and disorientated especially when receiving conflicting information from a number of professionals, whose specific roles in the child's life may not have been clarified. The therapist must be sensitive to the emotional feelings of the parents, as the reality about their child's ability and what the future holds for them becomes apparent. This could happen on several occasions through a child's life; for example, when the child moves from needing a baby buggy to requiring a major seating system or wheelchair. This is usually a difficult time for most parents as it emphasises that their child is 'disabled' and no longer a toddler who has not learned to walk.

Legislation

The therapist will need to be aware of current legislation that effects children. These include the following.

The Children Act 1989,

The Act[1,2] states that the welfare of a child is 'paramount' and that where possible children should be cared for within their own families. It uses the term 'parental responsibility' to sum up the duties, rights and authority which parents have in respect of their child. This responsibility continues even if the parent is not living with the child. Where possible both child and parent need to be involved with all plans regarding them.

One of the important provisions of the Children Act is to oblige Social Services and other agencies to provide services for 'children in need'. These include all children with disabilities, which will be a major part of the paediatric occupational therapist's caseload.

Children at Risk

The Children Act 1989[3] forms the main legal framework for child protection. A confidential register maintained by Social Services lists all children considered to be suffering or likely to suffer from significant harm and for whom there is a child protection plan. If at any time a therapist is concerned for the well-being of a child she should immediately seek specialist advice. Local authorities have a statutory duty to investigate where they have reasonable cause to suspect a child is suffering, or likely to suffer significant harm. The therapist must be aware of local procedures for reporting such cases.

Education Act 1981

This Act[4-6], which resulted from the Warnock Enquiry into special education, placed wider obligations on local education authorities to make adequate provision for educating children with special educational needs. This concept changed the focus away from the child's disability to that of their needs and abilities. It also emphasises the principle of children being educated in mainstream schools, wherever possible.

To gain an understanding of the child's special educational needs an assessment process is initiated following consultation with the parents. Advice in the form of reports is sought from the child's parents and all agencies involved with that child. The assessment aims to identify:

(a)   The child's strengths and needs, including an analysis of their learning difficulties.
(b)   Aims and objectives of the special educational provision.
(c)   Approaches, resources and facilities required to meet these needs, including non-educational provision.

A draft statement of these needs is drawn up at the conclusion of the assessment to which the parents must agree before the final one is issued.

A statement is subsequently reviewed annually to ensure the needs of the child are being met. Reassessment is required at the age of 14½ years, which begins the process of careers advice.

The therapist will need to be aware of procedures for reporting to their local education authority. Detailed information regarding the format for such reports is available in the references at the end of this chapter.[5]

Access to health records

Since November 1991 all clients have had access to their health records, although this can be denied in some circumstances. Some areas are also introducing parent-held records so that parents are responsible for keeping records pertaining to their child. All professions are expected to contribute to these records, thus improving liaison between them.

Safety legislation

Paediatric occupational therapists are involved not only with active treatment but also with the provision of specialist furniture, cushions and making adaptations to existing equipment. It is therefore important that the therapist is aware of all current legislation regarding security and safety, which includes the use of fire retardant foam and material. Under no circumstances should alterations be made to car seats which might prejudice the security of the child in an accident. As a result of the EC Lifting and Handling Legislation the paediatric occupational therapist may be involved with their physiotherapy colleagues in recommending appropriate lifting equipment to other agencies and also advising parents, carers and colleagues on appropriate techniques.

Common conditions and difficulties

Many different conditions are referred to the paediatric occupational therapist. These may include the following:

Cerebral palsy

Cerebral palsy[7-11] is the term used to describe a disorder of movement, posture and balance which is due to non-progressive brain damage. This may be the result of hereditary factors or events during pregnancy, delivery or occurrences during the first 2 years of life. Some children may present with minimal difficulties and may be described as being 'clumsy'; while others have major and multiple problems including sensory defects. The picture and subsequent treatment regimes will vary with each child depending on which body parts are involved and the child's type of movement difficulties.

Learning disabled

The causes of learning disability (mental handicap)[11,12] vary but may be due to hereditary factors or some specific genetic syndromes; cerebral malfunction; injury or degeneration; chromosomal abnormalities, metabolic or endocrine disorders. The cause may not be apparent in approximately 40 per cent of cases of severe learning disability and relatively more with moderate learning disability remain undiagnosed.

Spina bifida

This defective development of the spinal cord and vertebrae may cause sensory and motor impairment below the lesion and can include paralysis of bladder and bowel. The child may also have hydrocephalus. Bony deformities, such as those of the spine, may occur due to muscle imbalances.[11,12]

Muscular dystrophies

These are progressive hereditary diseases causing weakness of the muscles.[11,12] Muscle fibres are progressively broken down and replaced by fibrous tissue and fat. The various types of dystrophy are grouped under labels depending on the age of onset, parts of the body affected, methods of inheritance and the rate of deterioration. The most common is Duchenne Muscular Dystrophy, which only affects males.

Spinal muscular atrophy (SMA)

This is similar to motor neurone disease in adults and also resembles muscular dystrophy. It is the progressive degeneration of motor nerve cells within the spinal cord causing muscle weakness and wasting. The motor nuclei of the cranial nerves may also be defective. There are various types of SMA,[11,12] which differ according to age of onset, severity and prognosis.

Perceptuo-motor difficulties

There are a number of descriptive names for the group of symptoms described under this heading, such as clumsy child syndrome, dyspraxia and minimal cerebral palsy.[13,14] These children have difficulty with planning and organising movement. On close examination they may have other difficulties which include laterality, body awareness, visual perception, sequencing, attention, mid-line crossing and stereognosis. Psychological assessment usually reveals a discrepancy between verbal and performance IQ scores.

Juvenile rheumatoid arthritis

This autoimmune disease causes inflammation of joints and sometimes other body parts.[11,12] Arthritis usually ceases eventually after a fluctuating course of remission and activity. In some children the disease will cease soon after onset resulting in little or no deformity, while in others it will continue for several years, leaving the child with permanent deformities.

Children with absent limbs or congenital amputation

This defect is caused during the early stages of pregnancy when a foetal limb bud fails to develop.[11]

Achondroplasia

This inherited disorder is the shortening of long bones, due to defective bone and cartilage formation, so that the arms and legs are short and stubby relative to the head and trunk.[11,12]

Accidents and burn injuries

These injuries including head injuries are caused by a variety of accidents, which vary as the child becomes more exploratory. For example, at less than 2 years of age burn injuries are often associated with hot drinks; at 4 years by hot water; under 6 years by flame; and under 11 years chemical burns are more in evidence.

Treatment approaches

There are a number of treatment regimes and the therapist must be familiar with these, though she will require postgraduate training for any specialist training to be fully effective. These include Doman Delacato;[12,15] sensory stimulation;[9,12,15] proprioceptive neuromuscular facilitation;[9,15] and reflex creeping (Vojta).[9] However, the more common approaches are as follows.

Neurodevelopmental treatment (Karl and Berta Bobath)[8,9,10,16]

This approach is based on the knowledge that the child with cerebral palsy has abnormal development of postural control against gravity, together with abnormal patterns of co-ordination, postural tone and reciprocal innovation. To enable a child to experience more normal sensations, postures and movement, the therapist uses handling techniques including 'reflex inhibiting postures', to reduce spasticity; 'key points of control' to 'inhibit' abnormal activity, as well as 'facilitating' more normal sequences of movement. Children are treated in everyday situations with emphasis on parental training.

Conductive education (A. Peto and M. Hari)[9,15,16]

This is a system of education whose main aim is to stimulate the developmental process, enabling the child to be integrated back into his community. The therapist is called a 'conductor'. Conductive education is based on group work using simple wooden equipment, following a daily functional schedule, each child being motivated to obtain set personal goals. The conductor encourages 'rhythmic intention' to aid learning. Here the child verbalises the intended motion to himself and then the motion is achieved during rhythmic counting.

Sensory integrative therapy (J. Ayres)[16,17]

Sensory integration is the process that a normal brain uses to respond appropriately to the sensation it is receiving. Dysfunction of this process can lead to poor reflex inhibition and therefore delay motor development and the child's ability to interpret sensations. Therefore, the therapist organises the therapy environment to enable a child to receive controlled stimulation of his senses so that he might learn to adapt and respond to the stimuli effectively and appropriately. The child learns through self-directed spontaneous movement, such as climbing, swimming, spinning and rolling.

Assessment

It is important to have an understanding of what is 'normal'.[7,15,18] A visit to local nurseries, observing friends' children at play, or thinking back to one's own children's development can assist in establishing this. With these thoughts in mind, time needs to be spent investigating the child's previous relevant medical, social and developmental history; gaining current information on diagnosis; understanding the family situation and the child's strengths and needs as others see them. Despite this trawling for information the therapist must remain objective and avoid being over-influenced by others' thoughts.

Questionnaires sent to both parents and teachers seeking information on the child's abilities and difficulties at home and at school can be useful, especially for the older child. Providing they are carefully worded and appropriately used they enable parents and teachers to think through the child's strengths and needs in a logical fashion. They also enable them to express an

TEST TITLE	TEST AIMS	AGE RANGE (years)	APPROX. TIME TO ADMINISTER (minutes)
Aston Index	Screening assessment to assess language abilities. Tasks include: Picture recognition, vocabulary scale, word reading, spelling, laterality, copying, and geometric designs	5–14	60
Bruininks Oseretsky Test of Motor Proficiency	Test of gross and fine motor functioning. Tasks include running speed, balance, bilateral co-ordination, visual motor control and dexterity	4.5–14.5	45–60
Developmental Test of Visual Motor Integration (Beery and Buktenica)	Screening assessment to assess visual motor skills using pencil and paper. The child had to copy geometric figures which increase in complexity	3–18	30
Erhardt Developmental Prehension Assessment	Measures prehension development relating this to the child's age	0–1.25	Varies
Frostig Developmental Test of Visual Perception	Pencil and paper test measuring visual perceptual skills. Assessment includes eye motor co-ordination, figure ground, constancy of shape, position in space and spatial relationships. Used with a programme of development of visual perception	3–10	30
First Step Screening	Screening assessment to identify developmental delay in young children which includes picture completion, position in space, problem solving and discrimination, fine motor planning and balance	2.9–6.2	15
Goodenough Harris Draw a Man	Screening to assess performance by drawing a man. This may show problems with body image	3–15	Varies
Movement ABC	Assesses movement difficulties including manual dexterity, ball skills, static and dynamic balance. There is a checklist for teachers and guidelines for management and remediation	4–12	20–30
MAP (Miller Assessment for Preschoolers)	Assessment to identify mild to moderate developmental delay including neural foundations, co-ordination, verbal, non-verbal and complex tasks	2–6	25–30
Purdue Perceptual Motor Survey	Screening assessment to assess perceptual motor skills including perceptual motor matching, directionality and laterality	4–13	20–30
TVPS – non-motor (Test of visual perceptual skills)	To assess a child's strengths or weaknesses in a visual perception using a non-motor method. Includes assessment of visual discrimination, shape constancy, figure ground, spatial relationships and visual memory	4–13	30

Fig. 15.1 A selection of standardised tests available

SKILLS TO BE ASSESSED	PRESCHOOL Basic skills	SCHOOL AGE Additional skills included as appropriate	YOUNG ADULTS Additional skills included as appropriate
DAILY SKILLS			
Eating and drinking	Food and drink consumes Implements and equipment Child's position Method of feeding	Activities such as: pouring, stirring	Food preparation Making drinks Carrying items
Toiletting	Training or not Equipment using	Transfers Wipes bottom Washing hands	Flush toilet Personal hygiene
Communication	Indicates needs Verbal/non-verbal Method and equipment using		
Sleeping	Bed/cot Time asleep Behaviour at night	Independent transfers	
Bathing	Method Equipment using	Independence Cleaning nails/teeth Brush hair Blow nose	General hygiene Personal presentation Shaving
Mobility	Independently – roll crawl walk Car seat Buggy/wheelchair	Around home and school Adaptations made Use of bike Independent transfers	Around the community Accessing public buildings Shopping
Dressing/ undressing	Position Method of dressing Style of clothes used	Managing – fastenings – laces	Appropriate clothing for occasions Knows own clothes sizes
PHYSICAL SKILLS			
Supine/prone/ sidelying	Posture in these positions Ability to change position Tone Movements of limbs Pull to sit (check head control)	Ability to plan and organise movement Co-ordination Strength Concentration Balance Skip, hop, jump Ball skills	
Sitting	Saving reactions present Type of sitting – supported – propped – independent Equipment using		
Standing	Equipment in use Ability to high kneel		

Fig. 15.2 A basic checklist of observations useful during assessment

SKILLS TO BE ASSESSED	PRESCHOOL Basic skills	SCHOOL AGE Additional skills included as appropriate	YOUNG ADULTS Additional skills included as appropriate
HAND SKILLS	Ability to – reach – grasp – release	Hand preference	
Use of hands	Unilateral Bilateral Crossing midline of body Transferring Type of grasp Isolation of fingers – poke – pinch	Use of scissors Eye/hand co-ordination	Able to open jars, tins, sealed items
General dexterity	Interdigital manipulation		
BODY AWARENESS	Labels body parts	Copies gestures Moves without visual cues Stereognosis Left/right discrimination	
PLAY/COGNITIVE SKILLS Positions	Used for play Favourite toys		
Performance skills	Non-verbal performance including – stacking – pegging – posting shapes – insert puzzles – construction – interest in books	Use of language Able to convey name, address, date of birth Follow set of instructions Memory Remembers messages Reading Perceptual skills Reasoning	Ability to organise self Follow directions – verbal, using a map, and/or diagrammatic instruction
Conceptual skills	Including colour, size, shape, position		
Symbolic/imaginative play	Small/large doll play		
PENCIL SKILLS	Grip used Preferred hand Ability to imitate, copy, draw independently	Handwriting – letter formation, print or cursive Drawing/painting Use of microtechnology	Ability to write letters, application forms, forms in general
ATTENTION	Length of time Distracted by what		
METHODS OF LEARNING	Trial and error By demonstration Ability to problem solve Motivation/attitude Memory – visual, auditory		

Fig. 15.2 cont.

opinion and contribute to the assessment. It is important, however, to be aware that some parents may be illiterate or have a poor command of English and, if the parents wish, time needs to be set aside to complete them within the assessment session.

At the initial assessment, the parents' overall concerns regarding their child's progress and consequent expectations of occupational therapy should be documented. These will need to be addressed by both therapist and parents when a plan of intervention is drawn up and a useful tool when measuring outcomes of treatments. The method of assessment will vary depending on the child and their perceived needs, but wherever possible standardised tests should be included as these provide valid, reliable and objective information. They also enable an easy comparison to be made of the child's performance with their peers and allows subsequent therapists to repeat the test using the same objective tasks. Other information can be gained by documenting observations, such as how the child approached the test, tackled each problem and what their behaviour was during the administration of the test. Some of the more commonly used standardised tests are charted in Fig. 15.1.

The assessment should be relaxed, and in most cases take more than one session. It must begin as soon as the child and/or parents enter the room. Observations should include how the child is held; parent/child interaction; their attention and alertness; how the child sits, undresses; and the child's ability to play alone.

Once permission has been gained from the child or their parent, providing it is appropriate, confident handling enables the therapist to physically feel what is happening as the child moves, sits and plays giving further information on possible methods of intervention.

Where the assessment is held can vary; nevertheless, a useful start may be in a local clinic room in which the therapist is familiar with equipment and space. Follow-up sessions concluding this initial assessment could take place at school, home, nursery or wherever seems appropriate to maximise the potential sources of information. Naturally it should be remembered that an assessment is continuous as it may take several sessions to build up the true picture of the child's abilities and the therapist's initial views may change with time.

A simple checklist of activities which the therapist may need to investigate and/or seek further information about can be found in Fig. 15.2.

Recording

Each department will have its own method of recording.[15,18] Nevertheless, information should include the following.

(a)   All essential details such as name, address, date of birth, consultant, GP and school.

(b)   Child's parents' names, as these may differ from the child's.

(c)   Carers' names and addresses if the child regularly receives respite care.

(d)   Other professionals and agencies involved including Social Services, education and community health staff. (Usually the latter have already provided a great deal of input to these families and therefore constitute a great source of information.)

(e)   Other family members.

(f)   The child's 'social life'. (Some children have extremely full social diaries, some none.)

(g)   Previous occupational therapy involvement.

(h)   Access to transport. (This is especially important if the child is to attend regular therapy sessions.)

It is important that all contacts with the child, their parents/carers and other people involved with their care are recorded, including telephone conversations. These need to be concise, accurate and informative. Treatment notes need to refer to the treatment aims and therapeutic plan.

Therapeutic plan

Following assessment the therapeutic plan should be developed with the child's parents, taking into account the family's expectations of therapy, as well as their ability to attend treatment sessions and then to continue the advice given to them. The resultant collated report, which briefly includes the views of relevant agencies and the occupational therapist's observations, gives a good baseline for therapy as it details the child's strengths and needs.

SKILLS TO BE ASSESSED	PRESCHOOL Basic skills	SCHOOL AGE Additional skills included as appropriate	YOUNG ADULTS Additional skills included as appropriate
SOCIAL INTERACTION	Eye contact Interaction with parents, siblings, others, in play	Self-esteem Social skills Ability to make friends Telling time	Use of money/ budgeting, transport, telephone Crossing road Self-control Social etiquette Able to ask for help
LEISURE	Attends playgroup, musical groups	Attends local clubs, sports activities	Able to use sports and leisure facilities in community Hobbies and pursuits

Fig. 15.2 cont.

Intervention

A therapist should not attempt to treat a child in isolation, but must be aware of what the parents and her colleagues are doing.[18] Preparing joint aims for the child and holding sessions with another therapist are useful. For example, a play session can be tailored for preschool children who have little sitting balance and expressive communication so that work on balance, hand skills and developing their awareness of concepts can be undertaken alongside learning to use their communication book. Dorothy Penso[18] emphasised the importance of the therapist being an 'enabler' by training parents and other carers to become the therapist. The occupational therapist's role should only be a small part of that child's life because they have enabled parents, through thoughtful preparation and careful management, to become confident handlers of their child's therapy. Nevertheless, it needs to be recognised that there are times when the parent cannot be therapist and teacher as well as parent.

   The following selective activities could form part of a programme devised for a child, but must not be thought of as being complete in themselves.

Play

Children learn through play because it is fun, and they use it to practise social and sensory motor experiences. A young child will repeat, experiment and solve problems many times on an activity or movement, trying to make sense of it and to refine it until acceptable.

   Play also enables the child to develop relationships with people, expand language and allow social situations to be practised and roles explored. Therefore throughout childhood the child will be building a reservoir of experience which they will utilise as necessary in future.

   Therapy has to allow the child to play and consequently learn new experiences. To do this, the therapist needs to recognise anything which may interrupt the learning process. This may include physical and sensory difficulties, inappropriate positioning; use of language; a distracting environment; or less easily observed problems such as difficulties with perception, comprehension and sensitivity.[19]

Toys

Therapists are often asked by parents and carers for advice and ideas about toys that they can use with their child. Several factors need to be considered before suggestions are made.

(a)   Weight – preferably lighter ones for children with muscle weakness and for those with co-ordination difficulties.

(b)   Height – if the child is sitting he needs to be able to see the whole toy.

(c)   Developmental level – activities need scaling to suit the child's ability level, bearing in mind their chronological age.

(d)   Accessibility – these should enable those with poor motor control to use them. Adding an electronic switch to battery toys may allow a child to use that toy independently.

(e)   Sensory experiences – toys using a range of textures and with visual and auditory stimuli provide a variety of experiences for the child.

Parents may need reminding that their child learns from how they use a toy rather than what the toy is; therefore simple toys and day to day objects usually provide the stimulus required.

Listening and attending

A child's ability to play will naturally influence his ability to learn. To facilitate concentration distraction should be reduced, with the therapist sitting opposite the child in order to gain eye contact. By starting with short periods and gradually increasing these and by using exciting materials assists in this. Regaining attention can be achieved by calling the child's name, pausing and regaining eye contact or gently touching them. One or two clear concise instructions should only be given at one time, pausing to allow comprehension. Each new task will need to be tackled by breaking it down into small achievable parts, and giving praise when deserved. A child will need to maintain attention in order to develop the skills needed for language and communication.

Communication

Communication begins from the start of a child's life when it cries for attention because it is hungry.[20] Rapidly this becomes more sophisticated as the child smiles, watches, appreciates facial gestures; makes eye contact; initiates, copies and takes turns during play; enjoys nursery rhymes and stories, and under normal circumstances develops language, words and sentences.

For those children who are unable to communicate verbally or use non-verbal methods there are various forms of augmentative or alternative communication systems, which include Makaton, BLISS symbols, picture communication symbols and technological communication aids. The occupational therapist working closely with the speech and language therapist needs to be familiar with these and involved with positioning to facilitate good eye contact and purposeful vocalisation. When using other communication systems, she may be involved with developing an electronic switching accessing system and training the child in its use. Throughout therapy, time must be allowed for the child to participate fully and communicate their wishes.

When positioning the child consider the reasons and the therapeutic implications for each position and aim to have:

1.   The head in midline.
2.   The arms forward with hands visible.
3.   The body symmetrical.
4.   A straight extended back.
5.   The shoulder girdles protracted.

PRONE

Why prone? Because the position encourages:

1.   Extension of hips, neck and spine.
2.   Protraction of shoulders which is needed for function.
3.   Weight bearing through arms to stabilise shoulders and improve head control.

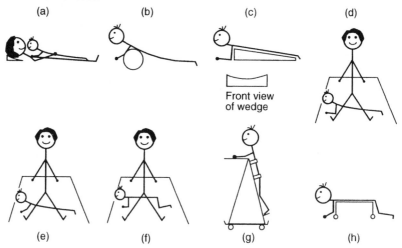

(a)   Lying on a parent's body allows lovely eye contact and sensory input.
(b)   Lying over a roll enables movement to reduce spasticity and provide sensory input. This may also encourage hips and knees to flex for crawling and kneeling.
(c)   Lying over a wedge. These vary in height, length and if the upper surface is slightly shaped helps to prevent the child from rolling off. Some wedges have straps to maintain the child's position. A longer wedge will support the child's legs, but the feet need maintaining in dorsiflexion. While the thicker end will enable the child to weight bear through straight arms, a second smaller wedge at the base of the front will allow him to weight bear through flexed arms.
(d, e)   Lying across adult's legs enables parental contact and play as well as movement and sensory input.
(f)   Lying across adult's legs – enables weight bearing through elbows and knees.
(g)   Using a prone stander – enables trunk and limbs to be held symmetrically and slightly forward.
(h)   Lying over a scooter – promotes reciprocal crawling motion.

Fig. 15.3 Positioning a child for play and work – positions will vary according to their needs and abilities

Perception

Perceptual skills will develop during play and exploration along with an awareness of body image. These are difficult to assess in a younger child but are essential for the development of normal motor activity. A child will need to be aware of shape, size and form constancy, figure ground, position in space and spatial relationships; along with sequencing and discrimination. Consequently the therapist will need to initiate play which will practise these skills and give children a base for further learning.

Positioning for play and work

A child needs to be enabled to play or work in a variety of positions.[21–26] Examples are given of equipment pieces available which may assist this positioning (see Fig. 15.3–15.8). Once the child feels secure against the effects of gravity he will be more able to overcome the abnormal patterns of movement that may dominate his life as well as be able to perform tasks and activities. A child affected by cerebral palsy often has difficulty isolating and processing the information they are receiving. Consequently they may not be able to concentrate on sitting upright as well as listening to the instructions for a task. Therefore, time needs to be set aside to work on such tasks as sitting, by using a programme where the child is encouraged to maintain an upright posture with their hands down by their sides, feet on the floor, head up, and less emphasis on the task in hand. On other occasions the child should be supported so that they can concentrate fully on the activity that they are doing with their hands rather than on their sitting.

SIDELYING

Why side-lie? Because the position:

1. Encourages the use of both hands for play.
2. Encourages the child to see his hands.
3. Allows the child to take toys to their mouth.
4. Prevents side flexion of the trunk.
5. Supports the head.
6. Prevents abnormal abduction at the hips.

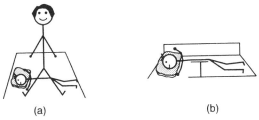

(a)   (b)

(a)   Sidelying on the floor with adult support.
(b)   Using a commercially available board.

Fig. 15.4

SITTING

Why sit? Because the position encourages:

1.   Improved contact with the surrounding environment.
2.   Free hands for play and work.
3.   Extension of the spine and a lumbar lordosis (if developmentally capable).
4.   Improved head control.
5.   Equal weight bearing through buttocks.

Sitting:

(a)   Between adult's legs on floor – enables play with an adult in a secure position with legs straight and abducted stretching the hamstring muscles.

(b)   Over flexed leg of an adult – enables a strong extension thrust to be controlled using hip and knee flexion.

(c)   Against an adult's legs – enables physical interaction with parent and a reasonable secure seating position.

(d)   Astride an adult's legs – enables good hip abduction. (Commercially available seats achieve the same.[24])

(e)   In a corner seat on floor with table – enables floor play and the legs to be extended.

(f)   On a stool – enables training in sitting balance and a suitable position for dressing.

(g)   In a regular chair – enables hips to be flexed at 90 degrees or less with feet flat on the floor to enable greater stability of the trunk.
       If a child rocks their chair, screwing the chair to a board will stop this. Skies can also be used on the legs but these cause tripping in a classroom situation.

(h)   In a regular chair with foot box to provide a base for the feet.

(i)   Using a pommel – enables greater abduction and symmetrical positioning at the hips. These should not be used if it increases tone in the adductors or used to hold a child in the chair.

(j, k)   On an angled stool – enables hips to be tilted anteriorly encouraging greater extension of the spine.

(l)   In a commercially available angled seat enables greater security for the child and is multi-adjustable.

(m)   In a commercially available multi-adjustable chair – enables the therapist to provide the best supportive position for the child and help prevent deformity. These chairs provide knee blocks, trunk and hip pads, foot plate, tray and can be mounted on wheels.

(n)   Using a ramped cushion and sacral pad – enables the femur to remain horizontal, with consequent even weight distribution over the sitting base thus reducing the tendency to sacral sit by maintaining hips and knees at 90 degrees.

(o)   In a moulded seat – enables a child with poor trunk and head control to be in a more upright position.

(p)   Using a waistcoat with straps over shoulders and (down over) hips helps to maintain an extended trunk position and reduce forward and side flexion. Care has to be taken not to full the shoulders into a retracted position. Protect the child's neck by placing the strap under a collar or covering it with a soft sheath. The hip strap needs to be carefully angled and if the waistcoat is too tight it will inhibit breathing and digestion.

Fig. 15.5

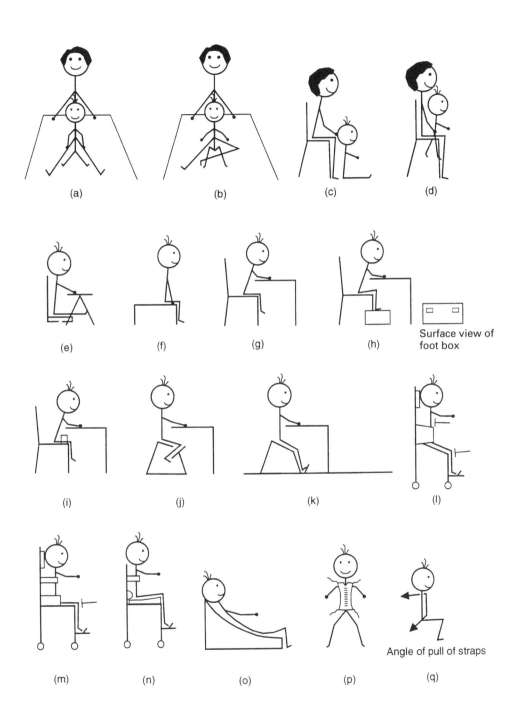

(a) (b) (c) (d)

(e) (f) (g) (h) Surface view of foot box

(i) (j) (k) (l)

(m) (n) (o) (p) Angle of pull of straps (q)

Fig. 15.5

STANDING

Why stand? Because the position encourages:

1.   An extended weight bearing posture.
2.   Frees the hands for play.
3.   Allows the child to participate in activities with other standing children.
4.   Weight bearing which provides proprioceptive input to the joints.

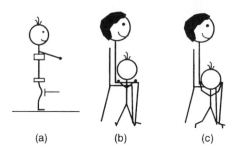

(a)   (b)   (c)

(a)   Commercially available frames with hip, knee and trunk support – the knees are held in slight flexion.
(b)   Using adult support – toys can be played with on an adult's lap.
(c)   Kneeling at an adult's legs.

Fig. 15.6

Equipment provision

The following points need to be considered before using any equipment.

1.   Handle the child first to find the best position to align pelvis, trunk and head as well as promoting active balance in trunk and neck before trying any activity.
2.   Is the equipment necessary and why is it being provided?
3.   Is the equipment placing the child in a comfortable, functional position allowing him to experience normal movement and posture?
4.   Can their hands come forward for play while the head remains in midline?
5.   Is the equipment clean, safe and stable? Are there siblings who may interfere with knobs, velcro fastenings or castors?
6.   Is it duplicating another provision?
7.   Is there space in the child's room or classroom?
8.   Are parents/carers aware of why the equipment has been provided and are they fully trained in its use?
9.   Can the equipment/position be tried out for a period of time to avoid expensive mistakes?

WORK SURFACES

Work surfaces are integral parts of most commercially available specialised chairs. Surface heights can vary depending on the needs of the child. For example, higher ones encourage the child to have a more extended posture and provide more stability to the trunk, and lower ones encourage greater use of the hands allowing weight bearing through the arms and reduce hyperextension of the trunk.

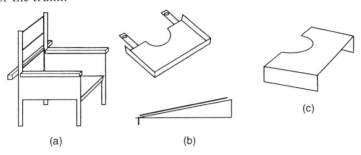

(a)

(b)

(c)

(a)   A tray added to a regular chair using a strut screwed to the back. Check the stability of the chair and tray before issuing.

(b)   Angling the work surface encourages a more upright posture but the child will stand out in the classroom as being different. It also takes a great deal of desk space. A metal board and a ruler with magnetic strips is useful for children who cannot hold a ruler still to draw a line.

(c)   A low table for floor play.

Fig. 15.7

Daily skills

Eating. Ideally, as soon as the child is able and the parents feel ready, they should be encouraged to eat sitting in a chair preferably at a dining table. Sitting offers a position which encourages the child to feel more actively involved with eating and it frees one parent from holding him, thus allowing more family orientated meals.

Careful investigation should take place if there are concerns about feeding. Mealtimes can be stressful and time consuming because of the child's difficulties. Some Child Development Centres organise feeding clinics run by local experts. These provide comprehensive assessment and can refer on to other professionals for further investigations and intervention if necessary.

Toiletting. A child cannot be trained until:

(a)   developmentally ready;

(b)   the child (and family) is motivated to learn; and

(c)   the child is secure in seating with feet well supported.

Grab bars and fold-down rails are useful for older children, providing they do not inhibit access. Moulded seats, specialist commodes, training seats and

STABILITY BARS

Why use stability bars? Because a child can grasp this to maintain trunk stability. The position, angle and length of the bar will vary according to the child's needs.

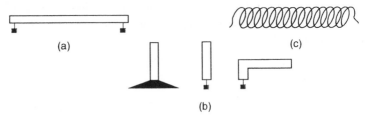

(a)
(b)
(c)

(a)   Across a tray – can be held by one or two hands in a pronated grasp. It does, however, get in the way of work.

(b)   Single bars held to a table by suckers or screws. The child holds this using a semipronated grasp. They are easier to use, providing the child can hold them, because they do not obstruct the child's work.

(c)   Elastic bungicord – a more mobile position so avoiding increasing tone in arms.

Fig. 15.8

footstools are all commercially available. A child may also be trained using a timed toiletting programme, for example placed on the toilet every 2 hours.

Bathing. If bathtime is fun then the bath is a great place to encourage play. Nevertheless, under all circumstances the bath needs to be warm and the child safe, secure and supervised. A variety of specialist seats are available although some require a great deal of water in the bath and a hoist may be necessary for the older child. A shallow bath placed over the existing family one reduces the need for the parents to lean over a bath to wash a child, although storage can be a problem. A thermostatically controlled shower is useful for older children, but careful consideration must be given regarding the shower tray or specialist floor covering and the position of rails, bars and seat.

Dressing/undressing.[27] Children with any form of balance problem need encouragement to sit to dress and use loose-fitting clothes. Backward chaining is a useful behavioural tool to teach dressing along with visual cues, such as labels and the position of pictures and pockets for those who have difficulty getting clothes on the right way round. Other children need a strict structure and routine to enable them to concentrate sufficiently to complete the task. Children who need to sit for long periods of time will be more comfortable wearing natural fibres, as they absorb moisture.

Sleeping. Like everything else the child and the family's needs regarding sleep will vary and similarly the consequent solution. Some families find high-sided travelling cots or beds useful. Others use commercially available harnesses which once strapped to the bed allow the child to sit up but not stand, and some children need specialist mattresses or sheepskins. Placing the mattress on the floor may be all that is necessary for a child who will not stay in bed!

Handwriting.[28,29] This is one of the most precise tasks the hand performs and therefore careful preparation is necessary to achieve a successful end result. Before a child can write or draw he will need to be able to sit correctly, use his hands for co-ordinated activity, and be aware of perceptual concepts such as space, direction, shape and form constancy. The child will need to know how to construct a shape from several parts as well as be motivated to develop the skill.

A child may be experimenting with random marks and scribbles from as early as 15 months of age and should be encouraged to do so, for drawing allows them to refine the movements of their hands; experiment with various grips and different drawing media. They need to have fun making patterns and shapes, and should be encouraged to develop these creatively. Also, a child learning from a variety of sensory experiences such as drawing in sand or shaving foam, finger painting, using large rollers or paint brushes and streamers to make shapes in the air, will be well prepared to use a pencil for handwriting in a classroom having had a wealth of prewriting activity which has refined his gross and fine motor movements.

To conclude, the therapist's involvement in a child and the family's life is varied, but nevertheless she must remain available for support and direction and accept the challenges, pleasures and heartaches that this may bring. The therapist needs to be aware of what the local community will provide relating to information, support and practical resources for the child and his parents, and as a consequence complement and work alongside them, thus giving the child a comprehensive plan of care.

References

1. *The Children Act 1989*, NAPOT, London: College of Occupational Therapy, 1992.
2. Department of Health, *An introduction to the Children Act 1989*, London: HMSO, 1991.
3. *Joint Policies and Procedures for the Protection of Children*, Issued by Norfolk Area Child Protection Committee, 1992.
4. Joint Circular 1/83 (Department of Education and Science), Health Circular HC (83)3, Local Authority Circular LAC (83)2, Department of Health and Social Security, 1983.
5. NAPOT, *The 1981 Education Act: Contributing to statements of special educational need guidelines for occupational therapists*, London: College of Occupational Therapy, 1988.

6. *You can help*, London: Preschool Playgroups Association, 1985.

7. Cogher, L., Savage, E. and Smith, M. *Cerebral Palsy, the Child and Young Person*, London: Chapman and Hall, 1992.

8. Bobath, K. *A Neurophysiological Basis for the Treatment of Cerebral Palsy*, Oxford: Spastics International Medical Publications, 1980.

9. Levitt, S. *Treatment of Cerebral Palsy and Motor Delay*, Oxford: Blackwell Scientific Publications, 1983.

10. Bobath, K. and Bobath, B. *Motor Development in the Different Types of Cerebral Palsy*, London: Heinemann Medical Books, 1987.

11. Forfar, J.O. and Anrell, G.C. *Textbook of Paediatrics*, Edinburgh: Churchill Livingstone, 1984.

12. Bleck, E.E. and Nagel, D.A. *Physically Handicapped Children – A Medical Atlas for Teachers*, New York: Grune and Stratton, 1981.

13. Gordon, N. and McKinlay, I. *Helping Clumsy Children*, Edinburgh: Churchill Livingstone, 1980.

14. *Praxia Makes Perfect*, produced by the Dyspraxia Trust, PO Box 1270, Gerrards Cross, Bucks, 1991.

15. Clancy, H. and Clark, M. *Occupational Therapy with Children*, Melbourne: Churchill Livingstone, 1990.

16. Scrutton, D. *Management of the Motor Disorders of Children with Cerebral Palsy – Clinics in Developmental Medicine*, London: Spastics International Medical Publications No. 90, 1984.

17. Ayres, J. *Sensory Integration and the Child*, California: Sensory Integration International, 1989.

18. Penso, D. *Occupational Therapy for Children with Disabilities*, London: Croom Helm, 1987.

19. Lear, R. *Play Helps*, London: Heinemann, 1980.

20. Cooke, J. and Williams, D. *Working with Children's Language*, Oxford: Winslow Press, 1991.

21. Finie, N. *Handling the Young Cerebral Palsied Child at Home*, Oxford: Heinemann Medical Books, 1990.

22. Mulcahy, C. An approach to the assessment of sitting ability for the prescription of seating, *British Journal of Occupational Therapy*, Vol. 49(11), 1986.

23. Mulcahy, C.M. and Pountney, T.E. The sacral pad - description of its clinical use in seating, *Physiotherapy*, Vol. 72(9), 1986.

24. Stewart, P. and McQuilton, G. Straddle seating for the cerebral palsied child, *British Journal of Occupational Therapy*, Vol. 50(4), 1987.

25. Wisbech, A. *Positions for Play*, London: Play matters/National Toy Libraries Association, 1982.

26. Cotton, E. *The Basic Motor Pattern*, London: The Spastics Society, 1994.

27. Klein, M. *Pre-dressing skills*, Tuscon, Arizona: Communication Skill Builders, 1983.

28. Klein, M. *Pre-writing Skills*, Tuscon, Arizona: Communication Skill Builders, 1982.

29. Sasson, R. *Handwriting, the Way to Teach it*, Cheltenham: Stanley Thornes, 1990.

Further reading

Chisholm, J. A rising hazard, *Paediatric Nursing*, vol. 2 No. 9, November 1990.

Erhardt, R.P. *Developmental Hand Dysfunction*, Maryland: Ramsco Publishing, 1982.

Equipment for Disabled People – Children with Disabilities, London: The Disability Information Trust, 1993.

Fink, B. *Sensory Motor Integration Activities*, Tuscon, Arizona: Therapy Skill Builders, 1989.

Levitt, S. *Paediatric Developmental Therapy*, Oxford: Blackwell Scientific Publications, 1986.

Morris, S. and Klein, M. *Pre-feeding Skills*, Tuscon, Arizona: Therapy Skill Builders, 1987.

Richardson, A. and Wisbeach, A. *I Can Use My Hands*, London: The Toy Libraries Association, 1976.

Warner, J. *Helping the Handicapped Child with Early Feeding*, Oxford: Winslow Press, 1984.

Useful addresses

NAPOT (National Association of Paediatric Occupational Therapists), c/o College of Occupational Therapy, 6–8 Marshalsea Road, Southwark, London SE1 1HL.

APCP (Association of Paediatric Chartered Physiotherapists), c/o Chartered Society of Physiotherapy, 14 Bedford Row, London WC1R 4ED.

LDA, Duke Street, Wisbech, Cambs.

Nfer-Nelson, Darville House, 2 Oxford Road East, Windsor, Berks SL4 1DF.

Psychological Corporation, Footscray High Street, Sidcup, Kent DA14 5HP.

Psycholocial and Educational Publications Inc., 1477 Rollins Road, Burlingame, California, 94010–2316, USA.

Chapter 16

The challenges of community integration for people with learning difficulties

JANE DOLAN
*Senior Occupational Therapist, Richmond, Twickenham and Roehampton Health-
care NHS Trust*

Confusion over terminology around this client group continues, but the term
'learning disabilities' used by the Department of Health and adopted by the
Occupational Therapy National Learning Disabilities Special Interest Group
in 1991 will be used throughout this chapter.

Community care for people with learning disabilities

Community care for this group of people was first discussed by the Royal
Commission on the law relating to mental illness and deficiency (1954–7),[1]
and the debate and question of the effectiveness and necessity of institutional
care has continued for more than 30 years with the publication of various
documents advocating community care. *Better Services for the Mentally
Handicapped*, published by the Department of Health and Social Security in
1971[2] began to effect the change from institutional to community care, and
more recently the Griffiths Report (1988),[3] the government's White Paper,
Caring for People (1989)[4] and the National Health Service and Community
Care Act 1989[5] have attempted to make a reality of the implementation of
community care for many people, including those with learning disabilities.
Many of the old institutions are now closed or in the process of closing, and it
is widely recognised that service providers should be working towards developing services that recognise the rights of people with learning disabilities
to live as full and valued a life as possible within the local community.

Philosophy/value base

In the early 1970s the term normalisation was used by Wolfensburger[6] to
describe his ideals of people with learning disabilities living within ordinary
communities benefiting from normal daily routines and participating in
normal community activities with the same rights as anyone else. However,

the term normalisation was frequently misinterpreted as the need to make people normal using no specialist services, and consequently in 1972 Wolfensburger redefined normalisation as Social Role Valorisation (SRV) in order to avoid further confusion and encompass the necessity of valued social roles via the enhancement of people's social images and personal competencies. The principles of Social Role Valorisation advocate that people with a learning disability have the same rights and needs as the rest of humanity, and demand that they be enabled to live an ordinary life in the community receiving whatever support and assistance they require, and provide the background philosophy for the development of new community-based services.

Professionals and all those involved in care are urged to consider some of the reasons for the low value and expectations society places on people with a learning disability. Restriction of privileges, opportunities, freedom and ordinary expectations of adult life compounded by self-fulfilling prophecies, such as 'the eternal child', all result in perpetuation of the widely held belief that people with a learning disability are deviant, different, difficult and need different forms of care and patterns of life.

The implications of SRV for occupational therapists and others working with people with learning disabilities are clear, and therapists should always consider these when planning any interventions, ensuring that activities or goals selected reflect the normal expectations of other people of the same age, sex and culture. People need special support, not special places, and wherever possible activities should take place in ordinary, easily accessible community facilities where the individual can be given the necessary support to achieve success.

When designing a therapy programme it may help to consider the five accomplishments defined by O'Brien[7] which provide the broad areas in which services should work to enhance the quality of people's lives. The five accomplishments are as follows.

1. *Community presence:* the right to take part in community life, and to live and spend leisure time with other members of the community.
2. *Relationships:* the right to experience valued relationships with non-disabled people.
3. *Choice:* the right to make choices, both large and small in one's life. These choices include where to live and with whom.
4. *Competence:* the right to learn new skills and participate in meaningful activities with whatever assistance is required.
5. *Respect:* the right to be valued and not treated as a second-class citizen.

The multidisciplinary team for people with learning disabilities

In order to ensure that people receive an effective and efficient service many professions and agencies now work as part of multidisciplinary community teams for people with learning disabilities. The benefits of teamwork include the following.

1.   Improved communication leading to consistency of approach, a sharing of knowledge and improved care.
2.   Ease of access for clients and carers who can reach the whole team with one referral.
3.   A broader perspective in care provision.
4.   Mutual support in times of stress.

There is no set formula for the pattern or diversity of professions within a community team for people with learning disabilities (CTPLD). This depends largely on local policy and resources, but it may be multi-agency and include care managers, social workers, community nurses, psychologists, psychiatrists, occupational therapists, speech therapists, dieticians, providers of day and residential services, community support workers and administrators. The new role of care manager advocated by the Griffiths Report[3] has responsibility for ensuring the provision of individual care packages. This includes the assessment of individual need and the design, planning and implementation of the package, monitoring effectiveness and providing support to ensure success. Local authorities have been encouraged to take the lead role in co-ordinating the input of other services into the community care initiatives, and thus the community team may be Social Services-led with social workers often also being given care manager responsibility.

There has been much discussion relating to skill-mix and role blurring as it becomes clear that various professions share some of the same skills or have developed and put into practice some other professions' skills. An occupational therapy skill-mix study by the Kings Fund consortium in 1989[8] states that overlaps in role should be seen as beneficial to the service user, and makes recognition of the essential or core skills or each profession an important issue. Essential skills are those that are central or possibly even unique to the practice of that profession. Clear statements and negotiation of skills, roles, attitudes, knowledge, values and contributions are needed in order to produce the most valuable, efficient and effective service for the individual. Furner[9] defines the role of occupational therapy for people with learning disabilities as being 'an holistic, problem solving approach to facilitate an individual's adaptation to and with his environment by providing functional assessment and treatment in areas of human occupation and their skill components'.

What then are the essential skills of an occupational therapist working with people with learning difficulties? Again, there has been much debate over this and many of the skills identified here are applicable to the whole profession, while being highlighted as being of particular importance within this field.

1. The use of activity for assessment and treatment or intervention is central to the practice of occupational therapy. Whether for assessment or intervention the activity selected should be appropriate to the age, culture and interests of the individual, being carried out in a real and appropriate setting at normal times.

2. Assessment of an individual's functional performance and independence skills identifying and evaluating motor, sensory, cognitive, intrapersonal and interpersonal skills in the areas of self-care, education, domestic skills, leisure, work and community integration.

3. The use of activity to maintain or improve function and quality of life assisting the individual to attain the maximum independence possible within their environment. For some profoundly disabled clients this may be very limited but none the less important, for example, using a simple single-switch environmental control to attract attention or control music.

4. Activity analysis: the breaking down of activities into their physical, cognitive, interpersonal, social, behavioural and emotional components enabling the therapist to identify the various steps and skills that an individual will need to master in order to perform the activity.

5. Problem identification and solving skills: if the individual is unable to achieve the task in its original or usual form, the activity may be changed by adapting the sequence, the teaching method, the equipment, the environment or the client's approach and behaviour.

6. Knowledge of specialist equipment and adaptations that may facilitate participation or independence in a wide range of activities including self-care, mobility, domestic activities, leisure, communication and work.

7. Communication, interpersonal and teaching skills. People learn in many different ways, at different rates, and use different methods to obtain the same goal. Many people with learning disabilities also have limited communication and comprehension skills and the occupational therapist is able to design a programme based around all these factors to facilitate the acquisition or maintenance of skills.

8. The application of a wide spectrum of knowledge concerning medical, social and psychological diagnosis and issues. Many people with a learning disability also have additional physical, sensory and psychological disabilities or handicaps to overcome and the wide scope of occupational therapy training and practice is extremely valuable when assessing, designing programmes and teaching new skills.

Transition from institution to community

One of the first challenges of community care is the transition from institution to successful integrated community living. Occupational therapists are often involved in gathering and providing information to be used in the resettlement process. This may include the following.

1.   Compatibility of proposed groups considering factors of age, friendships, physical abilities, common interests and practical and emotional support needs.
2.   Type of housing required considering individual needs, e.g. physical and sensory disabilities, personal space and location.
3.   Present skill levels of each individual which will affect their support needs, e.g. bathing, dressing, eating and drinking, using the toilet, cooking, shopping, road safety and making simple choices.
4.   Advice on suitable furniture and equipment, e.g. chairs, bathrooms, electrical appliances and safety features or measures to minimise risk.
5.   Assessment and advice on special equipment, e.g. hoists, access for wheelchairs, kitchen design. Checking that equipment is installed correctly and teaching clients and carers how to use it safely.
6.   Transport needs, e.g. garage, parking area with sufficient space for wheelchair access, distance to public transport.
7.   Induction training of the new support team covering a wide range of issues, e.g. lifting and handling, designing training programmes and encouraging participation.

Once profiles of individual and group service needs have been completed, and housing design finalised, occupational therapy staff are often involved in the transition process supporting people emotionally and practically as they move from institution to their new home. In the light of current thinking large old-style institutions may appear forbidding, repressive and isolated, but for some long-stay clients they may represent safety and security; with other residents and staff providing real, valued and indeed possibly the only relationships available. Compliance with a lack of control, privacy, initiative and possessions are common effects of institutionalisation. For the individual who may have little experience or memory of any role other than that of patient, resident or client, and who has had all aspects of his life controlled, there are huge adjustments to make and an enormous range of new roles to understand and explore: as being tenant, housemate, neighbour, citizen.

Areas to consider within the transition process include the following.

1.   New rights and responsibilities, e.g. shared space and domestic tasks; personal space and privacy with respect of these for others; safety, and personal choice.
2.   Acknowledgement that some aspects of the institution will be missed

and consideration of ways in which valued areas can be maintained, e.g. leisure activities, social clubs and links with staff and other residents who will not be moving into the new home.

3.   Building of positive relationships among the new group.

4.   Compilation of life books using photographs and personal stories to ensure that the past is not lost or ignored when people move. These books can also help build positive relationships with new staff members.

5.   Familiarisation with the new home and local area with a gradual introduction if possible.

6.   Participation wherever possible in choosing furnishings, decor and equipment for the new home.

7.   Individuals' current interests, ways of maintaining these and other leisure and employment opportunities in the new area.

Simply living in a house sited within the community does not signify community living, and the client will usually require support accessing local facilities and activities. For some clients this may mean simply providing information about availability, and introducing them to the location, route, formal or informal rules and supporting them in the short term. For others this may mean looking at ways of providing long-term support in order that they might participate in any chosen activity.

Transition is not a process or issue limited to people moving out of hospital. Individuals moving from the parental home, or group home to more independent living, will also require emotional and practical support in order to achieve and enjoy a successful move.

Occupational therapy interventions

Occupational therapy intervention with people with a learning disability living in the community covers many areas, a few examples being:

1.   assessment of functional independence skills to make recommendations about future placement and support needs for individuals wishing to move away from the parental home;

2.   assessment and advice to clients and carers, e.g. aids and adaptations to assist with seating, eating and drinking, lifting and transfers, access, wheelchair kitchens, new housing projects and bathing and personal hygiene;

3.   support and teaching for carers working with individuals who have additional physical or sensory disabilities or challenging behaviours; and

4.   support in accessing local community facilities: this may take the form of advice for carers and support workers or direct intervention with individuals whose behaviour, physical disability or other

problems make community activity and integration potentially difficult.

Programmes can be designed to maintain or improve:

- community living skills;
- road safety, use of public transport;
- personal hygiene;
- kitchen skills;
- domestic skills;
- participation in leisure/social skills;
- self-confidence and social skills;
- work skills;
- self-advocacy;
- personal dignity in public places.

Assessment

There is a wide variety of assessment options, methods and tools available, but before selecting any one, the therapist must first consider the purpose of the assessment and information required; the means of assessment most likely to succeed with the individual; time-scale available and any other constraints that may limit choice.

Various commercially available standardised assessments are used by many occupational therapists as a way of ensuring that a wide range of information is consistently gathered and recorded in a methodical and ordered way. However, this information may then be inaccessible to other professions unfamiliar with the assessment, and therefore usefulness may be limited as to specific skills levels, constraints and support needs of an individual. In order to make information more accessible and tailored to meet the needs of the individual, many therapists use their own checklists and forms to obtain the information required, which can then be used as a basis for a comprehensive report.

Reasons for referral for an occupational therapy assessment may be varied, with the therapist being asked to decide:

1. whether intervention is necessary;
2. whether occupational therapy is the most appropriate form of intervention;
3. the individual's support needs in terms of housing, occupation, leisure and staffing levels to support and facilitate maintenance or improvement of skills and promote quality of life;
4. individual needs for specialist equipment or adaptation;
5. who else might need to be involved; the skills these people would require, and how they might be supported to develop them;
6. priorities of need, and where and when intervention should start;

7.   the individual's potential for learning with the original assessment then being used as a baseline to evaluate future progress.

Assessment can be carried out in a number of ways, with a combination of several often being the most successful.

1.   Direct observation.
2.   Standardised assessments.
3.   Interviews with the client and carers.
4.   Asking carers to record the information using checklists or forms provided by the therapist.

When using any or all of these methods consideration should be given to the effects of the presence of a stranger if the therapist is a new face, and possible constraints or reasons for lack of skill, poor performance or non-compliance. For example, institutional routines which may have limited opportunities for experience, negative expectations of others present during the assessment, or fear and anxiety.

The information contained within an assessment report or profile will vary according to the reasons for referral, but should contain all or some of the following information.

1.   The current situation – where the person lives, who they live with, how they spend their time, how they and others involved feel about all of this.
2.   Reason for referral.
3.   Method used, contributors to, and time-scale of assessment.
4.   Current skills and abilities with any constraints recorded.
5.   Personal strengths, likes, dislikes and motivating factors for the individual.
6.   The individual's thoughts and feelings about the assessment and future goals.

Having completed an assessment the occupational therapist is then able to use this as a basis to make recommendations about the future and any further action required. There will certainly be occasions when these recommendations do not involve further occupational therapy intervention and the individual can be referred to another agency or discharged. Where occupational therapy is considered to be the most appropriate intervention, the therapist should then involve the clients and carers, wherever possible, in decisions about goals, aims and objectives. Many of the tasks traditionally seen within the role of occupational therapy may carry little or no reward for the individual. For example, there seems little intrinsic reward in improving table manners, brushing teeth or learning to get dressed independently. Success is much more likely if the person is enthusiastic and motivated by the task and its end result. Consequently, it may be better to start elsewhere until a good relationship has been built between client and therapist, or look for some way of building in extra rewards.

Teaching new skills

A skill can be defined as 'an ability acquired by training', and in order for the person with a learning disability to acquire a new skill the principles and practice of good training and teaching are essential. When designing a new training or teaching programme the following pointers are useful.

1. Success or acquisition of the skill is not solely the responsibility of the learner. Responsibility lies with the therapist in ensuring that the programme is tailored around individual needs and uses methods most likely to succeed.
2. All people are capable of learning; this does not mean that anybody can be taught anything, but that the therapist must select a suitable activity and design a programme to meet individual need. People with severe learning disabilities can learn fairly complex skills given good teaching and enough time.
3. People should not be excluded on the grounds of behaviour or assumptions about their ability. If the activity is one in which the learner has shown interest, or would benefit from, it may be that the training programme needs to build in more support, change the level of achievement, or change the way in which the activity is usually taught.
4. Using activity analysis the task can then be broken down into a series of steps and sequences. Initially the activity should be taught in a normal sequence using the natural equipment and cues. Specialist adaptations or training methods may be unnecessary and will draw attention, labelling or stigmatising the learner as different. The least conspicuous way will help community integration and acceptance. If this is not successful then adaptations or alterations can be made to the programme using the steps of the task analysis to pinpoint the areas needing change.
5. People with learning disabilities find it difficult to generalise skills by using pieces of information learnt elsewhere and applying them to new areas or tasks. To provide the best chance of success teaching should take place in the same environment and using the same equipment that the learner will eventually use once the skill is acquired. Consequently, role-playing exercises may not be suitable or successful.
6. Success is most likely if the learner is given frequent opportunities to practise. This may mean that the programme should be carried out with a variety of trainers other than the therapist. Steps and se-

quences of the task will need to be recorded clearly with instructions for the trainers about when and how to give prompts and rewards. Record keeping is important and needs to be accurate and consistent in order to help identify success; pinpoint areas of difficulty; demonstrate progress and help make future training decisions. It is tempting to 'help' by doing some of the task, ignoring small mistakes, giving half a tick, or rewarding effort rather than achievement, but it is important that all those involved in the training programme realise that in the long term this does not help the learner and may even place them at risk if the training is stopped early, in the belief that the task has been learnt.

7.   Giving too much information or direction verbally at one time should be avoided as this can be distracting and prevents the learner from focusing on the task. Giving too much praise may also be detrimental in the long term as the learner may come to rely on this rather than the intrinsic reward of successfully completing the activity.

8.   Demonstration is useful to give an initial idea of what the task and its end result look like.

9.   Physical prompts may be less complex and of more use than a whole series of verbal instructions. As the learner becomes more adept at the task these can be reduced from hand-over-hand guidance to a gentle nudge in the right direction, and eventually to a nod or gesture in the air.

10.   People learn more quickly if they get into a rhythm or routine of performing the task. Errorless learning means that the trainer must be near enough to ensure that each step is performed correctly and intervening immediately if the learner is about to make a mistake. This creates a positive learning environment: no one likes to be told 'no'.

11.   If the learner does not succeed the idea should not be abandoned, but teaching methods altered, the task changed in some way, or more support included.

12.   Teaching new skills will not always be limited to the therapist working directly with a person with a learning disability. It may also involve teaching carers more effective ways of working with the individual, or the use and safety of a new piece of equipment.

Maintenance of skills

It is not enough to simply ensure that a new skill is learned and for the therapist to then withdraw. In order to maintain the skill the individual will need regular opportunities to practise it. Within the occupational therapy programme it may be necessary to examine ways of facilitating, supporting or enabling the individual to continue to practise the task once the therapist has closed the case and moved on.

Participation

For some severely disabled clients participation will be much more important than the acquisition of new skills. Participation is doing things with, not for, people and gives severely disabled people a chance to interact with others in meaningful and purposeful ways, creating a more equal balance between carer and client and increasing quality of life. Activities, education and training programmes for people with severe learning disabilities often focus on special equipment or take place in specially designed and designated areas where there is great emphasis on special sensory stimulation. This emphasis on special procedures can mean that individuals continue to be seen as different and childlike, and consequently are given little opportunity to participate in age-appropriate activities that would enable them to live more ordinary and fuller lives within their community. Sensory stimulation is certainly valuable, but can be adapted to encompass age-appropriate, functional activities that relate directly to the client's life at home and in the community.

Participation means that even though the individual will never be independent at the task, they are given whatever support is needed and are fully included throughout the activity by watching and participating in various steps, using physical help, specialised equipment and engagement procedures. For example, many people with a severe learning disability may never prepare a meal for themselves, but will enjoy participating in meal preparation by: making choices about the menu; selecting and fetching ingredients from around the kitchen; smelling and tasting various ingredients as they are used; stirring, chopping and measuring; using the oven timer and watching kitchen activity. Many tasks involving the use of electrical equipment can be accessed using simple switches which can be linked to any appliance, thus allowing people with only limited movement or motor control to turn their washing on, chop the vegetables or turn on the light. The steps involved in washing up and putting away crockery and cutlery include many of the activities that might be seen in traditional, but separate 'sensory stimulation' programmes, such as: water play, a variety of colours, shapes, sizes and textures and plenty of opportunities to practise sorting and stacking.

Occupational therapy intervention may take the form of working with carers to demonstrate ways of including these people in many everyday activities that have hitherto been done for them as they have been seen as too difficult, too dangerous, or simply as easier for the carer to do alone. By using a very simple plan where activities of daily life are broken down into their component steps, using the principles of task analysis, the therapist can identify in which steps the individual may be able to participate, what equipment is required and how much assistance is needed. Remaining steps can then be identified as needing to be done solely by the person assisting. Within each step it will be necessary to specify strategies and techniques for introducing the task, engaging the person in the task, minimising unwanted or negative behaviours and inhibiting spasticity and promoting co-ordination, body awareness and motor control through good positioning and use of specialist equipment.

As people frequently use a wide variety of different services, such as special care units, respite care facilities and home-based care, it is important to ensure that all staff are made aware of any programme being used and its progress, thus giving maximum opportunities to practise, participate and enjoy new and familiar tasks.

Evaluation

All occupational therapy intervention should be evaluated and updated regularly. In order to ensure that occupational therapy is available to as many individuals as possible it will be necessary to make decisions about the length of involvement, case closure and future recommendations or possibilities for the individual. This will be made easier if clear aims and objectives are made at the beginning of intervention. The occupational therapist will never 'cure' anyone of a learning disability, but it is possible to close a particular piece of work having enabled the individual to improve their skills in a particular area, or having facilitated an ongoing programme of support which can be passed onto other carers enabling that person to participate in an activity or task.

Evaluation may incorporate the use of quality standards, peer audit and client or customer satisfaction surveys.

References

1. *Report of the Royal Commission on Mental Illness and Mental Deficiency*, London: HMSO, 1957.
2. Department of Health and Social Security, *Better Services for the Mentally Handicapped*, London: HMSO, 1971.
3. Griffiths, R. *Community Care: Agenda for Action*, London: HMSO, 1989.
4. *Caring for People: Community Care for the Next Decade*, London: HMSO, 1989.
5. *National Health Service and Community Care Act*, London: HMSO, 1989.
6. Wolfensburger, W. *The Principle of Normalisation in Human Services*, Toronto: Canadian National Institute for the Mentally Retarded, 1972.
7. O'Brien, J. *The Principle of Normalization: a Foundation for Effective Services*, London: Campaign for Mental Handicap, 1981.
8. Kings Fund consortium, *Occupational Therapy Skill Mix Study*, London: Kings Fund, 1989.
9. Furner, L. *British Association of Occupational Therapists Reference Book, 1988*, London: BAOT/Parke Sutton Publishing, 1988.

Further reading

Bracegirdle, H. Occupational therapy with mentally handicapped people, *British Journal of Occupational Therapy*, Vol. 50(10), 1987.

Brown, H. and Benson, S. (eds) *A Practical Guide to Working with People with Learning Disabilities*, London: Hawker Publications, 1992.

Clarke, D. *Mentally Handicapped People: Living and Learning*, Ballière Tindall, 1986.

Compton, A. and Ashwin, M. *Community Care For Health Professionals*, Oxford: Butterworth-Heinemann, 1992.

Fraser, W., MacGilveray, R. and Green, A. (eds) *Hallas Textbook for the Mentally Handicapped*, London: Butterworth-Heinemann, 1991.

Garnham-Hooper, L. *British Association of Occupational Therapists Reference Book 1992*, London: BAOT/Parke Sutton Publishing, 1992.

Harris, J. (ed.) *Innovations and Educating Children with Severe Learning Difficulties*, Chorley, Lancashire: Brothers of Charity.

Isaac, D. *Community Occupational Therapy with Mentally Handicapped Adults*, London: Chapman and Hall, 1990.

Kings Fund consortium, *An ordinary life: comprehensive locally based residential services for mentally handicapped people*, London: Kings Fund, 1982.

Renton, L. Occupational therapy core skills in mental handicap: a review of the literature, *British Journal of Occupational Therapy*, Vol. 55(11), 1992.

Stewart, A. EDURP, mental handicap project, *British Journal of Occupational Therapy*, Vol. 49(4), 1986.

Sutton, E. (ed.) *Older Adults with Developmental Disabilities: Optimizing Choice and Change*, Baltimore: Paul H. Brookes Publishing, 1993.

Thorner, S. The essential skills of an occupational therapist, *British Journal of Occupational Therapy*, Vol. 54(6), 1991.

Wilson, M. *Occupational Therapy in Long Term Psychiatry*, Edinburgh: Churchill Livingstone, 1983.

Working for Patients, London: HMSO, 1989.

Chapter 17

The head injured adult

AMANDA J. COUSINS
Co-ordinator, Norwich Head Injury Project

Head injury or traumatic brain injury (TBI) is a common problem and is mainly caused by road traffic accidents, falls, assaults, workplace accidents and sporting activities such as horse riding. A wide variety of problems can follow injury including physical, sensory, cognitive and behavioural, resulting in disabilities which benefit from occupational therapy intervention.

Britain has a population of up to 70 000 disabled survivors of brain injury, most of whom have a normal life expectancy,[1] with the majority ultimately being cared for at home by families and friends.[2] However, those who are more severely disabled may require long-term nursing care in hospital, younger disabled units or specialist nursing homes for young adults. A few patients in each health district survive in what is called persistent vegetative states (PVS) or in a permanent coma. Often these patients never leave hospital or nursing home care although a few have been successfully managed at home with a well-supported and dedicated family.

Head injured people are statistically most likely to be young men. For many, a severe head injury results in shattered dreams and aspirations, as they find themselves having to deal with complex problems and permanent severe disability. In the long term head injured people have to rebuild their lives and re-establishing social and family relationships which, while important, can be difficult.[3] Families with young children are seen as particularly vulnerable as the needs of a head injured parent compete with those of the children.

The problems of head injured people and the lack of specialist services for this group have been well documented. The Royal College of Physicians,[4] the Royal College of Psychiatrists[5] and the British Society for Rehabilitation Medicine[1] have all produced reports on the severity of this problem. Head injury problems are not limited only to those clinically defined as severely head injured, for people with seemingly mild injury have been shown to experience measurable neuropsychological deficits and problems which can severely impair their ability to return to work.[6] Post concussional syndrome

(PCS), as it is sometimes known, is a recognised diagnosis with a range of symptoms including headaches, fatigue, memory problems, inability to concentrate, emotional lability and loss of drive.[7] People with minor head injury often show great insight into their poor performance but little understanding of the reasons for it. The anxiety, frustration and anger caused by their failure to return to work can be great and cause depression, irritability and emotional burn-out. Given early advice and support these individuals can do well and often make a good recovery, although in some cases it may take several months.

All head injured people have unique combinations of disability, social circumstances, premorbid personality and environmental factors. For a therapist, head injured people can pose a fascinating challenge requiring multidisciplinary co-operation to enable them to achieve their maximum potential.

The head injury rehabilitation team

Many health districts now employ head injury care co-ordinators or specialist care managers. These care co-ordinators organise and oversee the care of head injured people in the early stages; advising on early management, care plans, rehabilitation and community reintegration.

The team involved with the patient may be a combination of the therapists working within a specialist brain injury team together with local community and/or hospital-based therapists. The team frequently consists of any combination of the following, as available:

care co-ordinator,	occupational therapist,	physiotherapist,
speech therapist,	social worker,	psychologist,
community nursing,	dietitian,	technician,
medical consultant or general practitioner,		home care,
HEADWAY support staff and volunteers.		

When treating patients who have behavioural problems in the community it is often difficult to co-ordinate activities and ensure consistent approaches. The use of client-held multidisciplinary records has been used in some cases to good effect. Regular team reviews are essential to establish consistent goals for all treating an individual and to help form positive coping strategies where needed.

The determined strategies for dealing with cognitive and behavioural problems should be understood and reinforced by all team members and taught to the family, as teamwork is essential.

The National Head Injuries Association (HEADWAY) has made enormous strides in improving support services for head injured people. They offer support through meetings and groups and may provide day care, sheltered workshops or drop-in centres in some local districts. Some HEADWAY groups employ welfare workers who act as advocates and providers of information for those injured and their families.

The problems of head injured people

Head injuries produce infinite combinations of a wide range of impairments including the following.

1. *Physical impairments:* paralysis, increased spasticity, sensory loss including the ability to taste and smell, visual disturbances, visual loss, tremor; loss of co-ordination, communication skills, and swallowing ability.

2. *Cognitive impairments:* amnesia and memory problems, disorientation, perceptual disorders, difficulty in thinking, planning and sequencing, learning deficits.

3. *Behavioural and emotional problems* including uninhibited or inappropriate social behaviour, loss of emotions, aggression, anxiety, lability, irritability and restlessness, apathy and loss of drive.

The most troublesome group of problems to deal with in the long term is often seen as the behavioural and emotional ones.[8]

The assessment of people with severe head injury

Assessment should be a multidisciplinary process. The occupational therapist has a vital role in this by assessing the impact of physical, cognitive and behavioural disability on the individual's ability to perform and function within their given environment and previously held roles. However, in order to complete an overall picture, assessments must be made alongside other team members, with information gathered from the patient, family and others who are important to the patient. Gaining a true picture of family relationships and a patient's past life and personality, may be difficult and take time to piece together for it takes time for people to open up and be able to give very personal and accurate information to a therapist. Developing relationships and building trust between families and the therapy team is not only an important first step, but essential if very difficult issues are to be faced as time progresses. For example, a spouse may find that he can no longer relate to his head injured partner or cope with her behaviour and consequently may want a separation. Both parties need support to get through that difficult time.

Assessment of skills and the coping mechanisms used are important to record. Basic information required includes: a detailed social history with analysis of relationships; record of pre-accident health; employment; personality traits; roles and previously held responsibilities; hobbies and interests. Such information gathering is crucial to understanding the way the individuals and their family may react to severe trauma and the way they develop coping mechanisms.[9] Radical changes in personality following a head injury can change relationships between patient and family members and those with very fixed roles of homemaker or breadwinner may find the inability to resume those roles very difficult, resulting in negative feelings of self-worth. The occupational therapist will therefore not only need to be concerned with improvement of function on a number of levels, but encourage positive attitudes and help to build up confidence.

Assessment of confusion and disorientation/post-traumatic amnesia

Post-traumatic amnesia (PTA)

What is it?	PTA describes the state which patients experience before regaining reliable short-term recall and continuous memory. Some patients do, however, suffer from permanent amnesic states in which they never score within normal ranges. The longer PTA lasts the more severe the brain injury is seen to be.
How to measure it.	The most common method is with the Galveston Orientation and Amnesia test (GOAT).[10] This gives a series of simple questions that test memory function. Other tests are also available.[11]
How to deal with it.	Orientate the patient as much as possible to time, place and person with clocks and reminders.
	Give clear short instructions and allow time for responses.
	Keep the session short with much reassurance, especially if the head injured person becomes agitated.
	In the early stages, rest and quiet is often the best remedy, and regular rest periods, structured during the day, avoid increasing fatigue.

Cognitive problems following head injury

What is it?	This is a problem of disordered thinking which may occur after head injury. Cognitive or communication problems can make people appear confused and disorientated.
How to test.	Many therapists use a mini-mental state test[12,13] to assess general orientation and the level of confusion. They need to work with a speech and language therapist to ensure that expressive and receptive language problems are identified, if they exist. Practical problems caused by the patient's head injury need to be highlighted and explored as to whether they are the outcome of resulting cognitive, attention, concentration, memory or communication problems.

How to deal with it.   Orientate the patient to time, place and person with each session. Habit-train personal care routines and be consistent.
Explain things carefully, slowly and simply.
Do not rush the patient for answers to questions but give time for thought and the reply.

Assessment of a patient's level of insight

It is extremely difficult to work with an individual who does not appreciate that changes have occurred as a result of the head injury and that they have a problem. Families faced with an irrational member who does not appreciate that they are behaving abnormally find life particularly stressful. In such cases the family become very much the focus for care and support and need to be engaged in a programme of rehabilitation in which they are often the main facilitators. Coping strategies and teaching relatives how to help the patient recognise their problems without confrontation, and making the patient feel persecuted, are difficult. How much a therapist can achieve depends on previous family relationships and strengths, the nature of the patient's problems and its effect on their ability to cope.

Communication and interaction skills. Head injured people may display a whole range of levels in communication, from some very basic displays of frustration through biting and screaming to minimal levels of expressive dysphasia. The ability for a patient to express feelings and frustrations and understand incoming communication is important to achieve, even on a very basic level. Pictures, symbols and signing are one means of helping to improve basic levels of communication.

It is important for the occupational therapist to establish a basic level of communication with the patient through touch and tone of voice, if necessary. Visual demonstration of activities and assisted movement sometimes work with a very impaired patient to get the required response.

As patients are discharged home the occupational therapist may need to develop strategies for coping with communication difficulties in the home and workplace.

Memory and learning difficulties. Head injured people commonly suffer from a wide range of memory problems. Some lose blocks of long-term memory which can be filled in by relatives and friends, to some extent, who can tell them what happened in the past. It can take some time for them to realise that they have lost these memories and, as a result, they can become devastated. For example they only find out they are divorced by asking where their wife is.

Difficulties in recall, retaining and storing information in learning processes are more difficult to overcome. A few patients suffer from very severe memory impairment and have no recall at all and start each day not knowing who or where they are. Trained therapists can assess memory function deficits using standardised memory testing, commonly in a joint assessment with a clinical psychologist.

Mood and motivation levels. A severely head injured person will often experience great feelings of loss, anger, guilt, frustration and deep depression. In some cases, where insight is lacking the patient will set totally inappropriate goals for themselves and present as excitable, restless individuals. Moods and motivation levels may change significantly as they progress through time. Initially there can be euphoria at having survived a potentially lethal accident; then motivation is often high to effect a fast return to normal. When people fail to recover this starts a slow and often painful period of adjustment and acceptance which depends much on the individual patient. Many younger patients go through periods of denial, anger and depression and their motivation for treatment can vary accordingly. Token systems and positive rewards for progress can help to motivate and focus some individuals but this can be difficult to introduce into a home situation.

Behavioural problems. Therapists need to work with families to identify changes in an individual's behaviour compared to premorbid levels. The most usual behaviours to assess are as follows.

Social and sexual behaviour.	Inappropriate touching, loss of social skills, e.g. manners, inappropriate conversation, inappropriate sexual behaviour.
Aggression and irritability.	Rages and temper tantrums, physical or verbal aggression.
Apathy and lack of drive.	The loss of ability to perform tasks not because they are unable to do them physically, but because they cannot initiate the task. Some individuals become exhausted, apathetic and will in consequence neglect themselves completely.

Assessment of concentration and distractibility

In the early stages very short concentration spans are evident. The length of time can be measured by observation during therapy and assessment sessions. Patients unable to concentrate become distracted, give up, become irritated or switch off. Concentration often improves slowly and then motivation takes over and rules the length of time an individual will persist with an activity.

Head injured people do find it difficult to concentrate selectively on one thing and may find group work or treatment in a busy environment difficult.

Patients who are distractible and lack concentration find it difficult to complete activities successfully at home. Initially one-to-one activities are often the answer, starting with short activity sessions and gradually building on these.

Working towards independent self-care

General head injury assessments of basic levels of functioning can be used, such as the Disability Rating Scale which looks at a range of items including the cognitive ability to perform tasks and employability.[14] Many now use standardised activities measures, including the Functional Activities Measure (FAM),[15] the extended ADL scale[16] or the Barthel Index.[17] Scales can be helpful to engage patients actively in discussions about their problems and if repeated over periods of time can illustrate improvements and set ongoing goals. Most standardised assessments, however, should not be used in isolation but accompanied by other information and observations.

When assessing someone at home for the first time a therapist needs to note and observe how the head injured patient and their families cope. This includes such things as acceptance of the accident itself, the willingness of all family members to adapt to the needs of the head injured person and the strategies which have developed to deal with any problems. People can become extremely bitter about what has happened, caught up in court proceedings and compensation. Difficult feelings can be stirred up and need to be worked through. Some families encounter enormous difficulties, with parents and partners at loggerheads and family infighting occurring over the perceived needs of a particularly severely head injured individual. Counselling skills are needed in dealing with such situations, which may be prolonged.

Occupational therapy for head injured adults living at home

Occupational therapy can be seen within four key areas.

1. Independence and life skills training.
2. Assessment for aids, equipment wheelchairs and seating systems.
3. Working with families and developing strategies for behavioural modification and ways of coping.
4. Life planning, exploring long-term opportunities for leisure, employment and in extending home-based activities.

The fields of independence and life skills training, and the assessment for equipment and wheelchairs, are common to the treatment of all groups with physical disability, and the occupational therapy skills of analysis and problem solving apply. Encouraging independence with positive feedback and rewards for appropriate efforts are also the same as for clients who have some forms of learning difficulty.

Working with head injured people and their families

The occupational therapist, together with other team members, needs to develop the skill of working with families, for being able to help them to develop coping strategies when the patient returns home is important. The costs to carers in choosing to care for their loved one at home can be emotional, physical as well as financial and therefore families need a great deal of support from health and Social Services, voluntary agencies and others to succeed.

Working particularly with colleagues in clinical psychology and speech therapy is crucial. Head injured people are often discharged home after long periods of in-patient hospital care and rehabilitation may have taken years. Old relationships need to be renewed and in some cases rediscovered. Discharge from hospital should, in the ideal world, be a gradual, carefully planned process observing the hospital's discharge planning guidelines and protocols. Trial placements at home prior to discharge can be very beneficial, especially as home care for some simply may not work. There are important considerations when working with families for a successful return to home.

1.   An honest and open relationship between therapist and family members.
2.   Families need support and care in their own right with opportunities for respite and consideration of their own needs.
3.   Families need education and training to look after their head injured member and contribute to their rehabilitation.
4.   All need information and be enabled to make their own choices. The use of independent advocates can be one solution to ensure that their interests are upheld.

Developing management strategies

It is crucial that the family is involved with the behavioural management and retraining of appropriate social behaviour. Occupational therapists and clinical psychologists working together need to identify strategies to keep a patient's behaviour within acceptable limits for life at home. Families need to have some understanding of the underlying trigger mechanisms which may increase the level of inappropriate behaviour such as frustration, anxiety, anger, fatigue, attention seeking, depression or a patient's misinterpretation of given cues. For some, it is as if the social rule book has been lost: such as the lessons learned as a child about what behaviour is tolerated. An adult having to regain those skills from the beginning has a hard task. However, through role play, discussion, experience and talking through a situation many can relearn the skills. Families are crucial in helping them to relearn behaviours and social skills; however, the family with internal problems can exacerbate it. Positive rewards and encouragement for controlled behaviour can work well. When they display unacceptable behaviour, 'time out' – that is, where he is left alone in a safe environment until he calms down – can be used effectively.

All individuals form coping strategies for dealing with emotional difficult-ies and the frustrations which life presents, and many head injured people appear to carry these strategies over post-injury. The post-traumatic coping strategies are often dependent on the cerebral damage which dictates the sophistication of the coping strategy; mental trauma caused by the accident; environmental factors; the social structure within which the individual inter-acts; and the premorbid personality.

Providing long-term emotional support for head injured patients and their families

Partners may need someone to talk to about very personal issues around the reforming of relationships and their ability to cope with the changes which a head injury may have brought about. This requires the forming of a relation-ship with one or other member of the team selected usually by the relative themselves, with whom they feel comfortable. Opportunities for carer coun-selling should be defined to tackle all sorts of issues which may cause enormous problems if left unresolved. Other agencies, such as Relate and HEADWAY, may be able to offer help to individual partners.

Other emotional support can be given in arranging regular breaks and respite. This may include any of a number of options dependent on local availability.

Training and education for carers of head injured people

Carers need training and support to enable them to cope with the demands of their head injured family member. Training may be needed to help them understand the problems experienced by the head injured person and a great deal of therapist time is often spent in this. There are a number of good books written for families[18,19] which can help them to learn to become extremely expert in the care of their loved ones. Training in the use of equipment, lifting and handling techniques and the use of communication aids is vital. Nursing skills such as monitoring fluid intake, gastrostomy feeding, bathing and catheter management is possible with the help of training from the nursing services. All is possible for families to take on if they so wish.

Exploring respite options

Opportunities for a break from caring are important and families should not feel guilty if they need to take one. Options need to be explored with the patient's GP, social worker and care manager, if they have one. These could include the following.

1.   Sharing care within the wider family.
2.   Home-based respite, such as Crossroads schemes, Night nursing/home care input to give carers a good night's sleep, voluntary services befriending schemes.
3.   Day care, such as activity centres; HEADWAY houses; Social Services day care facilities.
4.   In-patient respite within a younger disabled unit or other independent sector respite provision.
5.   Holiday schemes and outward bound courses for disabled people.

Case study: Martin

Martin, a 30-year-old builder, fell 14 feet while fixing his own garage roof and sustained a severe head injury, with post-traumatic amnesia lasting 4 days. He was treated on a general surgical ward and discharged home after 10 days. Martin developed post-traumatic epilepsy, which responded well to treatment. The community occupational therapist was called in to see Martin to help with his continued problems.

Social situation

He lives with his wife and two young children aged 18 months and 4 years. His wife Jayne works part time as a secretary. They have regular contact with Jayne's parents.

Head injury problems

On Assessment. Mobility – independent in getting around with no dizziness or instability.
Self-care – independent with prompting.
Communication – talked a great deal, but did not always follow through a conversation as his concentration failed. He changed subjects rapidly, repeated himself and when stressed became verbally aggressive, swearing and shouting.
Driving – unable due to epilepsy, short term.
Cognitive problems – Martin found it very difficult to concentrate for longer than 10 minutes. His memory showed some deficits in short-term recall, particularly with retaining verbal instructions. He would not remember things and became anxious and agitated when he felt he was being made to look foolish.
Martin's thinking was often disjointed. He could not cope with problem-solving situations or planning.
Behaviour – Martin was restless and sleeping badly. He complained of feeling exhausted but was unable to 'switch off'. He was often seen pacing around the house or garden and becoming increasingly short-

tempered. He could not tolerate the noise the children made and Jayne was worried that they were making him worse.

Emotional status – Martin was frustrated, depressed and agitated, unable to understand his problems and felt the whole world had gone mad. Jayne felt stuck in the middle with the needs of the children on one side and Martin on the other. She felt lost in dealing with his restless and demanding behaviour, which she also failed to understand. Jayne and Martin both understood their need for support and help.

Plan. The occupational therapist completed an initial home visit to explore and discuss Martin's problems. She then gained consent from Martin's GP to refer him to a speech and language therapist and a clinical psychologist to form a core team to help Martin to progress.

Aims
- to help Martin understand and control his agitation and restlessness;
- to help him understand and come to terms with his problems;
- to enable him to participate and contribute to his treatment sessions;
- to enable him to maximise his skills and rebuild a life for himself with his family;
- to help Jayne to gain greater understanding of the underlying head injury problems and the coping mechanisms which they could employ to enable them to cope much better.

Action. A therapy programme was established to include the following.

Relaxation sessions – to teach Martin how to consciously unwind and also to provide structured sessions to spend time in the bedroom alone thus giving Jayne a rest.

Simple familiar activities – to establish appropriate planning and problem-solving skills, e.g. doing the washing up, making the bed when he got up from his afternoon rest.

Counselling – explanations of head injury and the problems it causes and the reasons for his agitation. This was done with both Martin and Jayne and notes were taken for Martin to refer to.

Daily plan. The occupational therapist and clinical psychologist worked up a list of strategies for the following.

Coping strategies; for example, becoming agitated – go to bedroom, put on relaxation tapes or do simple deep breathing exercises.

Daily routine of activities with a timetable on the kitchen wall to act as a reminder; a weekly programme of appointments was also put up to make things easy to remember. The daily routine incorporated self-care activities, gentle exercise (a walk in the local park), rest periods with time for a relaxation session to help 'wind down'. It also allowed for helping in the home, starting with some short duration easy tasks and building these up.

Progress. With support Martin regained control and settled down at home,

Jayne learned to drive and returned to work, and the children were cared for at a local nursery while Jayne was at work. This gave Martin space at home to relax alone and complete a set of activities on his own. He progressed enough to feel confident about doing the shopping and going back to see his old workmates. He is currently doing some voluntary work in a storehouse for a charitable agency. His epilepsy made it difficult for him to do his previous job working on ladders and scaffolding, but he hopes to be able to return to some sort of long-term job, possibly in local industry, with the help of the Shaw Trust. Martin has also taken up bowling and swimming with a local group, where he helps out with other disabled people.

References

1. Medical Disability Society, *The Management of Traumatic Head Injury*, London: Development Trust for the Young Disabled, 1988.
2. Brydn, J. How many head injured? in *Models of Brain Injury Rehabilitation* (eds Wood, R. and Eanes, P.), Chapman and Hall, 1989, pp. 17–27.
3. Oddy, M., Humphrey, H. and Uttley, D. Subjective impairment and social recovery after closed head injury, *Journal of Neurosurgery, Neurology and Psychiatry*, Vol. 41, pp. 611–16, 1978.
4. Royal College of Physicians, London, Physical disability in 1986 and beyond, Journal of the Royal College of Physicians, London, Vol. 20, pp. 3–37, 1986.
5. Working Group of the Research Committee of Royal College of Psychiatrists, Services for Brain injured adults, *Bulletin of the Royal College of Psychiatrists*, Vol. 15, pp. 513–8, 1991.
6. Bruckner, F.E. and Rande, P.H. Return to work after severe head injury, *Rheumatology and Physical Medicine*, Vol. 11, pp. 344–8, 1972.
7. Goldstein, J. Post traumatic headache and post concussive syndrome, *Medical Clinics of North America*, Vol. 75, pp. 641–51, 1991.
8. Thomsen, I.V. Late outcome of very severe blunt head trauma. A 10–15 year second follow up. *Journal of Neurology, Neurosurgery and Psychiatry*, Vol. 47, pp. 260–8, 1984.
9. Cronholm, B. Evaluation of mental disturbance after head injury, *Scandinavian Journal of Rehabilitation Medicine*, Vol. 4, pp. 35–8, 1972.
10. Levin, H.S., O'Donnell, M.A., Vincent, M. and Grossman, R.G. The Galveston Orientation and Amnesia Test, *Journal of Nervous and Mental Disorders*, Vol. 167(11), pp. 765–84, 1979.
11. Fortuny, L.A.I., Briggs, M., Newcombe, F., Ratcliffe, G. and Thomas, C. Measuring the duration of post traumatic amnesia, *Journal of Neurology, Neurosurgery and Psychiatry*, Vol. 43, pp. 377–9, 1980.
12. Hodkinson, H.M. Evaluation mental test score for assessment of mental impairment in the elderly, *Age & Ageing*, Vol. 1, pp. 233–8, 1972.
13. Folstein, M.F., Folstein, S.E. and McHugh, P.R. Mini Mental State, a practical method for grading the cognitive state of patients for the clinician, *Journal of Psychiatric Research*, Vol. 12, pp. 189–198, 1975.
14. Rappaport, M., Hall, K.M., Hopkins, K., Belleza, B.S. and Cope, D.N. Disability

rating scale for severe head trauma. Coma to community, *Archives of Physical Medicine Rehabilitation*, Vol. 63, pp. 118–23, 1982.

15. Santa Clara Valley Medical Centre, *FAM: Functional Activities Measure*, San Jose, California: Santa Clara Valley Medical Centre.
16. Lincoln, N.B. and Gladman, J.R. Extended ADL scale; a further validation, *Disability and Rehabilitation*, Vol. 14(1), pp. 41–3, 1992.
17. Mahoney, F.I. and Barthel, D.B. Functional evaluation the Barthel Index, *Maryland State Medical Journal*, Vol. 14, pp. 62–5, 1965.
18. Gronwall, G., Wrightson, P. and Waddel, P. *Head Injury. The Facts*, Oxford: Oxford Medical Publications, 1990.
19. Fussey, I. and Muir Giles, G. *Rehabilitation of the Severely Brain Damaged Adult, a Practical Approach*, London & Sydney: Croom Helm, 1988.

Information for families and professional staff

HEADWAY (publications list available), National Head Injuries Association, King Edwards Court, 7 King Edward Street, Nottingham NG1 4EW.

Chapter 18

Maintaining mental health

CATHERINE WELLS
Lecturer in Occupatinal Therapy, School of Occupational Therapy and Physiotherapy, University of East Anglia

Working within the framework of mental health, as opposed to mental illness, is very much the remit for the occupational therapist in the 1990s. However, change does not occur overnight, and in many areas of the country there is a legacy of large old psychiatric hospitals, responsible for the asylum of those with mental illness, alongside the development of flourishing mental health teams working within the community. This situation has been brought about in part by the government reforms which have pervaded the whole working of the National Health Service. In every area, change and development seem to take on a different perspective, making the picture of maintaining mental health a confusing one for both the patient and the professional. Reforms have led to mental illness being treated more on a parallel with physical illness; specialist units housed within general hospitals, and patients more likely to experience short admission periods and then be returned to the community for continuing treatment and support. In this way, patients suffering from mental illness are no longer caught up within institutional care but are encouraged to use a hospital base only when necessary, receiving the remainder of their care from the team of professionals working with their own general practitioner (GP). This change enables the GP, who may be the professional with more knowledge and understanding of the patient than anyone else, to monitor and oversee care thus making it not only easily accessible and appropriate, but also providing a continuity of involvement.

It would be useful at this stage to clarify what is meant by mental illness, to explore its incidence and place these data against diminishing bed numbers and the increase of community involvement.

The Mental Health Act 1983[1] states mental disorder as:

> mental illness, arrested or incomplete development of mind, psychopathic disorder and any other disorder or disability of mind.

This term encompasses two main categories of disorder, namely mental illness and learning disabilities, previously known as mental handicap. However, mental illness cannot be seen as a single condition, as it ranges from a relatively minor disorder of a temporary nature to a severe and entrenched disorder, which is likely to have more permanent symptoms of illness.

It is acknowledged that accurate data on the incidence of mental illness are hard to find. This is partly due to changes in the collection of data – from discharge figures to completed episodes of treatment – thus giving differing statistical evidence, and to the fact that many incidences of mental illness are not recognised and recorded with accuracy.[2] The government has responded to this situation by commissioning a national survey of psychiatric morbidity, which should be completed by 1995. Official figures suggest that there are between 2 and 6 million adult sufferers of mental illness at any one time.[2] These figures, however, conflict with research studies,[2] which suggest a greater number of adults who are in touch with their GPs presenting with symptoms of mental illness.

One of the far-reaching changes which reflects health strategy is the overall reduction of hospital beds as the larger institutions close down and are replaced by purpose-built smaller units. This can be seen by the total number of hospital beds reduced during the 1980s – hospital bed numbers were 85 000 in 1981, reducing to 50 000 in 1991–2.[3]

The White Paper *Caring for People*,[4] which preceded the National Health Service and Community Care Act 1990,[5] clarified the government's policy of

> developing locally-based health and social services for people with a mental illness, enabling many who would previously have had to be in hospital to be treated in the community.

In consequence, together with the preceding Griffiths Report,[6] formal recognition was given to the formation of a multidisciplinary team approach for delivering health care in the community. For many people, however, 'care in the community' resulted in 'transinstitutionalisation', a term used by Bean and Mounser[7] whereby one form of institutional care is merely changed for another. Patients may move to hostels, community homes or residential care, but may not have the personal resources or support to enable them to live independently. Often in this situation discharge from hospital tends not to mean discharge from the mental health care service. In fact, it may be difficult to work out exactly when, or indeed if, a patient is ever 'discharged'. To allow effective treatment to be carried out following the move from an admission environment, professionals and carers must be involved to ensure that efficient communication and collaboration exist to assist the patient through this transition.

Community mental health care teams (MHCT) are becoming established throughout the country, although many are still at a formative stage with the actual structure varying according to area. The essential focus, however, is to see the patient as the central figure around whom the team will function. MHCTs are concerned with the prevention and treatment of chronic illness, the needs of an ever-increasing identified population of the 'worried well', those suffering from emotional or situational disturbances[7] and with the needs of those people who care for the sufferers of mental illness within their own homes.

Mental health care teams revolve around the GP practice, rather than the hospital ward, so that the community becomes the place for treatment, with the hospital becoming the 'back-up' facility. The team usually includes community psychiatric nurses, occupational therapists, psychologists, social workers and other appropriate disciplines. Each team have their own structure allowing for the core skills of its members to work together in providing a comprehensive package of care for the patients. Many establish a 'key worker' policy, where an identified member of staff takes on the role of liaising on behalf of the patient, co-ordinating treatment plans, monitoring these to confirm effectiveness and reporting accordingly. The key worker then becomes the person to whom the patient and/or the carer relates as being there to support and assist them, taking the responsibility of seeing the programme of care through to discharge.

Legislation

It is important to consider the legislation which underpins working in the community as in a climate of constant change an understanding of related legislation is now required by all working in mental health.

The Acts which most concern the occupational therapist are the Mental Health Act 1983[1] and the National Health Service and Community Care Act 1990,[5] the community care aspect of which was implemented in April 1993. Summaries of these Acts are given in Appendix I, but therapists need to refer to the entire documents for further clarification.

The effective therapist

The occupational therapist working within a community mental health care team will be required to use core skills in a different and unpredictable environment and therefore needs the ability to think creatively. The essential features underpinning the work will focus on communication skills; time management; resource management; continuing training and education; support and supervision.

Communication

No therapist is able to work effectively with patients unless they are skilled at both instigating and receiving communication. Community therapists may be working alone, need to be highly mobile and thus will be difficult to track down. This gives a contrasting picture to the traditional hospital setting where informal and formal communication follows established routes and with built-in procedures for establishing contact. Despite this, therapists working in the community have to ensure that they communicate with all members of the team, patients and their carers, and any other professional involved with the referral.

There should be an awareness of the possible difficulties involved in communicating with this client group, and the rapport which must be developed to ensure that contact is maintained and identified needs are met. This communication is not only verbal but extends to the responsible management of paperwork, including confidentiality, and the development of the team's network of communication in dealing with each referral. To ensure that no one person is working in isolation it is important that all team members attend regular meetings, and that the needs of the patient are constantly being addressed.

Time management

The occupational therapist working within the community needs to develop a sophisticated system of time management with a balance between patient contact time and other management tasks. Patients may be geographically distant, while treatment programmes and meetings are held in a number of decentralised locations, involving frequent travel. There is an increasing need to provide weekend or evening sessions, especially for those suffering from a stress-related disorder, and who may be in employment or have family commitments which make it counterproductive for them to attend for treatment between the hours of nine to five. Flexible working arrangements therefore become relevant for them and for the longer-term patient, coping with a more severe disorder of mind or behaviour. Many lost social skills can be practised in a social setting by using leisure activities within the community, making treatment more realistic and enabling the patient to function in real situations.

Resources

The resources which are available to the community occupational therapist are likely to be very different from those found within a hospital environment. It is important to seek out resources which are used by other sections of the community, and are available within the patient's own locality.

An accessible base with a telephone, support services and storage space is essential, preferably with community rooms for group work and meetings. Although treatment may often take place in the patient's home, there are times when this is not appropriate and a change of environment is beneficial. Dedicated accommodation is not always necessary, but the hiring of church halls, village rooms, sports facilities and other venues that adapt themselves to the purpose required are often satisfactory. Cost implications must be considered, as well as the accessibility of the chosen treatment media (e.g. horse riding, social outings, or sports events), which may in part be governed by the financial resources of the team or the patient's ability to contribute.

A reliable car is essential, with a current road map, as the therapist who is constantly getting lost and arriving late does not present a professional image and does little to gain the confidence of the patient they are there to treat.

Continuing training and education

Therapists working within community health care tend to be those who have a range of experience and expertise to bring from previous clinical positions. However, because of the tendency to work in isolation, and as they may be the only member of their profession in the team, further training and education is extremely important. With increasing workloads time must be planned for this so that new skills are acquired and older ones consolidated. Time also needs to be allowed for meeting and sharing ideas with peers and colleagues working in other environments. At a time when there is a blurring of roles and skill-mix presents potential for conflict among different professionals within the team, it is especially important that core skills are identified and respected, thus ensuring a strong presence within the framework of the team.

Support and supervision

The subject of support and supervision for therapists has been addressed in Chapter 5, but it is important to consider the effect of community work upon the health of the therapist working with this particular group of people. No therapist will be able to work with consistent effectiveness on their own, dealing with increasing referrals, long unsociable hours, busy roads and the geographical spread between patients unless they are well supported by colleagues and their managers. Many will have the additional responsibility of being the identified key worker for a patient, and therefore may find themselves in a position of having to make decisions about the patient's safety in the absence of in-patient resources. Risks must be carefully assessed over problems such as deterioration, which may lead to a hospital admission. The safety of the patient and others must be paramount in this decision making. Research suggests[2] that 9 of every 10 suicides involve people suffering from a mental illness. Although the therapist does not carry sole responsibility it is essential that the line of responsibility for the patient is clear, and that help and support is accessed easily at times of need. The Mental Health Act[1] specifies clear categories for admission to hospital for a patient suffering from mental illness, and although the occupational therapist will not be required to give one of the two written medical recommendations required for compulsory admission they may have a significant role in assessing and advising on the health of the patient, especially if contact has been extensive and the patient is well known. In this way the therapist will not only provide support to those making the decision, but will have an important role in supporting and negotiating with the patient, giving reassurance during a time of difficult decision making.

Supervision of clinical work is essential, and should be seen as having a high priority. The widely diverse nature of conditions with which the therapists will be working, linked with the individual nature of the work, makes supervision vital. It will ensure the highest standards of intervention, and allow for the development of therapeutic skills. Whilst the occupational therapist may have opportunities to use reflection in self-supervision, they also need to ensure that the process goes beyond this into team or group supervision, so that this reflective process is carried through into action. In this way supervision becomes not only supportive but challenging, resulting in greater job satisfaction and allowing for growth and development of the individual and the team.

Assessment and treatment planning

Treatment to maintain and promote mental health in the community begins with the referral process. Every member of the mental health care team will receive large numbers of referrals which require prioritising in a manageable way to ensure that the patients receive the treatment they require. Therapists working within the team may find that referrals are received, discussed and allocated to the member of the team who is recognised as having the skills required, and who has the time available. Inevitably there will be areas of overlap in skills among members of the team. This raises opportunities for interdisciplinary work and co-leadership, giving different team members the opportunity of working and learning together. The ability to juggle referrals and keep long-term contracts in place while responding to the needs of the more acutely ill patient are key aspects of the referral process.

Allocation of the referral will lead to contact being made with the patient, and an initial assessment carried out to identify treatment needs. The National Health Service and Community Care Act[5] stresses the importance of assessment prior to the appointment of a key worker, and this is an important aspect of occupational therapy intervention. The assessment process may well differ from that used within a hospital department, but it is an essential precursor to successful treatment. It may form the basis of the initial interview following referral, and be the first time the therapist meets the patient. It can also be the time at which the patient chooses to become involved with treatment, and so it is essential that a working rapport is established as soon as possible to develop trust and commitment to the treatment programme. Assessments which take place in the patient's own home are likely to expose clues which contribute to the overall perception of the problem, and the occupational therapist needs to be acutely aware of information gained from other family members or carers, the surroundings or the general state of the home. The therapist must not be judgemental about any patient's home situation or their lifestyle, but be aware of this and allow clinical reasoning skills to build a comprehensive picture of each situation. It has been recognised that mental illness and social deprivation are linked,[2] and therapists will be able to observe lack of financial resources, isolation or poor housing conditions from this initial meeting.

Assessment must be thorough but concise. It is important to recognise that work within a multidisciplinary team requires paperwork and reports which need to be circulated among key members. Lengthy, ill prepared paperwork is tedious and time consuming, and could be misleading to other professionals involved with the patient. The initial assessment may well identify areas where the joint working of health and Social Services is required. The care plan which is then put into place will cover both aspects and include accommodation issues, day centres availability, out-patient treatment programmes and personal support. It should identify a 'seamless approach' where Social Services are responsible for the care needs of the patient in the community and the health service responding to the health needs. It is not helpful to be prescriptive about the types of treatment or client groups with whom the occupational therapist will work as these can, and will be, as broad ranging as the community itself.

Rehabilitation enables a person to adjust to the limitations brought about by the illness, and to regain lost skills through the development of coping strategies.[7] Therapy therefore may be limited to a short-term intervention, based on assessment of the problem, or become a long-term rehabilitative programme. The occupational therapy treatment programme planned for an individual should be based on their rehabilitation needs, having been agreed between both the patient and the therapist, and may include individual and/or group work. Treatment should take place in the most appropriate place, which could include the home, community group areas and day centres. Different mental health teams work with different criteria of mental illness, some offering a broad approach of short- and longer-term intervention, whereas others specialise in one area of involvement. These widely differing approaches may lead staff to seek out models of practice occurring elsewhere, enabling them to take up the challenge of establishing a new area of work. The following account of a city-based team, which was required to respond to the mental health needs of a rural community, together with a case study of a patient treated at this centre, illustrate this.

A city house

The treatment centre was based in a large, ordinary and homely house complete with garden in the centre of the city. It was well served by bus routes and in the main shopping area, thus making it easily accessible. The centre was staffed by a core team of occupational therapists, but others such as art therapists, dieticians, clinical psychologists, community psychiatric nurses and consultants arranged sessions there when facilities were appropriate and available. This encouraged multidisciplinary participation, and enabled patients to attend one place to see the different professionals involved in their treatment, rather than returning to the hospital base. The centre had a wide-ranging referral policy from consultants to general practitioners, or any other professional working within the field. It did not accept self-referrals simply as a means to limiting numbers, working on the premise that quality treatment could only be delivered within a manageable framework. Patients attended from all over the county, and were encouraged to travel independently as the location made it easy to reach, while those in employment within the city were able to attend with the minimum of disruption to their working lives. The overall philosophy was a needs-led service which reflected the wide range of treatments required, and operated a flexi-hour programme, thus ensuring that therapy could be available at times to suit the receiver.

Careful organisation and good management were required, as being away from a hospital site meant that day to day resources had to be organised differently. An important aspect of this was the communication needed between the staff and other members of the mental health service. Being isolated made it harder to achieve the different resources which were required. Ongoing support, especially from management, and supervision of the centre was essential for effective working and regular meetings were held together with training opportunities for the staff, which ensured a professional and high quality service.

The pattern of work for the occupational therapist within the team was initially the receipt of a written referral. This was carefully discussed at a team meeting and then allocated to a key worker, who would be responsible for contacting the patient, assessing their needs and developing a treatment programme with them. All aspects of communication relating to the referral would be dealt with by the key worker. The emphasis was always on working with the patient, developing commitment, motivation and trust. However, it was recognised that some patients would occasionally find it too difficult to attend for a variety of reasons.

Following assessment a treatment programme was selected from a range of options which included either group or individual work, or a mixture of both. There were also sessions at which it was appropriate to involve members of the patient's family, or close friends, as this would encourage support and understanding of the work undertaken.

Individual work

Patients were seen on a regular basis by the occupational therapist to recognise, explore and work with the problems affecting mental health. Important resources for this type of work focused on the skill and expertise of the therapist, with regular time-bound sessions in a location which was quiet and unlikely to be interrupted. This was followed by skilled supervision for the therapist involved.

Counselling took different forms in working with the patients, some therapists having gained further qualifications, and for many this type of involvement formed a large percentage of their patient contact time. Counselling involved ensuring congruence, empathy and unconditional positive regard with the patient, thus enabling him to understand and move forward from the present situation. Another type of individual work involved *social skills activities* such as shopping or leisure pursuits, where the patient initially required the close support of the therapist.

Group work

A wide variety of group activities needed to be available throughout the week, including some evening sessions. The following examples give an indication of the types of group work which could be undertaken, and the specific advantages and requirements of each.

Relaxation, stress or anxiety management. There were always large numbers of referrals for these groups and they needed to have a regular place within the programme. The groups were co-led where possible, allowing a more junior member of staff to gain experience, or to share expertise with other professionals. By having two members of staff continuity of sessions was ensured. The content of the sessions varied according to the staff and patients involved, but the emphasis was on understanding the symptoms of anxiety and developing subsequent coping strategies.

Psychotherapy groups. At this centre a group was held on a weekly basis for mothers with parenting or family problems. The group was supported by a supervised crèche for preschool aged children, which was an important part of making the activity available to those in need. The dynamics of the group allowed for the involvement of all members, facilitated by the staff who led the sessions, and encouraged the identifying, sharing and understanding of problems which mothers were experiencing at that time. The group developed a supportive network of its own, allowing members to move on and yet retain contacts they had made.

A younger person's group. Referrals for these sessions were for patients who had frequently experienced admission to hospital, or who were maintaining tenuous independent existences. Some would be in hostel accommodation, others in their own flats or family homes. Many of these patients would have been spending greater proportions of their time as in-patients were it not for the development of resources in the community. The group activities focused on aspects of independent living and decision making, such as budgeting, cooking and personal care, or social, leisure and sports activities. There was a place for creative therapies within the group, thus ensuring a wide menu of activities from which a day could be planned. A similar programme was available for older patients, which took place 1 day per week.

Social skills or assertiveness groups. One of these groups would be included according to the needs of the referrals. The group would be co-led, closed, and ran to a specified programme with an agreed a number of sessions.

Agoraphobic programmes. With the co-operation of the patient, their family or carers, agoraphobic programmes centred around their home and the immediate vicinity. It proved more effective for the occupational therapist to go out on regular home visits, setting manageable targets and planning treatment around a familiar environment, than to bring a patient into the treatment centre. Walking out and gaining local confidence could then be extended to short public transport trips, leading eventually towards independent travel into the centre for group support. In this way problems were worked with in a specific and meaningful way, with a contract of independent working being established to give the focus of control back to the patient.

The vocational guidance group. Having identified the clear need to develop skills which could lead towards purposeful employment, either in a voluntary or salaried capacity, the centre worked closely with other employment opportunities within the city. It also provided a safe environment within which to learn and develop work skills, ranging from clerical work to computing. This led to the development of acceptable working practices, such as time keeping, responsibility, accuracy and perseverance, as well as the ability to work alongside others. The equipment, although well used, was expensive and needed to be updated regularly, thus accounting for a large percentage of the available budget.

The garden. A private garden with the house enabled a wide range of activities to be undertaken out of doors. A greenhouse provided a focus for gaining and developing horticultural skills, as did the maintenance of the flower borders and lawn area. Interests were shared, and for many people the therapeutic effects of working with plants, as well as being able to socialise and enjoy outdoor pursuits, were an important part of their day.

Other sessions. Visiting professionals would run sessions as required, for example art therapy or problem solving with the psychologist. The groups would be co-led with an occupational therapist when appropriate, thus enabling the patient to receive different treatment sessions within a familiar environment.

Whatever type of treatment programme was chosen for the patient there was a need to constantly re-evaluate this to ensure that the centre was proactive in what it was providing. All contacts had to be reported efficiently and feedback and report writing took on an important emphasis as the staff rarely saw the referrer, or other professionals involved with the patient. It was important to see the centre as a resource, available to any patient referred, and that growth and change could take place to reflect the changing environment of mental health care.

An example of a case study of a patient referred to the centre illustrates an actual treatment programme.

Case Study

Miss A. was referred to the city community team following a series of lengthy admissions for a depressive illness. Her history showed deep depressive episodes following her inability to cope with academic pressures, the deaths of both parents and rejection from various career opportunities which she had attempted. She lived alone in a council flat, had no friends and lived an extremely frugal existence. Now in her forties Miss A. was barely able to maintain an independent life outside an institution, but she was adamant that she would not return to hospital for treatment, and would only consider out-patient treatment within a non-hospital setting at the insistence of her consultant.

Miss A. had established contact with a community psychiatric nurse (CPN) and had tenuous links with a mental health support group in her area, which was run by Social Services. She had regular contact with her GP for medication, and continued to see her consultant on an out-patient basis. She therefore had contact with different agencies providing care in the community, and was an excellent example of the need for collaboration and co-operation between different professional groups.

On assessment Miss A. was virtually mute, of very low body weight and was still experiencing periods of extreme depression, when she retired to bed until her mood lifted. It was obvious that she needed help to maintain an independent lifestyle away from the hospital, but one within which she felt at ease and secure, and one where the quality of her life became important.

Miss A. agreed to attend the mental health centre on a regular basis, starting with individual sessions with the occupational therapist who had completed the initial assessment. These sessions required her to get out of bed, dress and leave the flat; then, as she refused hospital transport, to travel by public transport to keep her appointment. The stress of this commitment was so great at the beginning that treatment consisted solely of a supportive and accepting counselling session, where her achievements were acknowledged and her anxieties explored. It was about a year later that Miss A. expressed an interest in other activities available at the centre, and was able to contemplate including some in her treatment programme. Her confidence, physical and mental health improved sufficiently to allow her to attend a relaxation group, which led to an interest in yoga, and eventually an art therapy group.

The treatment plan for Miss A. was interrupted when she suffered a stroke. As an intensely private person, she was able to receive a domestic assessment and subsequent adaptations by her community occupational therapist working in physical medicine only through the support and liaison of her mental health therapist. However, as her mobility improved she returned to the centre to continue her treatment programme. She received help from the dietician working in mental health, and was able to accept a gradual weight gain. Individual work continued, but at this stage activities in the community were explored allowing her to extend an interest in art and yoga by attending day classes away from a therapeutic setting. She enrolled for swimming lessons, and began to build up some contacts around her home environment.

As Miss A. improved support from the centre was gradually withdrawn, always with her co-operation and understanding, and she reached the decision that she was now able to manage an independent life away from it. Although she had been attending for 4 years the quality of life which she achieved at her discharge was so great compared with that on her referral that the staff commitment and the resources required were seen as a very valuable intervention.

This case study illustrates the value of community resources. The patient did not have to return to hospital, she gained confidence and self-esteem in the world by involving herself in everyday contact, and she was able to receive and benefit from specialist treatment input. Despite periods when she was unable to attend Miss A. remained an 'active case' and so there was no danger of professional contact being lost. Throughout the treatment time her consultant was unfailingly supportive and encouraging. When she was ready discharge arrangements were made with her, thus ensuring that the occupational therapy involvement finished appropriately, and at her own pace.

This chapter has considered the aspects of professionalism which contribute to enabling an occupational therapist to work effectively within the mental health team in the community, and has explored a treatment centre which provided a cornerstone for such intervention. It is clear that a knowledge of the legislation and current policies which affect working with patients in this client group is important in underpinning the work in which the occupational therapist will be involved.

As a profession occupational therapy is well equipped to play an important role within this area of health care, contributing core skills and complementing the work of other professionals within the team. There remains some tension in running community care alongside the closure of the hospitals, and it should be clearly recognised that community care is not a cheap alternative. Only if resources are available and fully utilised will a service be established which truly meets the needs of the patients and where occupational therapists can demonstrate their skill and commitment to working in this clinical area.

References

1. *Mental Health Act*, London: HMSO, 1983.
2. Thompson, D. *Mental Illness: The Fundamental Facts*, The Mental Health Foundation, 1993.
3. Department of Health, *Social Trends*, Central Statistical Office, London: HMSO, 1994.
4. *Caring for People*, London: HMSO, 1989.
5. *National Health Service and Community Care Act*, London: HMSO, 1990.
6. The Griffiths Report, *Community Care: Agenda for Action*, London: HMSO, 1988.
7. Bean, P. and Mounser, P. *Discharged from Mental Hospitals*, London: Macmillan, 1993.

Further reading

Davies, B.M. and Davies, T. *Community Health, Preventative Medicine and Social Services*, London: Baillière Tindall, 1993.
Dimond, B. Mental health law and the occupational therapist, *British Journal of Occupational Therapy*, Vol. 51(9), pp. 307–11, 1988.
Jones, K. *Asylums and After*, London: Athlone Press, 1993.
Thompson, D. *Mental Illness: The Fundamental Facts*, London: The Mental Health Foundation, 1993.
Tomlinson, D. *Utopia, Community Care and the Retreat from the Asylums*, Milton Keynes: Open University Press, 1991.
Tyrer, P., Higgs, R. and Strathdee, G. *Mental Health and Primary Care*, London: Gaskell, on behalf of the Mental Health Foundation, 1993.

Chapter 19

The ageing population
(i) Common problems amongst the elderly

ANNE C. M. GALLEY
Consultant Occupational Therapist

The philosophy of geriatric medicine and care of the elderly person cannot be encompassed in one simple definition, for it is very wide ranging. However, there is an absorbing range of diagnostic and remedial opportunities that exist with old people. Enormous rewards can be reaped from unexpected recovery after critical illness, in the successful management of protracted disabilities, or in assuring comfort and dignity in their last hours. People who survive to a 'ripe old age' usually do so through their own genetic make-up combined with the fundamentals of survival – warmth, food, fluids and companionship.

Few old people ask for help unless they feel really ill, if their mobility has created a significant loss of independence, or if they become so handicapped that outside support is essential for ordinary standards of hygiene and self-care to be maintained. Invariably the problem is that the elderly person, or relative, waits too long to ask. All community practitioners are now involved in preventive medicine in order to maintain good health, and the general practitioner (GP) is no exception; the 1990 GP contract includes offers of screening to those over 65 years of age every 3 years, and annually for those over the age of 75 years, in order to ascertain problems that may occur. These programmes have increased the workload of community occupational therapists by as much as 17 per cent, mainly for minor specialised equipment such as bath seats.

The growing elderly population is having enormous implications on the workload of community occupational therapists. By the year 2000 it is estimated that 25 per cent of Europe's population will be over 60 years of age. However, this is providing the occupational therapist with the opportunity of using the widest variety of skills, with some GPs asking them to be involved with the annual screening process. The pace may be slower than working with other care groups, but there is scope and opportunity for assessment and problem solving in a truly multidisciplinary environment.

Multiple pathology and loss of senses

The majority of elderly people referred to the community occupational therapist present with multiple pathological problems and are often referred as 'generally frail'. In old age both precise diagnosis as a basis of treatment and the assessment of disability are often compromised by a number of active or inactive pathological processes affecting the outcome. Degenerative and locomotor disorders are pre-eminent in the elderly. The outstanding limitations are imposed by cardiovascular disease, restricted exercise tolerance in ischaemic heart disease, transient cerebral ischaemia, postural imbalance and strokes, intermittent claudication, gangrene and amputations due to peripheral vascular occlusion, arthritis, neuromuscular disorders, cancer and the tendency to resistant pulmonary infections and thromoboembolism. Common respiratory diseases resulting from the ageing process are pulmonary thrombosis, carcinoma of the bronchus, pulmonary embolism, concurrent respiratory disease and failure.

Growing old automatically affects the locomotor system, resulting in loss of physical strength, reduced range of movement, stooping and loss of height. The senses are also affected, resulting in reduced vision, hearing, smell and taste. These systems/senses will be affected to a varying degree but there will also be a continuous decline.

Specific medical problems of which to be aware

Cerebrovascular disease

'A stroke is an acute disturbance of cerebral function of presumed vascular origin with disability lasting more than 24 hours.'[1] A stroke is only one of four main presentations of cerebrovascular disease. The others are: transient ischaemic episodes; disorders of postural fixation and balance; and dementia. Acute cerebrovascular accidents (CVAs) are covered in detail in medical textbooks but some points are emphasised here, as follows.

1.   At least 20 per cent of patients with CVA also have ischaemic heart disease.
2.   About 7 per cent of cerebral tumours present as hemiplegia of sudden onsets but strokes attributable to vascular disease can appear gradually with headaches.
3.   Stroke patients are at risk of hypothermia because the onset is often early in the morning and the patient may lie uncovered for several hours after collapsing before being found.

Points of management to be remembered

(a)   The elderly person cannot be expected to have a better mental or physical level of activity after a stroke than before it. It is essential therefore to have an estimate of former capacity.

(b)   No two hemiplegias are alike and thus any rehabilitation programme must be flexible and designed to meet the individual's needs.

(c)   Emphasis must be on remaining ability rather than disability as the tendency of many people who have suffered a stroke is to bemoan their loss.

(d)   Failure to progress indicates that it is important to develop a sensitive index highlighting causes of delayed recovery; for example, problem-orientated medical records (POMR).

A systematic assessment is essential to:

(i)   determine the person's progress;

(ii)   assess the person's and carer's needs and design an appropriate programme; and

(iii)   act as an index to effectiveness of treatment of the individual.

Mental barriers to recovery and response

1.   Inability to learn through
        (a) clouded consciousness;
        (b) aphasia;
        (c) memory defect; and
        (d) dementia.
2.   Disturbed perception through
        (a) anosognosia;
        (b) neglect of hemiplegic side;
        (c) denial of illness or paralysis; and
        (d) disordered spatial orientation.
3.   Disordered integrative action.
4.   Disturbed emotion.

A hemiplegic person seldom has insight to complain about these mental barriers, and it is usually an observant relative or neighbour who notices incongruous behaviour.

Faints and falls – control of posture, difficulty with walking

Balance exercises and constant practice are essential to encourage the best use of compensatory movements in the elderly after illness. However, no person can do better than their peak of activity before the illness.

Elderly people often complain of difficulty with walking. Disorders of gait fall into three principle groups (see also Chapter 12).

1.   Those attributable to 'old age', for instance, a shortened step, or loss of awareness of the vertical stance.
2.   Those accompanied by uni- or bilateral corticospinal lesions.
3.   Those related to peripheral neuromuscular disease.

Faints. Old people use a variety of terms to describe transient disturbances of consciousness, such as 'attack' , 'weakness'. They are also often embarrassed by their frequent 'attacks'/'accidents' and may be reluctant to volunteer information about them. Possible causes for these may include:

(a)   simple faints through stress, heat or pain;
(b)   postural hypotension, for instance, on standing up too quickly;
(c)   carotid–sinus syndrome; and
(d)   epilepsy.

Falls. It is thought that women are far more liable to falls than men, and that the incidence of these increases steadily with age in identical proportion to both sexes. Falls are easily classified according to intrinsic or extrinsic causes. Underlying most falls there appears to be an age-related defect in the control of posture and gait. Old people may *trip* and *fall* owing to senility, Parkinsonism, ataxic or apraxic disorders of gait; or to impaired eyesight, visual inattention or domestic hazards such as loose carpets, ill-lit stairways or loose wires. They may *stumble* because of clumsiness resulting from a physical disability such as arthritis. They may *sway* owing to deteriorating control of balance, or to vertigo caused by postural hypotension, adverse drug reaction or vertebral basilar inefficiency. Elderly people may suddenly *collapse* due to cardiac syncope.

Drop attacks. These are instantaneous falls occurring most commonly in women without warning or loss of consciousness. They are usually as a result of brain stem ischaemia and there is immediate recovery of function.

The elderly usually recognise their failing but realise there is little they can do about it other than to avoid sudden movements and protect themselves from environmental hazards. Help can be given by advice on proper clothing and domestic aids; for example, good lighting; hand rails; uncluttered rooms; well-placed furniture and floors without loose mats and clutter; or even highly polished floors.

Parkinsonism

Incidence in the over 65-year-olds in the United Kingdom is one per 100, but in the over 80-year-olds it is two per 100. In older people it occurs in association with cerebrovascular disease and phenotinazine intoxication. This disease follows a slow, unremitting course downhill towards total dependency. Old people often complain about slowing down, a sense of weakness, tremour or stiffness, and it is all too easy to dismiss incipient Parkinsonism simply as 'old age'.

Old people do not show a dramatic response to medication and although there may be a marked improvement in rigidity and bradykinesia the elderly person may still be heavily handicapped through loss of normal postural fixation, unpractised righting reflexes, weakness of disused muscles and loss of confidence. A programme of rehabilitation should include, in particular,

(a)   postural and balance exercises;
(b)   practise in turning in bed; getting in/out of a chair (raised to appropriate individual height if necessary);
(c)   walking exercises; and
(d)   washing, bathing and dressing practice.

In Parkinsonism associated with arteriosclerosis the instance of dementia is high and mental deterioration limits the possibility of re-education owing to impaired grasp, concentration and memory.

Late-onset diabetes

Age and obesity are the outstanding factors predisposing diabetes mellitus. Most, when first diagnosed, are well over the age of 50 years and the incidence increases with each decade over this age. The onset is sometimes as sudden and severe as in youth, but more often it is gradual and less dramatic. Diabetes in the elderly can be divided into three groups.

(a)   Those whose hypoglycaemia can be controlled by diet.
(b)   Those who need insulin.
(c)   Those who respond to antidiabetic drugs.

Accidental hypothermia

This has been recognised in Great Britain as a specialised hazard of old age. The endogenous causes for hypothermia are as follows.

(a)   Those directly related to old age such as impaired temperature regulation, infirmity and immobility, slowness.
(b)   Malnutrition.
(c)   Illness.
(d)   Reaction to drugs.

Mortality is high and therefore prevention is better than cure. Constant surveillance of old people at risk, provision of warm clothing and bedding, safe heating appliances and encouragement to activity are a few methods of helping to prevent this.

Incontinence and pressure sores

Incontinence is a symptom and not a disease, albeit a very worrying one to the elderly. Pressure sores are either superficial or deep. Some ageing skins are more prone to break down than others and when the elderly person is, for instance, malnourished, thin, or taking steroid therapy this is more true. Vigilance, careful handling and observation can prevent these superficial abrasions. Deep pressure sores are predisposed by:

(a)   lowered tissue vitality;
(b)   impaired peripheral circulation; and
(c)   sensory and motor deficits preventing mobility.

Prevention is far better than cure for all sores and acute awareness of susceptibility is critical. This is determined by general condition, mental state, physical capacity and incontinence.

Malnutrition

Old age can lead to physical and mental infirmity, social isolation or deprivation of one kind or another. Malnutrition is usually the consequence, *not* the cause, of such disorders as dementia or depression. Advanced signs are listlessness, hypothermia, pallor, slow pulse, low blood pressure and oedema. It is important to try to encourage old people to take the trouble to maintain a balanced diet and ensure that they are able to cook and prepare food with appropriate equipment such as a food blender, small microwave and built-up cutlery.

Social problems and loneliness

Many elderly people become labelled a 'social problem' as a matter of course. However, solutions often present themselves when the problems are assessed and analysed. As one grows older one generally experiences the need for a more restricted, but deeper, intimacy. Invariably those now old and alone will find boredom, fear and loneliness an increasing and very real factor. Under these circumstances regression, passivity and withdrawal crowd in. Frequent causes of becoming a social problem and/or lonely are as a result of:

(a)   antisocial behaviour, for instance unacceptable eating habits;
(b)   poor self-care and hygiene;
(c)   loss of hearing or sight which leads to isolation, withdrawal and unresponsiveness (often resulting in the label 'demented' or 'confused');
(d)   bereavement through the loss of spouse, friend, pet or familiar surroundings;
(e)   financial resources;
(f)   transportation problems;
(g)   physical disability;
(h)   fear of going out and being attacked; and
(i)   reluctance to go somewhere new without a companion.

Relocating an elderly person will set up a chain of reactions; they may become confused, disorientated and appear unresponsive. However, with a little forethought it is possible to overcome to a degree, if not wholly, these problems. Elderly people must be treated with respect and dignity. Wherever possible the person who knows the individual best – perhaps the community occupational therapist or health visitor – should visit the elderly person to help them adjust to the difficult transposition, remembering that an elderly person will not change well-worn habits. If aggression, paranoia or withdrawal is apparent, rather than automatically labelling the individual the therapist should analyse the situation, review the information acquired and consult the individual. For example, the reason for 'incontinence' should be questioned, for it may be that judicious positioning of a bed or commode will enable someone with limited mobility to reach the toilet or aid in time. Constant review of the total situation and the elderly person/carers is essential.

In this competitive, materialistic society elderly people, particularly the very old, express a great anxiety of going out and of being rejected by the young because they feel 'crabby', 'wrinkled', 'slow' and 'uninteresting'. Fear is also generated because they feel particularly vulnerable to abuse and attack. These fears result in the old staying indoors – frequently alone. An elderly person's expectation of success or failure differs somewhat from that of younger people. Older people are more prone to both overestimate and underestimate their abilities. This has been interpreted as a protective mechanism: overestimation of ability maintains self-esteem while underestimation protects the individual from loss of self-esteem in the event of failure. To counteract these, the elderly need to be encouraged to participate in activities now available specifically for them. There has been a great increase in leisure activities over recent years specifically organised for the over-sixties: for example, the University of the Third Age, where there are autonomous groups with a local tutor covering such subjects as art, history, languages, music, theatre, creative writing enhancing the experience of shared learning; the Sports Council supports locally organised mobilisation activities for the over 65-year-olds; and there are many other locally organised activities.

Through an appropriately designed programme, and with previous careful assessment, specific group and individual treatment to help overcome these problems can be applied. For instance, individual counselling and discussion regarding a specific bereavement or fear will enable the older person to become more objective as well as feel less isolated. Group activities such as a quiz on the highway code with pictures of the appropriate symbols, a cookery group related to the season, and self-help activities – such as what to do/not to do when a stranger comes to the door – will establish self-confidence, retain memory and sensory patterns and provide social interaction. Instead of evading an expressed or discovered problem it is important that the occupational therapist devises a means or activity to reach a solution. For example, unhygienic home surroundings which have resulted in an elderly person being labelled 'a social problem', unable to carry out self-care hygiene activities and being admitted to hospital with a multitude of problems could

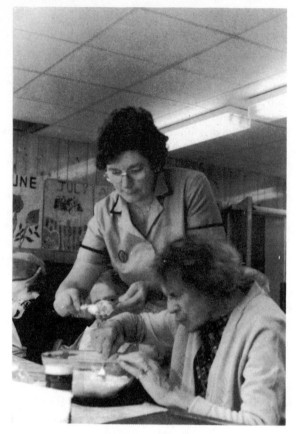

Photo. 19.1 Cookery sessions stimulate innate skills and form a useful social activity.

have a very simple solution. A home visit in such a case revealed that due to the flushing mechanism of the toilet being extremely stiff, similarly the sink taps, it was impossible to flush the toilet or wash anything. This elderly, immobile woman had resorted to using any receptacle, had become confused, malnourished, withdrawn and lost all self-esteem through her own self-degradation. Simple and careful reorganisation of her home situation, continual occupational therapy and physiotherapy at the day hospital, designed to meet her specific needs, facilitated progress and enabled her to return home both physically and psychologically strengthened. Group activities for the elderly should encompass well-known tasks and stimulate the senses, as well as being designed to stimulate social contact, physical activity, induce confidence and reinforce independence (see Photo. 19.1).

Meaningfulness of one's values is derived from occupations which meet basic needs and which provide intrinsic pleasure. The following are values which are commonly held by elderly people and considered meaningful to them:

- independence;
- social acceptance;
- adequate resources;
- ability to cope; and
- having significant goals.

There is a great variety of equipment on the market, enabling elderly people to remain at home with greater confidence and independence; for instance, communication devices to the front door so that keys need no longer be left in the latch or dangling from a piece of string (see Photo. 19.2). Such equipment enables the identity and business of the visitor to be ascertained before the door is opened – thus preventing, to a great extent, unsolicited visitors, and making the elderly person feel more secure.

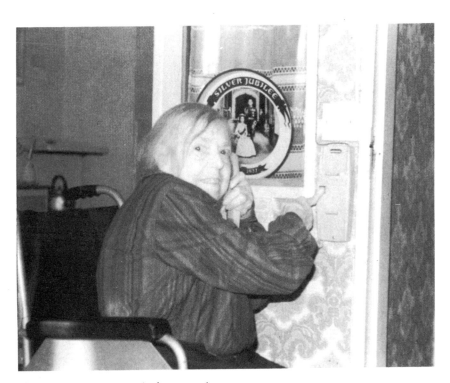

Photo. 19.2 An automatic door-opening system.

Functional assessment

The occupational therapist in the multidisciplinary setting is able to indicate how well, and at what level of independence, an older person can manage – for example, whether they can return/stay at home; require help from community services in the form of meals on wheels or home care, because they cannot manage the more complex tasks of shopping and cooking, or require constant support.

The ideal assessment tool for ascertaining the nature and extent of the problems is one that is specifically designed, valid and standardised for the elderly. The main principles of assessment of the elderly person are as follows.

1.   The assessment process must be a positive experience for the individual, not one that highlights deficits.
2.   Caution should be used interpreting results gained from assessment tools which are not designed for the elderly.
3.   Account should be taken of the elderly person's vulnerability to fatigue, slow response time, slowed change of mental comprehension and difficulty in dealing with more than one item at a time.
4.   Cognitive assessment tools should be used which provide a range of choices from which the patient selects a response.
5.   It should be noted that seemingly casual conversation can elicit useful information about habits and volitional activity. It is not necessary to assess each area of activity in a formal manner.

Occupational therapists frequently design their own assessments of Activities of Daily Living (ADL) function. These are often in the form of a checklist or a rating scale. However, these assessments have rarely been tested for reliability or validity. There are a number of rehabilitation assessments, mostly of ADL function that have had extensive testing and yield scores that are related to rehabilitation outcome.[2]

After assessment a programme is established and, to be effective, must be modified, reviewed and reassessed frequently as the individual progresses, improves or indeed deteriorates. The programme should concentrate on personal, physical, psychological, social and domestic needs; for example, exercise tolerance, motivation, mental capacity, motor and sensory deficits and postural control, the aim being to restore the individual to maximum ability.

The complexity of social, psychological and physical factors contributes to the following areas:

1.   personal independence;
2.   domestic skills;
3.   mobility; and
4.   social and leisure activities.

Whatever the prognosis, personal independence, confidence and harmony are paramount. Using a specific assessment form acts as an *aide memoire*. However, all the activities must *actually* be assessed before any accurate comments can be made. It is not necessarily good enough to accept only verbal responses and the recording should be exact; for example, 'Mrs. E can walk 50 metres with a frame and no physical assistance', rather than 'Mrs. E can walk independently with a frame'. The latter enlightens no one as to the true capability of Mrs. E who may, as a consequence, be placed in a situation totally unsuitable for her.

In order to help establish the level of cerebral function a test can be carried out, and repeated regularly (see Fig. 19.1). The outcomes of this test facilitate programme planning and, in part, define how confused a person is. An elderly person labelled 'senile dement' or 'confused' may prove to be 'confused' due to the fact that they are in a different environment. A test will establish this over a period of time. Once the elderly person has adapted and settled they will function at their usual accustomed level.

Maintaining independence

The occupational therapist may be, and should endeavour to be, involved in ensuring that the environment fosters independence. For instance, the therapist may advise on appropriate furniture, wheelchairs, special equipment and heights of rails. If a family understands the elderly relative's capabilities and has been instructed by the therapist in the ways in which to provide help, then maximum co-operation and harmony interfamilia is likely to be achieved. An awareness of how they can best help themselves should be included in this education; for instance, avoiding back strain through correct use of bathing equipment. On admission to any unfamiliar environment well-established patterns of behaviour are disturbed. This can affect body functions, sometimes contributing to incontinence and constipation. Disturbance of sleeping and eating patterns may increase confusion, and may indeed lead to frustration and aggressive behaviour. Any intervening personnel should work together to achieve a basic level of independence so that essential tasks, such as moving about in bed, walking or wheeling to the toilet/bathroom, dressing and feeding can be performed. The occupational therapist, as she develops a rapport with the elderly person, must get to know the pace at which tasks can be achieved and share this vital information with others. It is important that the individual is allowed enough time to master difficult tasks and thus build up self-esteem and confidence.

In many instances the therapist will need to advise the relatives and other relevant people on methods by which tasks are most easily achieved as a result of functional assessments, programmes, reviews and conclusions. A specific programme may be devised in conjunction with others, for instance community speech or physiotherapists, or residential home staff, to overcome

Simple tests of cerebral function	
Name..Age....................Ward......................	
Date of admission.................................Right- or left-handed.................................	
Date test performed..Time..	
Observer's name	

Tests	Score
Memory	
1. Name.	2 1 0
2. Age.	2 1 0
3. Address or last address before admission. (Q. Where did you live before you came into hospital?)	2 1 0
4. Ask patient to remember address – enquire after 10 minutes exactly.	5 4 3 2 1 0
Vocabulary	
5. Define the meaning of: ship, fabric, remorse, reluctant, sanctuary.	5 4 3 2 1 0
Calculation	
6. Subtract 17p from 50p.	2 – 0
Orientation	
7. State time of day (morning, afternoon or evening).	1 0
8. State whereabouts (room or hospital).	1 0
Speech	
9. Name objects on a tray. Five should be held up separately – coin, button, pencil, key and scissors.	5 4 3 2 1 0
10. Obey simple commands e.g. 'Put out your tongue'.	1 0
11. Read simple instructions e.g. 'Raise your arms'. Can instructions be obeyed?	1 0
12. Read aloud.	1 0
13. Write name spontaneously.	1 0
Practical tests	
14. Copy patterns with right hand using three matchsticks.	1 0
15. Copy patterns with left hand using three matchsticks.	1 0
16. Copy patterns with right hand using five matchsticks.	1 0
17. Copy patterns with left hand using five matchsticks.	1 0
Toy tests	
18. Posting box.	6 5 4 3 2 1 0
19. Pyramid rings.	6 – 4 – 2 – 0
Check answer to memory test (question 4). Total score	

To score: circle the appropriate figure under the 'score' column, according to the patient's ability to get the answer, or parts of the answer, right. Add up the score at the end.

Fig. 19.1 Cerebral function test

particular problems. For instance, when a person with a stroke becomes absorbed in a creative activity familiar expressive speech may be elicited which does not occur in a formal speech therapy session; or the taking of an elderly person into a residential home for a social activity prior to admission can alleviate fear and apprehension.

Each elderly person makes social contact in different ways. They may want to be able to listen and talk to others, feel useful, or simply be left alone. Through the earlier devised programme a situation is created in which the elderly can be encouraged to gain confidence and self-esteem. Special equipment can help with leisure, hobbies and interests; for instance, wooden card holders. Attendance at a day centre, luncheon club, adult education centre or local club helps to maintain social contacts for the individual. Regular day care provided by some homes, offering a hot meal, company and a change of environment gives opportunities for regular communication to be maintained with those at risk. Of the increasing number of elderly people, the majority do not go into care but remain in their own homes. The Community Care Act 1990 positively encourages this and care managers have responsibility to ensure that this happens. In consequence, there are increasing numbers of early discharges from hospital and therefore the community occupational therapist must make herself familiar with hospital discharge policies. Various building societies now offer financial packages to assist in this venture if financial difficulties exist. For instance, the building society purchases the home and in effect gives the person involved a mortgage.

Complications likely to occur with ageing have already been mentioned. However, many small aids and adaptations to and within the home will enable an elderly person to retain his independence and reduce risk. For those elderly people unable to look after themselves at home any longer a residential home may be the only reasonable alternative. Community occupational therapists may be involved with the care manager when deciding on the most suitable home and provide advice on appropriate aids and adaptations, as well as the individual's pace and capabilities. In addition they or their assistants should work with the staff in the home to develop activity programmes aimed at increasing and maintaining independence of the residents, or providing mental and physical stimulation.

Housing managers and occupational therapists

In most districts occupational therapists work very successfully with housing managers to ensure that, through their knowledge of an individual's capabilities, special housing is properly allocated. This sometimes includes occupational therapists working closely with architects on designing appropriate housing for the disabled elderly (Chapter 13).

Continuing care

Elderly people are referred for continuing care only as a final resort when they are unable to maintain sufficient independence, in spite of assessment, treatment, review and support. In many cases short-term care/respite care is attempted – this has increased considerably over the last decade – before continuing care is considered the final solution. Respite care is also of great support to carers and enables them to cope with an elderly person for much longer. A critical element of the therapist's role is to become involved in activity programmes which provide intellectual stimulation and encourage mobility and physical activity. Creative projects will enable those with varying handicaps to make a valid contribution. There is endless scope to using creative and educative media, for taking part in social activities, gardening and outings. Volunteers, relatives, handcraft teachers and others can all be involved to help provide these activities and encourage maximum participation and stimulation. In this way the elderly person retains a meaningful life.

The intervention of the occupational therapist in the rehabilitation of the elderly in various settings does not necessarily lead to dramatic results, but affords rich rewards in the responses and progress achieved as well as being a decisive element in maintaining or developing the self-confidence, independence and self-esteem for an elderly person.

(ii) The elderly mentally ill

GILLIAN ASPINALL
Head Occupational Therapist, Elderly Directorate, Norfolk Mental Health Care NHS Trust

During the past 10 years there has been a linear increase in the number of areas that have specialist services for elderly people with a mental illness. One of the primary reasons for this development is the increase in the elderly population and the prevalence of dementia. Establishing a discreet service for this client group has definite benefits as there are a number of conditions that present in old age for which specialist assessment, diagnosis and treatment are vital. An example of this is disorientation, a feature of dementia, which may also be due to Vitamin B12 deficiency and toxic confusional states. Specific conditions seen in the community include Alzheimer's disease, multi-infarct dementia and depression.

Alzheimer's disease

This condition is characterised by an insidious onset and gradual decline in mental abilities. Memory difficulties, especially those involving dealing with new information, are often the first symptoms to be noticed. Disorientation in time, place and person becomes more evident as the disease progresses, both of which may lead to restlessness and wandering. Insight gradually becomes impaired and communication problems are common due to expressive and/or receptive dysphasia. As the disease progresses, apraxias may develop in skills such as dressing and washing or the motivation to perform these tasks may fade. Some well-learned or familiar skills may, however, remain for some time. The person often retains parts of his personality, such as a sense of humour. The progressive nature of this disease eventually makes independent living in the community very difficult for the sufferer and carers, making this one of the greatest challenges for occupational therapists and others working in this area.

Multi-infarct dementia

This form of dementia is associated with multiple cerebral infarcts. The onset is usually sudden and the disease follows a step-wise progression. There are signs of vascular disease and a link with Parkinson's disease has also been found. The patient characteristically retains more insight and often emotional lability is found with depression. Some variation in mental ability is found as, due to the focal nature of the lesions, some skills remain intact. There may be variation throughout the day, with a particular tendency to increased confusion at night.

In order to understand the aetiology, presentation and treatment of these forms of dementia a more thorough study is necessary and the reader is referred to a medical textbook.

Depression

The presentation and management of mental illness such as depression, is different in old age from that occurring at any other age. An example of this is that physical illness can be associated with a depressed mood in some old people. Another important feature is that of social factors especially those associated with loneliness and loss. The proportion of elderly people living alone is high, with half of all women over the age of 75 years in Britain living alone. Older people are continually experiencing loss of various elements in their life – loss of a job and the difficulties associated with adjusting to retirement and reduced income may lead to depression; bereavements involving the loss of a partner, friend, a valued pet or a lower limb may follow each other over a period of time thus causing depression; losing a son or daughter seems especially difficult, as few people expect to outlive their children. Loss of independence or having to give up a home are major stresses and may lead to the elderly person becoming lonely and isolated. Depression is under-diagnosed in the elderly and is actually more common than dementia.

Ongoing support and treatment in the community have been found to be effective in preventing hospitalisation as many depressive episodes reoccur in the elderly. Severe depression may be life-threatening, either due to the risk of suicide or through self-neglect and treatment as an in-patient is then often required.

Community teams

Characteristic methods of working with elderly mentally ill people by a specialist team are as follows:

- Initial assessments are undertaken in the client's own home environment, in contrast to other medical specialities where initial contact is more often in a clinic.

- Community-based assessment ensures that difficulties are identified within their context and that carers and family members are involved from the outset.
- Links with other statutory and voluntary agencies are important if intervention is to be community focused and comprehensive.

To be effective and available to clients and carers, the team needs to employ flexible working patterns and ensure good communication and critical thinking between all professional groups. The team is typically made up of a consultant in old age psychiatry, community psychiatric nurse, clinical psychologist, social worker, physiotherapist and occupational therapist. A number of models of practice reflect the varying levels of contact and co-operation between community team members, for example:

1. The team is merely a number of individuals with responsibility within a given geographical area. Referrals are received by the consultant, and after medical assessments are passed on to an appropriate member of the team. Reviews are held with that team member and the consultant.

2. Referrals are discussed by all team members where it is decided who is the most appropriate person to undertake the initial assessment. This is then presented at the next team meeting and a treatment plan agreed. Training is required to enable all team members to undertake initial assessments and flexible hours are needed in order to respond to urgent referrals.

In some cases, referring agencies, such as general practitioners, will need information on the specific roles of group members in order to refer appropriately to the team. For example, a GP anticipating difficulties in the home will wish to refer his patient to the occupational therapist for preventative work before a crisis occurs.

Core skills specific to the occupational therapist for this group of people therefore need to be outlined and other skills which may lead to shared roles within the team agreed.

The role of the occupational therapist

A major focus of community occupational therapy is to help the client to restructure previous activities and adapt the environment to allow for maximum independence. In the home setting family members and others are intimately involved in the treatment process, as family dynamics are deeply affected by the client's illness and must be considered in the therapy process. Where a client is unable to adapt his or her behaviour to increase independence the main emphasis will be on the restructuring of the environment.

The assessment process should focus on the strengths and difficulties of the client and carer in the context of their particular environment taking into account their goals and values. If, for example, the goal is to remain in their own home following a bereavement then, with the client, the occupational therapist will need to identify areas of difficulty and design an appropriate treatment programme.

The assessment of independence in activities of daily living should include all relevant activities for the client, the interaction between physical, psychological and social factors and the impact of these on the client's independence. For example, a client suffering from depression may have significant difficulties in preparing a meal due to a sense of hopelessness and difficulty in concentration. Having developed a skills deficit in this area due to repeated difficulty, the client will need to relearn the skill or adapt it to a new environment. The approach, therefore, will need to focus on the mental health difficulties underlying a particular behaviour, but at the same time taking note of any associated physical problems.

Another important area to be included in the assessment process is that of socialisation. A supportive network of friends and social contacts is an important factor in maintaining life in the community. Conversely, isolation and loneliness play a significant role in difficulties encountered in coping with mental health problems. The occupational therapist will need to suggest strategies to increase opportunities for socialisation.

Treatment approaches in occupational therapy

There are a number of treatment approaches which are briefly described. However, more detailed texts will be required in order to fully understand them.

Loss and bereavement counselling. Individual counselling or supportive psychotherapy is helpful to enable the client to work through the emotional impact of losing a loved one. Loss groups are run on an out-patient or sessional basis and focus on coming to terms with losses and sharing experiences and strategies in a supportive environment. The occupational therapist should undertake further training and receive clinical supervision for such work.

Stress management. Carried out individually or as a group this focuses on educating clients in the causes and identification of stress and in the adoption of strategies to prevent and reduce it.

Relaxation training. Using a number of different forms of relaxation techniques, the therapist can train the client to adopt a method which will prevent stress or reduce it.

Reality orientation. This approach aims to give information about the environment in order to reorientate a client. It includes adapting the environment and the behaviour of carers. Simple measures such as providing a large clock and labelling doors are examples of this. Carers need to be taught how to reinforce routine and familiarity.

Validation therapy. This approach concentrates on the feelings behind the reality as expressed by the client. It takes a counselling approach rather than an emphasis on relearning information.

Creative arts therapies. Art, music and drama therapy undertaken by qualified creative arts therapists are all helpful in assisting a client to identify strengths and difficulties, to work through the emotion relating to problems and to provide an alternative form of communication.

Leisure, work and creative activities. A variety of pastimes may be used to encourage clients to identify a balance of activity, particularly following retirement. This may include paid or voluntary work and the encouragement to develop existing skills or learn new ones.

Special considerations

Wandering. As identified earlier, wandering may be found as a clinical feature of Alzheimer's disease and other forms of dementia. Wandering may have identifiable causes, such as a person's desire to find a meaningful place or person from the past, a person's need for security or a wish to perform previous work or roles. It may also result from the need to use excess energy, ease anxiety or to distract from pain. Wandering is often difficult for carers to deal with and advice should be available for them. Once the causes are known, the therapist is able to suggest strategies for dealing with it. For example, the client may respond to supervised exercise to reduce boredom and use up excess energy or may be diverted through the use of an activity that is safe for the client to perform. Sometimes, however, the client will need to be allowed to continue to wander within a safe environment.

Safety and the environment. This is a major consideration, particularly in relation to those living alone who have a form of dementia. Without insight, clients continue to perform activities such as cooking or DIY activities beyond the time that it is safe for them to do so. Hazards in the home are numerous and it is difficult to protect clients without withholding their rights. A common situation might be of a client who lacks the skills to use a gas cooker safely and frequently sets fire to pans, or stores newspaper in the oven but refuses to stop using the cooker. Relatives may choose to have the cooker disconnected in spite of the client's wishes but it becomes a difficult ethical issue for a therapist to do so. The occupational therapist will need to make a thorough assessment of the client's abilities and act with the support of the community team, while upholding the best interests of the client. An advocate will need to be appointed to assist in decision making for these difficult judgements (see Chapter 2).

References

1. Adams, G.F. *Essentials of Geriatric Medicine*, Oxford: Oxford University Press, 1981.
2. Kottke, F.J. (ed.) *Krusen's Handbook of Physical Medicine and Rehabilitation*, 3rd edn, Philadelphia: Saunders, 1982.

Further reading

Arie, T. (ed.) *Recent Advances in Psychogeriatrics*, Edinburgh: Churchill Livingstone, 1985.

Cornish, P.M. *Activities for the Frail*, London: Winslow Press, 1983.

Current Awareness Bulletin – Occupational Therapy with Older People, College of Occupational Therapists, 1994.

Gray, J.A.M. and McKenzie, H. *Take Care of Your Elderly Relative*, London: Allen and Unwin, 1980.

Holden, U.P. and Woods, R.T. *Reality Orientation: Psychological Approaches to the Confused Elderly*, London: Churchill Livingstone, 1982.

Jackson, O.L. *Physical Therapy of the Geriatric*, Edinburgh: Churchill Livingstone, 1983.

Kiernat, J.M. *Occupational Therapy and the Older Adult; A Clinical Manual*, Gaithersburg, Maryland: Aspen Publishers, 1991.

Lishman, W.A. *Organic Psychiatry*, Oxford: Blackwell Scientific Publications, 1986.

Murphy, E. Social origins of depression in old age, *British Journal of Psychiatry*, Vol. 141, pp. 135–42, 1982.

Rimmer, L. *Reality Orientation*, London: Winslow Press, 1983.

Royal College of Physicians and British Geriatrics Society (London) *Standardised assessment scales for elderly people*, 1992.

Shaw, M.W. *The Challenge of Ageing*, Edinburgh: Churchill Livingstone, 1983.

Wattis, J. and Church, M. *Practical Psychiatry of Old Age*, London & Sidney: Croom Helm, 1986.

Chapter 20

Quality assured

EILEEN E. BUMPHREY
Consultant/Adviser in Occupational Therapy and Rehabilitation

Concern about quality of care has always been apparent within health and Social Services; however, it is only recently that methodological assessments leading to reliable evidence have been considered necessary. In 1990, with the onset of the NHS reforms, regular, objective and critical monitoring of standards became important to meet the requirements of the internal market and the realisation by managers and professionals alike that, by these measures, a more effective service could emerge.

Standard setting is not new. Centuries ago the Livery Companies were established to ensure quality of workmanship, and goldsmiths' hallmarks similarly guaranteed quality. Today the manufacturing industries have British Standards – or kitemark – to ensure quality not only for themselves, but also for their customers. Within the service industries, however, there are no such standards, apart from the state registration requirements for some professions, and yet it is within these services, where people 'do things' to people, that the requirement of a 'kitemark' is even more important.

In 1983 the government launched a National Quality Campaign aiming to achieve the recommendations of its White Paper *Standards, Quality and International Competitiveness: 1982*. This White Paper promoted the importance of quality and encouraged the use of standards within all industries, including the service industries. It is against this background that the NHS, Social Services and education are judged.

In 1991 the government published the Patients' Charter[1] as the NHS element of the Citizen's Charter, which was to further its policy of improving standards. Three new rights were introduced within this Charter, namely information; guaranteed admission to hospital within 2 years for those on the waiting list; and complaints investigated properly and promptly. The public were also reminded of the previous nine standards, those relating to community care addressing the following.

- Respect for privacy, dignity, religious and cultural beliefs.
- Ensuring that everyone who needs the service receives it.
- Information given to relatives and friends.
- Waiting times.
- Discharge arrangements from hospital with a locally named contact person.

What is quality assurance?

The British Institute defines *quality* as 'the totality of features or characteristics of a product or service that bear on its ability to satisfy a given need' – or more simply, 'quality is that which gives the customer complete satisfaction'.

Bearing in mind that the customers' needs are extremely diverse and their 'complete satisfaction' subjective, there will inevitably be enormous variances that measurable quality will bring especially when this is related to health and social care. The perceived needs of patient/client and that of the professional practitioner will vary, for each have different perspectives. There is still the strong belief among both that 'the doctor knows best' and 'the nurse does her best' – whether or not the patient is satisfied.

Assurance means 'making sure', inferring that this is a continual process and that quality is maintained throughout.

The purpose, then, of *quality assurance* is to identify quality standards and to ensure that appropriate actions are taken to correct deficiencies or to make changes to meet service needs. Quality assurance embraces *quality control*, which implies compliance with predetermined standards such as accredited educational programmes.

The United Kingdom is committed to quality assurance (QA) in health and social care and as a member of the World Health Organisation (WHO), follow their objectives of quality assurance programmes which have four particular components:[2]

- performance;
- resources used;
- risk management (including the avoidance of injury and illness);
- patient satisfaction.

No single approach to QA is appropriate for all situations and types of health and social care. They must have clear objectives if they are to mean anything and these should be in terms of service users' experience rather than managerial statistical procedures. The WHO have suggested that after identifying the problem or task, each component should include monitoring, assessment and improvement.

> *Monitoring* – a system of continuous monitoring to identify potential problems; however, if it becomes a laborious procedure it will be counterproductive.

Assessment – this can mean many different things from a short initial process to the major part of intervention in care management. Assessing management issues such as waiting times and available resources also needs to be part of the process.

Improvement – that being implementation of what has been analytically and critically reviewed and evaluated. Unless implementation of the findings is carried out improvement in care is lost.

It is all too easy to keep the status quo – sometimes for very valid reasons; however peoples' expectations change, technology progresses, resources are shifted thus leaving the status quo option vulnerable. QA is about doing the right thing at the right time; the difference between success and failure, and asking why one procedure is more successful than another.

Quality assurance criteria

The criteria used for quality assurance within the care sector can be based on the British Standards Institute system, which includes:

1.   knowing the customer's needs;
2.   designing a service to meet these needs;
3.   providing clear instruction including training;
4.   delivering the product punctually;
5.   providing an efficient back-up service;
6.   using feedback from the experience to modify the service.

While the author is not entirely at ease with the term 'customer' it may be easier to use it in this context applying it to both patient, client and carer, especially as one definition expresses it as a 'person with whom one is concerned'.[3]

Knowing the customer's needs

In delivering a holistic service which covers varying lifestyles, age groups, disabilities and social situations, common factors have to be found in order to identify needs. Disabled people themselves have identified these as self-care; communication; mobility; continence; fulfilling activities; choice of treatment; and finance. However, like professionals, they have aspirations which may not be achievable within given resources and therefore to improve quality of life it may be necessary to narrow the gap between aspirations and what is actually possible.

Measuring quality applied to human interactions must have a scientific approach to avoid subjectivity and at times this will need to draw on the science of behaviour, including thought processes and perceptions. Personal family, social, financial and environmental issues also need to be considered. It then becomes a complex interaction between the subjective judgement of the customer and the professional, technical issues of the provider.

The National Health Service and Community Care Act 1990 gave both health and local authorities a duty to consult users and carers of their service. The two authorities, however, have had differing perceptions of how this can be achieved – the Health Service view being 'consultation', whereas the Social Service view is 'empowerment'. These differences of emphasis have their origins in their differing histories and cultures, although there is now a movement by the Health Service towards empowerment.

Healthcare has been dominated by the 'medical model of care' giving it the authority and mystique which lay people find hard to challenge. *Consultation* has been an integral ingredient to health care as patients visit their doctor 'for a consultation'. Thus the 'consultation model' for measuring quality relating to patient needs has been a natural step. However, it has drawbacks as being a top-down approach with the service asking the questions and the customer giving a response. It can fail to gain a true picture and give customers real opportunities for involvement and challenge. Another factor that can be detrimental to this system is the tendency for the more articulate and least burdened patient's voice to be heard the loudest. Because of this, consultation can actually reinforce inequalities in service provision.

Empowerment, on the other hand, places emphasis on the users of the service and implies 'user involvement' in every aspect from personnel care to strategic planning. Advocacy is a key element in this process as it gives vulnerable people the necessary support to exercise their power. Empowerment is not easy, especially for those disadvantaged or in distress, nor is it easy for the professional who is able to look at problems more objectively and consider those issues that may arise in the future and which the client may not wish to recognise. Empowering activities *are* achievable and have worthwhile goals, as has been verified by the Community Care Force[4] and other studies. Customers want better information and to be included in discussions on matters that directly affect them.

The customer may also be the purchaser – either the Health Authority or Social Services. Conflicts may arise as the practitioner endeavours to satisfy all – their patient/client, their employer's requirements as well as themselves with their own professional standards. All need to be satisfied and the balance right, with the views of all three taken into consideration.

Designing a service

All practitioners should be involved with designing the future direction of the service; however, this must not be based on personal whims and fancies or unquantifiable perceptions but on evidence and facts.

First, the practitioner needs to understand the framework within which they are expected to practice, including being familiar with the aims and objectives of the service, philosophy of care and departmental policies. The ability to carry out any intervention to a high professional standard will depend on the skill of the practitioner; the quality of equipment and facilities; management arrangements; and funds.

Practitioners are keen to perform well and gain job satisfaction and as such are well motivated to improve the service. However, this should not be achieved subjectively but, through a monitoring system which highlights strengths and weaknesses, and will meet the changing needs of society.

Setting standards. Central to quality assurance is the setting of standards. In the manufacturing industries standards are set by the customer for, at the end of the day, will they purchase the item or will they go elsewhere? In the public sector it is different, for often there is no alternative – there are simply providers and recipients, the providers being both professionals and carers.

Standards derive from the interaction between the provider and customer. Problems can arise through endeavouring to set standards using such interactions, for what of those recipients who are incapable of comprehending their own needs; the dominant carer with altruistic ideas; or the practitioner's own professional ideals. Often it is assumed that the provider knows best and therefore is left to play the greater role in setting standards. Providers will have their own professional standards which they will jealously guard and which managers expect them to follow, as these identify the roles of each discipline within the rehabilitation process. However, the first Griffiths Report[5] promoted the idea that the customer is the legitimate judge of quality.

A purchasing authority will state that they have a commitment to purchase services for their population that provides high measurable standards of care; uses systematic quality assurance as a method of ensuring high standards; and demonstrates improvements by outcome measures.[6] Fig. 20.1 illustrates the perceptual values used in agreeing such standards.

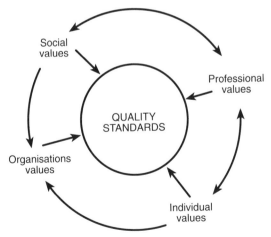

Fig. 20.1 Perceptual values used for determining standards

Standards therefore need to include those required by:

> purchasers – health and Social Services;
> local medical committees;
> education (when children and schools are involved);
> provider units;
> Patients' Charter;
> professions;
> customers

To comply, occupational therapists and other practitioners need to have clearly defined roles and responsibilities, customer requirements and standards of performance. Defining quality standards for a service as diverse as occupational therapy is not easy. It is therefore important that all staff, of whatever grade, are included in the writing of these for in this way they will own them and adhere to them. They also need to be set alongside those of the many disciplines and agencies with whom they relate and if possible, include a disabled person's viewpoint.

Terminology. The quality of information is determined by the uniformity of understandable concepts and terms that exclude synonyms and homonyms. There are several internationally recognised classifications, such as ICD, ICIDH, ICPM, ISO9999 – the majority emanating from WHO. However, many of these are complicated and too extensive for practical everyday use. Consequently, in 1990, the NHS established a Centre for Coding and Classification in order to devise a system that will be user-friendly. This centre is currently developing the Read coding system as a thesaurus of health care terms for all to use.[7]

The initial Read codes, developed in the early 1980s, had their origins in primary care to enable computerisation of patient records within GP practices and became the standard for primary care in 1988.[8] Later in 1992 the NHS Executive launched its Information Management and Technology (IM&T) strategy which will take this further, to include the needs of those working with Social Services, and the NHS number replacement programme which is due to commence in 1995.

The NHS project aims at producing meaningful clinical terms with common access across all branches of the NHS and throughout the country. This will assist in creating a more efficient service, as all will be able to communicate better and in the same language.

Within local authorities the current scheme is of data definitions associated with central requirements for the Department of Health and Local Government Management Board. There are many gaps in these especially relating to those clients who are transferred to and from the NHS. Consequently the Association of Directors of Social Services has commissioned the development of an Information Systems Strategy for Care Management.

As good clinical practice depends on the exchange of accurate information, it is vital that this interchange of information is understandable to all. Long written records, often in note form, are not only cumbersome but often unintelligible to the reader. A common language, understandable to all disciplines and patients, can only help to improve communication and liaison. Much work still has to be done; however, practitioners need to make a start towards this goal while awaiting the national codes.

Records. Individual records must be kept of all customers referred to the service and these need to conform to management as well as professional requirements. Purposeful documentation should include systematic and on-going records of the customer's condition and any intervention undertaken. These not only provide an essential record of events and communication with colleagues, but are a legal record. It is important therefore that these are clear, concise and accurate, especially in the event of the customer transferring to another agency or moving to a different part of the country.

Computerised information systems are becoming more common and an example of this is shown in Fig. 20.2.

Many departments are now using hand-held computers or light-pens with bar codes to help the itinerant practitioner. These have the advantage that records can be made immediately following a home visit rather than depending on the practitioner's memory after a long and possibly fraught day.

Instruction and training

All practitioners need regular training sessions and support when implementing quality assurance systems. As all those within the organisation will be on a similar learning curve, sufficient time, tolerance and patience are required for learning the chosen system, piloting and amending it.

Individual performance review (IPR) enables the practitioner to undertake their work effectively and is part of the QA process. It provides feedback on performance; clarifies job tasks and roles to meet changing service needs; identifies developmental and training needs; and provides an opportunity for setting performance objectives.

Clear instructions and training given to users of the service should also be included within a QA programme, whether it be in practical techniques such as mobility or handling, or the use of a piece of equipment, however simple it may be. Bearing in mind that only approximately 30 per cent of what is told to anyone is remembered by them, written instructions or leaflets can be a valuable *aide memoire*.

Delivery of service

There are many dimensions to consider in the delivery of a care service and perhaps Maxwell's six dimensions[9] are appropriate here, although others have produced additional dimensions. These are:

Norwich Health Authority Patient Profile

Patient Details

Mrs Alice Fynn   Fynnaf111210900
PONDEROSA   925392
DELL MANSIONS
NORWICH
NORFOLK NR8 5AB

GP - Fundholder DE Pickerson

Last Amended 09/09/91

Episode of Care OCCUPATIONAL THERAPY

Diagnosis   : CVA
Caseholder   : KHOT9 VAL MITCHELL
From   : 23/09/91   To: 29/11/91
Summary   : 10 contacts, totalling   575 minutes
Last Contact : 29/11/91
Discharged on 29/11/91 code DI Outcome PAT/THERAPIST SATISFIED

Treatment Record

Date	Staff	Main Activity	Duration	Outcome
Tue.24.09.91	KHOT9	FUNCTIONAL ASSESMENT	60	ONGOING
Thu.26.09.91	KHOT9	MOBILITY	120	ONGOING
Thu.26.09.91	KHOT9	TREATMENT-INDIVIDUAL	50	ONGOING
Thu.26.09.91	KHOT6	TREATMENT-INDIVIDUAL	50	ONGOING
Tue.01.10.91	KHOT9	HOME ASSESSMENT-WITH PATIENT	120	REFERRED TO SS NORFOLK
Wed.02.10.91	KHOT9	TREATMENT-INDIVIDUAL	30	ONGOING
Thu.03.10.91	KHOT9	HOME ASSESSMENT-WITHOUT PAT.	30	ONGOING
Tue.08.10.91	KHOT9	FUNCTIONAL ASSESSMENT	50	RESETTLED - OWN HOME
Fri.01.11.91	KHPT5	MOBILITY	60	PAT/THERAPIST SATISFIED
Fri.29.11.91	KHOT9	DISCHARGE WITHOUT CONTACT	5	PAT/THERAPIST SATISFIED

End of Profile.. Today's Date Wed Apr 8 1992

Fig. 20.2 Patient profile

By kind permission of Norwich Community Health Partnership (NHS) Trust

1.   Appropriateness.
2.   Accessibility.
3.   Equity.
4.   Effectiveness.
5.   Efficiency.
6.   Responsiveness.

Disappointment in a service often comes from unrealistic expectations, either on the part of the user or the provider. It is therefore important that the practitioner is familiar with the standards relating to these dimensions.

Appropriateness: are the referrals appropriate; have they been sent to the correct discipline; do they promote good health and healthy living?

Accessibility: are the services easily accessible for all sections of the community and are they timely?

Equity: is there equal provision for different social, geographical and disabilities groups?

Effectiveness: do outcomes indicate an achievement in improving quality of life, and prevention of ill health?

Efficiency: in terms of use of all resources, and delivery of service as appropriate, i.e. responding to emergencies.

Responsiveness: is the service sensitive to the needs of customers, demonstrating respect, preserving the rights and dignity of the individual?

Providing an efficient back-up service

In order to maintain any service, some form of back-up is required so that when an emergency occurs, such as staff sickness, patients and clients are not left in a quandary wondering whether or not they will receive the help promised. While this may of necessity have to be limited provision, at least the rudiments of the service can be maintained. All practitioners need to be conversant with the arrangements that management has made for such occurrences and the responsibilities that may fall upon them as a result.

Using feedback to modify the service

Unless everyone involved with providing care looks critically at what they are doing from time to time and modifies it as a result, no improvements will occur nor will the needs of the changing social situation be met. Life is constantly changing and so the service must adjust itself to meet these changes and the challenges that they bring.

Quality assurance programmes are a process – for example, the way goods are made, or how a meal is served in a restaurant. Feedback from customers is an important element of this process to ensure that the goods, or services, are what they want. Within the caring professions this process is less discernible as users are not sure what is available or what to expect and are often grateful for any help they receive. QA programmes can provide guidelines to reduce errors and engender confidence when in doubt, especially when practitioners are not always sure what they might have to provide when meeting a customer for the first time nor whether the service on offer is exactly right. For often, when undertaking a home visit they never know what may greet them when the front door is opened!

Audit is an integral part of quality assurance for it involves measuring standards against what happens in reality and then recommending changes to the service. Participation in audit is now a contractual obligation for all practitioners.

Audit is more often associated with accountants and finance; however, its principles have been brought into the wider field of examination of most public services to ensure that all resources are used effectively. In this context, there have been many definitions, often long and cumbersome. Maxwell[10] defined audit as a 'methodical review or investigation of resources and activities both clinically and managerially'. Others defining medical/clinical audit encompass similar concepts such as a critical analysis of quality of care including procedures used; the use of resources; the resulting outcome and quality of life for the patient, and colleagues reflecting on their work systematically. This definition can equally be applied to those working in social care situations.

The customer's involvement. Disabled people want the right to define their own needs and therefore need to be brought into the process. However, sometimes asking consumer and pressure groups gives bias. This may be overcome by asking local councillors for an unbiased opinion on behalf of the people they represent.

It is important that plain English is used and professional jargon avoided, as clear language fosters and enhances effective communication which in turn facilitates quality of care (Fig. 20.3).

The right time and method for talking to customers after they have experienced the service is crucial. If this is done too soon after intervention they may not know what the ultimate outcome will be, whereas discussing the service with them too late may present difficulties, as they may have already got into the swing of ordinary life and forgotten many details that were pertinent to the service provided. The place where the discussion takes place is also important in order to elicit thoughtful and useful responses and should preferably be either in their own home or in the reassuring presence of others, such as a focus group.

The audit process

This process is a cyclical one from agreeing standards through review to taking any necessary action. The British Standard starts with a 'mission statement' (BS4778) and then poses the question 'does your practice match up to this?' The results of any audit process must be objective, easy to analyse and understandable by others, including the public. All audit within this context must be customer focused, valid and appropriate. Difficulties may

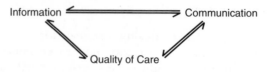

Fig. 20.3 Facilitating quality of care

arise with the overlap of varying agencies who apply different methods of auditing. Agreeing common aims and objectives by each will be the key to the success of developing integrated provision. Key elements to the process are as follows.

(a)   Setting objectives, standards and expectations.
(b)   Collect and present data.
(c)   Compare measurable performance.
(d)   Adjust performance via change to inputs (buildings, equipment, staff) and processes (clinical practice).

Ideally, audit should wherever possible be facilitated by a non-practitioner and be of a multidisciplinary nature, for rarely is intervention a 'one profession only' affair. However, single discipline audit is just as important, for by identifying the core skills of the profession before moving into multi-disciplinary activity, their identity is secure and dialogue with others can be entered into comfortably. Initially the tasks to be audited need to be broken down into small components, such as managerial groups or clinical specialties.

The audit cycle (Fig. 20.4) should not only allow for improvement to the service, but vision for the future.

Data collecting. This is an essential part of audit and different groups such as the epidemiologist, manager and clinician/practitioner will need different information. Ideally two data sets covering both clinical and managerial aspects will be needed. Inevitably, however, there are common factors which can be shared to give a common set of data which may include such information as age groups, sex, ethnic group, referring agency, GP and activity levels. From these data sets care plans, audit and research can all be undertaken (Fig. 20.5).

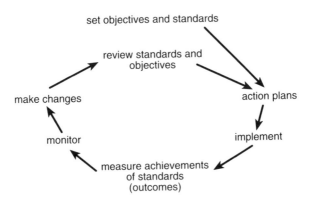

Fig. 20.4 The audit cycle

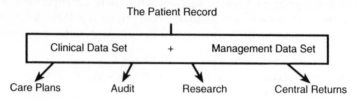

Fig. 20.5 The uses of data collection

Comparing performance – the audit tools. It is not easy to measure quality of services and thus make comparisons. Audit therefore has to be a mixture of attempts to measure effectiveness and the quality of inputs and processes.

There are a number of tools that can be used very effectively, from observation, peer group review, interviews, focus groups and standardised measurements to checklists and questionnaires. The following are of particular benefit to the process of audit.

Integrated Care Pathways (ICP) are a multidisciplinary case management tool as well as a clinical audit tool. They identify those activities that must occur in a consecutive and synchronised fashion to achieve an appropriate episode of care and set of outcomes for the customer. The care pathway, written by the team members for each condition or case type chosen (e.g. preoperative hip replacements) amalgamates into one document all the core elements of the care and treatment that a customer can expect to receive. It is not meant to account for all the ideosyncrasies of each individual customer, for these are accounted for in 'variances', but they do need to be recorded and analysed.

Surveys are useful in understanding local community needs. However, they should not simply encompass those who are receiving or who have recently received intervention, but need to include those who would benefit from the service. Surveys do not always work for all groups such as the homeless or itinerant travellers. Others may hold old suspicions and prejudices and therefore in these situations developing good communications is essential.

A useful checklist for designing *questionnaires* can be based on the 'Why, Who, How, When and Where' questions. For example:

Why?	Are the aims of intervention clear?
Who?	Who are the customers to be involved? Who are the recipients of care? Who are the givers of care?
By whom?	Who from within the organisation will obtain the information ensuring objectivity?
When?	When is the right time to undertake a survey?
How?	What method is to be used?
Where?	Where is intervention to take place?

Two factors need to be remembered when carrying out surveys – the 'vulnerable' and the 'gratitude' factors. The 'vulnerable factor' is, for example, asking the user for their views about the service while waiting to receive it and perhaps feeling apprehensive. They also may fear that any negative comment will adversely affect subsequent care. This factor can have a profound affect on those with a chronic illness unless they are reassured of anonymity and confidentiality.

The 'gratitude factor' is, for example, when the user is questioned immediately after receipt of care. Users are often extremely grateful for any help given, especially if it enhances their wellbeing. They may also fear the consequences of a negative comment.

Users need to be listened to and imaginative ways should be found for doing this. Additionally, it is important that practitioners endeavour to try to discern what the user is thinking and not simply depend on what they relate – or what they want to be known!

Outcomes

To ensure quality there must be *measurable outcomes* – an outcome being the consequence of an intervention related to stated goals. Assessing effectiveness of any intervention means examining the outcomes carefully. This is not straightforward for there may be a variety of outcome criteria with differing perspectives of care workers as well as those of users and their carers as to what an appropriate outcome might be. There is also the key issue of attribution – e.g. was the outcome brought about by the intervention itself or by some other means; would the patient have got better on their own given time? It is a well-known fact that the prospect of recovery and adapting to a newly acquired disability are improved if the person is happy about the care being provided.

'*Measures in outcomes*' is a phrase used to indicate how documentation of client programmes can assist the practitioner and manager to evaluate their service especially in relation to quality by showing:

- that intervention is appropriate and effective;
- that the service is responsive to needs;
- whether contractual and service agreements have been met;
- where changes to the programme may be indicated;
- where service developments should occur;
- that resources have been effectively and efficiently used.

These measurements will vary to meet the requirements of those needing them. For example, *purchasers* seek population-wide indicators such as mortality, morbidity, waiting times, and readmission rates. *Managers* concentrate on resource utilisation for achieving improvements of the overall health status of the population they serve; the number and strengths of complaints received – and compliments. *Practitioners* will be more concerned with the direct results of their interventions and satisfaction for both customers and themselves. *Customers* want relief from the presenting problems, reduced disability and impairment; choice of action with adequate information, and easy access to a personalised service. *Carers* look for adequate information and support. The *general public* want to know how to access the service, should the need arise, and to feel confident that it is of the best possible standard of care.

The NHS already collect a basic data set (the Körner data set). However, being a paper-based system which in itself has limitations, it is very limited and tells managers and practitioners alike little about the service provided. It is basically factual, including nothing about quality of the service, interactions between therapists and patients, or outcomes.

Roberts[11] identifies three major types of measure of outcome. These are:

- clinical indicators and measures, many of which are already available, such as the Barthel Index and Edinburgh Rehabilitation Status Scale (see Chapter 7);
- measuring health status which includes functional assessment and of wellbeing;
- patient satisfaction which not only includes perception of treatment received, but other factors such as hotel services.

When selecting measures for outcome of clinical intervention key questions need to be asked which should include the following.

1.   What is the ultimate purpose of the measure and how will it be used?
2.   What will be the content of the measure? While many concentrate on disability and impairment, handicap also needs to be evaluated as comprehensive rehabilitation focuses on the social effects of this dimension, which affects quality of life.
3.   How will the data be collected – paper or computer-based? How much staff time will be required and is user participation expected?

Many assessments give standardised outcomes for impairment, but none that measure how people adjust to their disability. How can a person's emotions of feeling better be measured, or indeed their anger and frustrations in not achieving? What is meant by 'good results'; what constitutes 'better'? It is therefore important to ask the right questions, with meaningful grades for the answers. It is also important to include lifestyle outcomes rather than simply those that relate to health gains, e.g. the affects of the disabled member of the family on others within the family unit.

Outcome measures for therapeutic intervention will vary depending on the problems presented by the customer and their carers and wherever possible standardised measures should be used (see Chapter 7). Obviously it will neither be possible nor appropriate to use these for all those referred to the service and therefore random sampling may need to be undertaken.

Satisfaction surveys must be designed to include features of the service that are important to the user and not only those that managers and professionals think are important to them. Most satisfaction surveys show that most people are satisfied with most things, most of the time! If these are therefore to be an intrinsic part of QA they need to target those aspects that can be changed. People need to judge a service in terms of the features they value.

Satisfaction can reflect numerous social influences, such as gratitude for help given while feeling vulnerable; anxiety that any expressions of dissatisfaction could jeopardise future care; sympathy for staff; and a desire to conform. Other factors that reflect the relationship between expressed satisfaction and actual quality of the service are psychological wellbeing, self-esteem and locus of control.

Complaints form an essential part of the monitoring process. The most common complaint within any public service lies in a failure of communication resulting in problems of misunderstanding and a lack of appreciation of what actually happened. Complainants want three things: truth and knowledge; things put right and an apology; and changes to take place so that others are not affected in the same way. People on the whole do not find it easy to complain, as first they need to feel confident enough to raise concern without feeling intimidated, or labelled 'complainant', and then need to find the right person to speak to. Both the Patients' Charter and the Community Care Act clearly set out the right to have any complaint investigated properly and promptly and therefore the practitioner needs to know the local procedures and ensure that customers are fully aware of their rights and the way to go about it. Those with comprehension or learning difficulties will need special help in this.

Complaints can be avoided by the sensitive practitioner being alert to the customer's needs and showing empathy. This can be achieved by:

- establishing a good rapport;
- involving the customer fully with their own programme;
- observing their activities carefully and giving encouragement;
- being enthusiastic, but at the same time realistic about perceived outcomes;
- determining achievable goals and so avoid failure;
- encouraging and supporting throughout the programme.

Complaints, whether formally written or informal, are a useful form of feedback and should be treated positively and not defensively.

Expected benefits

The practitioner should not consider that what is already being undertaken is ineffective or of a poor standard, for much of what is carried out is excellent practice. Quality assurance can confirm that is so and much more such as:

1. Improvement in the quality of care where it is needed and the support given to achieve it by improved teamwork and working relationships thus giving better co-ordination of care.

2.   Quantifying the perceived problem areas by knowing precisely what is going on and thus gain real evidence in those areas identified as needing attention, or with little resources.
3.   Constant review and updating of practice.
4.   Educating managers in the precise roles of therapists.
5.   Understanding more clearly the roles of colleagues and thus being able to integrate skills more effectively.
6.   Up to date detailed and accurate information for basing future requirements rather than on statistics that are out of date.
7.   Influencing how customer care is provided. Through empowerment, more knowledge and understanding of what can be expected, customers will be encouraged to become more involved in their own care.
8.   Influencing the internal market.
9.   Research opportunities.
10.   Promoting the best practice to other areas.

In order to achieve any benefits, the therapist must view the process positively and not be defensive about their individual professional practices but at the same time be willing to accept constructive criticism based on facts. Inadequate resources should not be used as an excuse – it is better to take the challenge and prove that the resources are simply not there to deliver the required service. Reduction of quality of service in order to meet demands does no one any good – it simply leads to dissatisfied customers and disillusioned staff.

Audit may be viewed as yet another task over and above the plethora of administrative 'niceties'; however, it is a most valuable tool to get a message across, to achieve and maintain high standards of practice, to have many satisfied patients and clients and motivated staff.

Audit does provoke new concerns and poses complex questions but it also improves quality and builds confidence.

References

1. Department of Health, *The Patients' Charter*, London: HMSO, 1992.
2. World Health Organisation, *The Principles of Quality Assurance*, Geneva, 1983.
3. *The Concise Oxford Dictionary*, Oxford: Oxford University Press.
4. Morris, J. and Lindlow, V. *User Participation in Community Care Services: Community Care Support Force*, Department of Health, London: HMSO, 1993.
5. Griffiths, R. *The NHS Management Enquiry*, London: DHSS, HMSO, 1983.
6. QUOTE – *Quality in Occupational Therapy Ensured*, Norwich: Norwich Health Authority, 1992.
7. NHS Centre for Coding and Classification, *Read Codes and Their Terms Project: A Brief Guide*, London: NHS Management Executive, Department of Health, 1993.

8. Information Management Group of the NHS Management Executive, *What are Read Codes?* London: HMSO, 1993.

9. Information Management Group of the NHS Management Executive, *Community Information Systems for Providers*, London: HMSO, 1993.

10. Maxwell, R. Quality assurance in health, *British Medical Journal*, Vol. 288(1), pp. 470–1, 1984.

11. Roberts, H. *Outcome and Performance in Health Care*, London: Public Finance Foundation, 1990.

Further reading

Chisholm, J. The Read Clinical Classification, *British Medical Journal*, Vol. 300, p. 1092, 1990.

College of Occupational Therapists *Standards Policies and Proceedings*, London.

Crombie, I.K., Davies, H.T.O. and Abraham, S.C.S. *The Audit Handbook – Improving Health Care Through Clinical Audit*, Chichester: Wiley, 1993.

Ellis, R. (ed.) *Professional Competence and Quality Assurance in the Caring Professions*, London: Croom Helm, 1988.

Ellis, R. and Whittington, D. *Quality Assurance in Health Care*, London: Edward Arnold, 1993.

Fricke, J. Measuring outcomes in rehabilitation, *British Journal of Occupational Therapy*, Vol. 56(6), 1993.

Jeffrey, L.I.H., Aspects of selecting outcome measures to demonstrate the effectiveness of comprehensive rehabilitation, *British Journal of Occupational Therapy*, Vol. 56, pp. 394–400, 1993.

Law, M., Baptiste, S. and McColl, M.A. The Canadian Occupational Performance Measure: an outcome measure of occupational therapy, *Canadian Journal of Occupational Therapy*, Vol. 57, pp. 82–7, 1990.

Local Voices. Involving the Local Community in Purchasing Decisions, London: NHS Management Executive Department of Health, 1992.

Measures in Outcome in Rehabilitation, Report to the DHSS on a preliminary enquiry about reviewing, London: Society for Research in Rehabilitation, 1980.

Øvretvert, J. *Co-ordinating Community Care: multidisciplinary teams and care management in health and social services*, Milton Keynes: Open University Press, 1993.

Quality in Action, Milton Keynes: British Standards Institute Quality Assurance, 1993.

UK Clearing House for Information on the Assessment of Health Outcomes, Leeds: Nuffield Institute of Health, University of Leeds.

World Health Organisation, *International Classification of Diseases, Injuries and causes of Death*, 9th revision, Geneva: WHO, 1977.

World Health Organisation, *International Classification of Impairments, Disabilities and Handicaps*, Geneva: WHO, 1980.

Wright, C.C. and Whittington, D. *Quality Assurance, An Introduction for Health Care Professionals*, Edinburgh: Churchill Livingstone, 1992.

Relevant legislation

National Health Service and Community Care Act 1990 (NHS and CCA)

This Act, together with the White Paper *Caring for People*, sets out government policy and framework for health and community care. Its overall aims are to enable people to live independent and dignified lives either in their own home or elsewhere within the community for as long as they are able.

The *key objectives* are:

1. To promote the development of domiciliary day care and respite services to enable people to live at home.
2. To ensure that service providers make practical support for carers a high priority.
3. To make proper assessment of needs and establish good case management in order to provide high quality care. Packages of care should be designed in line with individual needs and preferences.
4. To promote the development of an independent sector alongside the public services with Social Services being the enabling agency. It is their responsibility to make maximum use of private and voluntary providers and so increase the options for consumer choice.
5. To clarify the responsibilities of agencies and so make it easier to hold them accountable for their performance.
6. To secure better 'value for money' by introducing new funding arrangements for social care.

Key sections

Part I – The National Health Service, England and Wales.

> *Sections* *1 – 4* Local management
> *5 – 11* NHS Trusts

Part II – The National Health Service, Scotland.
Part III – Community Care: England and Wales.

Sections 42 – 45: Provision of accommodation and welfare services.
46 – 50: General provision concerning community care services.
Section 46 requires Local Authorities to consult with DHAs, FHSAs, housing departments and associations, voluntary organisations and others in preparing community care packages.
Section 50 states that grants will be available to assist Local Authorities in developing the voluntary sector contribution in improving care for alcohol and drug abusers.
This section also states that Social Services are required to continue to expand services for the mentally ill and those with dementia being treated in the community.

Part IV – Community Care: Scotland.
Part V – Miscellaneous and General.

While the policies set out in the Act and *Caring for People* apply to adult services, there is much in common between these policies and those that underlie the Children's Act as there is a particular need to consider the implications of what happens when a child reaches 18 years of age, and children's services are replaced by those designed for adults.

The Chronically Sick and Disabled Persons Act 1970 (CSDP)

A major Act relating to the provision of services for disabled people.

Section 1 – requires Local Authorities to inform themselves of the number and needs of disabled people as defined in *Section 29* of the *National Assurance Act 1948*. A disabled person is defined in terms of this Act as 'a person who is blind, deaf or dumb, or other persons who are substantially or permanently handicapped by illness, injury or congenital deformity, or such disabilities as may be presented by the minister'. This includes those people with mental disorders within the meaning of the Mental Health Act, and disabled people of any age including children and those over 65 years of age. They are also required to publish information on the services they provide under *Section 29*; and that disabled people using their services are informed of these.
Section 2 – relates to the 'arrangements' that can be made to promote the welfare of the individual. The level of provision made in any authority will depend upon its identification of needs.

The Disabled Persons (Services, Consultation and Representation) Act 1986 (DPA)

The 1986 Disabled Persons Act enhanced parts of the Chronically Sick and Disabled Persons Act (1959). Its primary objective is to give disabled people a greater say in the decisions that affect their lives. It intends for the person's needs to be fully assessed and appropriate services made available to meet these.

> *Sections 1, 2* and *3* provide for the appointment of authorised representatives and places duties upon local authorities to enable these people to make representations regarding the needs of the disabled person. The Community Care Act superseded these sections (official statement in March 1991).
>
> *Section 4* – confirms that the local authority must assess the needs of a disabled person if requested to do.
>
> *Section 5* – states that Local Education Authority and Social Service departments must arrange assessment of 'statemented' children leaving full-time education.
>
> *Section 6* – requires Education Authorities to establish procedures to keep under review dates when disabled children are expected to leave full-time education.
>
> *Section 7* – related to the discharge of patients from hospital after in-patient treatment for mental illness or a mental handicap lasting more than 6 months. This section is now covered by the NHS and CCA Act.
>
> *Section 8* – requires Local Authorities to make adequate arrangements for carers and to provide them and the disabled person for whom they care a range of choices.
>
> *Section 9* – extends the provisions made within the CSDP Act (*Section 1*) to require Social Service departments to inform disabled people of other relevant services which may be available to them.
>
> *Section 10* – opportunities are given for disabled people to be co-opted on to relevant committees.
>
> *Sections 12* and *13* – applies to Scotland and covers amendments to the CDSP Act 1970 and the Social Works (Scotland) Act 1968.

The Manual Handling Operations Regulations (1992)

These regulations come under the aegis of the Health and Safety at Work Act 1974 and implement the European Community manual handling directive, which aims to reduce the high level of injury and ill health associated with manual handling of loads within the workplace.

Employers are required to avoid hazardous manual handling tasks so far as is reasonably practical, assess those which cannot be avoided and reduce the risks of injury to the lowest level reasonably practicable.

The assessment and risk reduction should take an ergonomic approach and so consider the task, load, working environment and individual capability.

Mental Health Act 1983

The Mental Health (Amendment) Act 1982 made substantial amendments to the Mental Health Act of 1959, all of which are consolidated into the Mental Health Act 1983. The Act affects 'the reception, care and treatment of mentally disordered patients, the management of their property and other related matters'.

It defines mental illness as a mental disorder, arrested or incomplete development of the mind, psychopathic disorder and any other disorder or disability of the mind.

The Act provides for the following:

1. A Mental Health commission to protect the interests of detained patients.
2. Requirements regarding the treatment of detained patients including the provision of second opinions via an independent body.
3. Procedures for the admission to hospital and discharge procedures (*Section 117*).
4. Mental Health review tribunal procedure including an appeal mechanism to 'hospital managers' (as defined by the Act).
5. Powers for courts to remand to hospital for reports or treatment and to require from Regional Health Authorities details of what hospital places are available.
6. Informal patients in mental hospitals are able to make a declaration which allows their name to be included in the electoral register.
7. Part I defines criteria for admission to hospital which are that the patient is suffering from one or more of the following:
    mental impairment;
    severe mental impairment;
    psychopathic disorder;
    mental illness.
8. Both verbal and written information must be given to patients and their nearest relative (as defined by the Act) as to their reason for detention and their rights of appeal.

For detailed information see:

Biennial reports of the Mental Health Act Commission, HMSO.
The Mental Health Act Code of Practice, HMSO.

The Children Act 1989

This Act covers all aspects of child care, and relates to professionals working within Social Service departments, Health and Educational Authorities, private and voluntary organisations.

The Parts and Schedules of the Act relevant here are:

Part I   *Sections 1 – 7*: introduction which explains key terms.

Section 2: 'parental responsibility' replaces the former term 'parental rights' and aims to change attitudes towards children. All those with 'parental responsibility' must be consulted when any decision or action is taken about a child's welfare. This includes medical assessments.

Part II   *Sections 8 – 16*: orders with respect to children in family proceedings.

Part III   *Sections 17 – 30*: Local Authority support for children and families.

Section 27: co-operation between authorities.

The Act encourages inter-agency practice and empowers Local Authorities to request the assistance of others, especially health, education and housing.

Part IV   *Sections 31 – 42*: care and supervision.

Part V   *Sections 43 – 52*: protection of children.

Section 43: Child Assessment Order. This order can be used to gain an assessment of a child's health or development in order to determine whether or not the child is suffering or is likely to come to harm. This order only applies after reasonable attempts have been made to gain voluntary co-operation.

The Act requires all professionals working with children to consult parents and children on all aspects of the child's welfare. Adequate information about services and matters relating to the child must be given to the families.

Education Act 1981

This Act establishes a framework for the education of children with special needs and requiring special education provision whether in mainstream or special schools.

Key sections

Section I – identifies the special educational provision required for the educational needs of individual children. 'Special educational needs' are defined as:

(i)   having greater difficulty in learning than the majority of children of the same age;

(ii)   having a disability which either prevents or hinders the child from making full use of local educational facilities;

(iii)   is under the age of 5 years but will fall into one or both of the above groups by the age of 5 years.

Section II – introduces duties needed to accommodate the framework of special education and establishes the principle that all be educated in mainstream schools wherever this is reasonably practical, and are to be encouraged to participate with other children and the school's extra curriculum activities. This principle is subject to the views of the parents having been taken into account, and the ability of the school to meet the child's needs.

Section III – provides for special education to take place elsewhere other than in schools if it is assessed to be more appropriate and agreed by the parents.

Section V – Local Education Authorities (LEAs) have the responsibility for assessing the child's educational needs. The child's parents should be fully consulted and informed in writing of any decision made. Parents have a right of appeal.

Section VII – LEAs have a responsibility to make a statement of a child's special needs following assessment and that educational provision specified in the statement is met.

Section VIII – gives parents the right of appeal against the statement on their child.

For detailed information see:

> DES Circular 8/81, *Education Act 1981*.
> DES 1/83; HC(83)3; LAC1(2), *Assessments and Statements of Special Educational Needs*.

Local Government and Housing Act 1989

The most relevant part of this Act is Part VIII, Grants Towards Cost of Improvements and Repairs to Dwellings. This includes house renovation grants replacing the improvement grants of the 1985 Housing Act. It builds on established practice and reinforces the philosophy of community care by requiring housing and welfare agencies to co-operate in identifying needs and establishing that proposed adaptations enable any care plan to be implemented.

Disabled Facilities Grants (Section 114)

This grant applies to both public and private sector dwellings. There are mandatory and discretionary grants.

Mandatory grants are given for:

•   facilitating access into and out of the home, and to the principal living room, kitchen and bathroom;

- providing suitable bathroom and kitchen facilities;
- adapting heating and lighting controls;
- improving heating systems;
- making provisions for carers as well as the disabled person.

Discretionary grants may be provided for a wide range of works that go beyond the basic housing requirements in order to make the dwelling suitable for the accommodation, welfare or employment of the disabled person. This grant is subject to a means test.

Minor Works Assistance (Section 131)

Grants may be available for owner occupiers and private sector tenants in receipt of Income Support or other benefits. Two are particularly for the elderly (over 60 years).

1.   'Staying put' – to repair, improve or adapt the property so that they can remain within their own home.
2.   'Elderly resident' – to adapt a property so that they are able to stay or move in with the owner or tenant on a permanent basis.

Assistance may be given either in the form of a grant or the provision of materials. For detailed guidance refer to the following DOE circulars:

10/90 Housing adaptations for people with disabilities.
12/90 Housing renovation grants.
5/91 Local Government and Housing Act 1989, Parts VII and VIII.

Disabled Persons Act 1981

Much of this Act relates to adapting the environment for disabled people. The relevant sections are:

Section I – relates to roadworks throughout the United Kingdom. It requires local and highway authorities to have regard to the needs and safety of disabled and blind people when undertaking roadworks; considering providing ramps between carriageways and footpaths; and ensuring holes are properly protected.
Section II – relates to the use of Orange badges.
Section III – relates to public buildings and draws attention to the relevant sections of the CSDP Act 1970 and the Code of Practice for Access for the Disabled to Buildings BS 5810.
Section IV – is concerned with toilets for the disabled in places of entertainment.
Section V – this section replaces *Section 7* of the CSDP Act and requires those making provisions required by *Sections 4, 5, 6* and *8* to provide signs indicating facilities for disabled people and the appropriate route to those facilities.

Section VI – re-provision of buildings. In all sections of the CSDP Act which impose a duty to pay regard to the needs of disabled people in the provision of buildings. This means provision in accordance with BS 5810: (1979) or, for educational buildings, Design Note 18, unless the developer can demonstrate that it is not practical or reasonable to make such provision in that particular situation. This section applies only to England and Wales. (For Scotland there is similar provision within the Local Government (Miscellaneous Provisions) (Scotland) Act 1981.)

Section VII – relates to access to buildings.

The Disabled Persons (Employment) Acts 1944 and 1958

This act defines 'disabled person' for employment purposes as one 'who on account of injury, disease (including a physical or mental condition arising from imperfect development of any organ) or congenital deformity is substantially handicapped in obtaining or keeping employment, or in undertaking work on his own account of a kind which, apart from injury, disease or deformity, would be suited to his age, experience and qualifications'.

The main provisions of the Act are:

1. Keeping a register of disabled people at Job Centres.
2. Introducing the Quota Scheme on companies employing 20 or more staff. Of these 3 per cent must be registered disabled people.
3. Prohibit the recruitment of non-registered disabled staff if employers are below their quota, unless they have gained exemption from the Department of Employment.
4. Prohibit the dismissal of registered disabled employees without reasonable cause if this reduces the quota level.
5. Allow the Secretary of State for Employment to prosecute employers below the quota level.

The Companies Act 1985

Section 235 of this Act requires companies with more than 250 employees to publish information about their policy on the employment of disabled people. The statement should appear in the Annual report.

Data Protection Act 1984

This Act regulates the use of identifiable information which is held on computers. It requires all personal data to be secure and registered with the Data Protection Registrar. Disclosure of information can only be made in accordance with the terms under which it has been registered and individuals have the right of access to information about themselves.

Access to Personal Files Act 1987

This Act allows individuals the right of access to manually maintained records about themselves, held by Social Service departments. Information recorded before April 1989, when the Act was introduced, is not covered by it.

The legislation applies to personal information held by Local Authorities Social Service functions, but does not include records of voluntary organisations or other agencies even though they may be acting on their behalf. An individual is not entitled to know what is recorded about another person without their prior consent.

Requests must be made in writing by the individual and a maximum fee of £10 per request may be levied. The authority must respond to the request within 40 days of receiving it.

Although it is intended that applicants should have access to the complete record, the Act states that certain types of information can be excluded such as that about the individual which the department feels is likely to cause serious harm if accessed – for example, self-harm, or harm to another person.

Glossary

Advocacy	one who speaks and acts on behalf of the disabled person
Audit	monitoring the service
Business planning	process for planning future services
Care managers	those responsible for purchasing and co-ordinating services for clients
Care substitution	shift of services from hospital to primary care
Commissions	Joint Health Authorities and GP services for purchasing Health Care Services
Competences	adequately qualified for undertaking professional practice
Contracting	process by which services are purchased by Health and Social Services
Cost per case	method of costing services
Disability	restriction or lack of ability to perform an activity normally
Empowerment	giving the disabled person choices and opportunities for them to take control of their lives
Enablement	helping the disabled person to achieve what is important to them
FHSA	Family Health Services Authority
Generic	generalist
Handicap	disadvantage resulting from an impairment or disability which limits or prevents a normal lifestyle
Health needs assessment	process of assessing health status
Impairment	loss or abnormality of psychological, physiological or anatomical structure or function

Internal market	system whereby Health Authorities purchase services from any NHS trust or other agencies
IPR	Individual Performance Review
Key worker	practitioner responsible for co-ordinating treatment/care
Management speak	management terminology
Management values	code of conduct as defined by one's employer
Mapping	seeing how allied parts of the service fit together
Measures in outcomes	documentation of client programmes to record effectiveness of intervention
Medical/clinical audit	monitoring treatment/care process
Mission statement	statement of intent: vision and goals for the future
Multi-skilling	developing skills by professionals to avoid duplication or overlap between different disciplines
Needs-based assessment	assessment made for future service developments according to actual patient/client needs
Networking	linking of organisations especially by computer
NVQ	National Vocational Qualifications
Outcomes	measurable results of intervention
Output	number of patients/clients seen
Patient focus care	patient care organised around patients rather than around specialised departments/ organisations
Performance review	measurement of output of employee/ organisation
Primary care	first point of health care
Prioritising	putting in order of priority
Protocols	formal statement of actions/intentions
Provider units	organisations providing care to people
Purchaser	those buying the service on behalf of consumers particularly related to health and Social Services
QALYS	'quality adjusted life years'
Re-engineering	redesigning of business process
Role blurring	overlapping of professional skills
Seamless service	continuum of care between provider units
Secondary care	providing more intensive medical care often within hospital
Skill-mix	mix of differing staff types and grades required to provide a particular service
Standards of practice	written professional standards

Tertiary care	continuing/terminal care
Time out	time set aside from one's work for planning and other activities
TQM	total quality management
Veracity	speaking the truth

Index